Coronary Stenting:
Current Perspectives

Legends to cover images
1. Two dimensional intravascular ultrasound image of a Wallstent™ obtained in vitro.
2. Three dimensional 'fly through' reconstruction of intravascular ultrasound images of a Wallstent™ obtained in vitro.
3. Three dimensional 'fly through' reconstruction of intravascular ultrasound images of a Wallstent™ obtained in vivo.
4. Two dimensional intravascular ultrasound image of a Radius™ stent obtained in vitro.
5. Three dimensional 'fly through' reconstruction of intravascular ultrasound images of a Radius™ stent obtained in vitro.
6. Three dimensional 'fly through' reconstruction of intravascular ultrasound images of a Radius™ stent obtained in vivo.
7. Two dimensional intravascular ultrasound image of a Palmaz-Schatz™ PS-153 articulated stent obtained in vitro.
8. Three dimensional 'fly through' reconstruction of intravascular ultrasound images of a Palmaz-Schatz™ PS-153 articulated stent obtained in vitro.
9. Three dimensional 'clamshell' reconstruction of intravascular ultrasound images of a Palmaz-Schatz™ PS-153 articulated stent obtained in vivo.

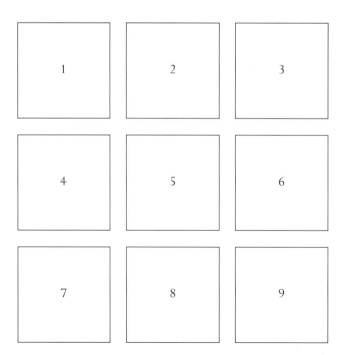

Coronary Stenting:
Current Perspectives

A Companion to the *Handbook of Coronary Stents*

Michael JB Kutryk MD PhD FRCPC
Catheterization Laboratory
Division of Cardiology
Heart Center Rotterdam
Academic Hospital Rotterdam-Dijkzigt
Rotterdam
The Netherlands

Patrick W Serruys MD PhD FACC FESC
Professor of Interventional Cardiology
Head of the Interventional Department
Division of Cardiology
Heart Center Rotterdam
Academic Hospital Rotterdam-Dijkzigt
Rotterdam and
Professor of Interventional Cardiology
Interuniversity Cardiology Institute
of the Netherlands (ICIN)
Utrecht
The Netherlands

MARTIN DUNITZ

©Martin Dunitz Ltd 1999

First published in the United Kingdom in 1999 by

Martin Dunitz Ltd
The Livery House
7–9 Pratt Street
London NW1 0AE

A CIP record for this book is available from the British Library.

ISBN 1-85317-693-1

Distributed in the United States by:
Blackwell Science Inc.
Commerce Place, 350 Main Street
Malden, MA 02148, USA
Tel: 1–800–215–1000

Distributed in Canada by:
Login Brothers Book Company
324 Salteaux Crescent
Winnipeg, Manitoba, R3J 3T2
Canada
Tel: 204–224–4068

Distributed in Brazil by:
Ernesto Reichmann Distribuidora de Livros, Ltda
Rua Coronel Marques 335, Tatuape 03440–000
Sao Paulo,
Brazil

Composition by Wearset, Boldon, Tyne and Wear

Printed and bound in Great Britain by
Biddles Ltd, Guildford and King's Lynn

CONTENTS

ACKNOWLEDGEMENTS

We are very grateful to Jan Tuin and Paula Delfos at the Thoraxcenter for providing us with superb photographs, sometimes at very short notice, and Dr Nico Bruining of the Computer Group for the intravascular ultrasound images. At Martin Dunitz Ltd, it was a joy to work once again with our commissioning editor, Alan Burgess, whose patience and encouragement helped rather than hindered us in completing the manuscript. His colleague, Clive Lawson, was instrumental in ensuring we met our deadlines.

PREFACE

The use of intracoronary stents has been increasing at a rapid pace since they were first used in clinical practice just over a decade ago. This increase is due in a large part to the conviction of the interventional cardiology community that stent technology can be applied to progressively more complex lesion subsets and unstable clinical situations. The success of coronary stenting is the result of the introduction of improved implantation techniques, a better understanding of the vascular response to injury, and advances in adjunctive pharmacology. The stent manufacturing industry has also contributed by providing more versatile and user friendly stents, designed specifically to address the problems of thrombosis and restenosis, and a host of custom devices designed for use in particular lesion types and clinical situations. In response to rapid progress, and fuelling the quest for new applications, is an ever increasing amount of basic science and clinical literature on all aspects of coronary stent implantation. Advances such as the development of intravascular brachytherapy, local drug delivery techniques, novel stent coating technologies and molecular biological approaches now represent the cutting edge of research.

With the enormous amount of newly published material and new advances in the field, it is becoming increasingly difficult to keep abreast of the new developments. *Coronary Stenting: Current Perspectives* was prepared as a review of the available literature on coronary stenting with the goal of identifying the indications for stent implantation and the use of adjunctive therapies which are supported by clinical evidence.

It has become commonplace to provide companion editions to all great textbooks of cardiology. In keeping with this custom, we felt that the technical information found in *The Handbook of Coronary Stenting (2nd edition)* and the contents of this book complemented each other so well that they be considered a set. We hope that these tandem publications will serve as valuable reference texts and provide a comprehensive overview of the current state of the practice of coronary stenting and coronary stent technology.

Michael J B Kutryk
Patrick W Serruys

1. Historical Overview

The use of percutaneously introduced prosthetic devices to maintain the luminal integrity of diseased blood vessels was initially proposed by Charles Dotter in 1964, who speculated that the temporary use of a silastic endovascular splint might maintain an adequate lumen after the creation of a pathway across a previously occluded vessel.[1] Dotter and colleagues were also the first to apply the term *stent* for vascular implants in their description of an experimental technique for the non-surgical endarterial placement of tubular coiled-wire grafts in the femoral and popliteal arteries of healthy dogs.[2] The etymology of the word "stent" is unclear. It has been associated with a device to hold a skin graft in position, with a support for tubular structures being anastomosed, and with an impression of the oral cavity made from Stent's mass. Stent's mass was concocted by Charles Thomas Stent (1807–85), an English dentist who developed it to form an impression of the teeth and oral cavity[3,4] (figure 1.1). Stent, as applied to endovascular scaffolding devices, may also have its origins from the verb "to stint", which means "to restrain within certain limits". The early stents used by Dotter were mounted coaxially on a guidewire and positioned with a pusher catheter. Since the pre- and post-implantation stent dimensions were identical, the graft diameter was limited by the size of the arteriotomy and the approach vessel, and only small coils could be passed percutaneously. Although these stents could be properly positioned, stent dislocations and significant narrowing within the stented segments occurred. These problems temporarily bridled any optimism that such a device might find clinical application in the treatment of vascular diseases.

In 1983, two preliminary reports showed the feasibility of transcatheter arterial grafting, and rekindled interest in the non-surgical placement of endovascular prostheses.[5,6] Using coil wire stents made of nitinol, a unique alloy of titanium and nickel, Dotter and colleagues[5] (figure 1.2) and Cragg and colleagues[6] (figure 1.3) described encouraging results of their transcatheter endoluminal placement in canine arteries. Nitinol has a unique heat-sensitive "memory", which allowed the coil stent to be compressed or straightened at room temperature and introduced through a catheter. When positioned properly, the coils were warmed to body temperature or higher. This caused the metal to lose its malleability, and allowed the stent to return to its initial configuration. These devices successfully maintained vessel patency at 4 weeks in

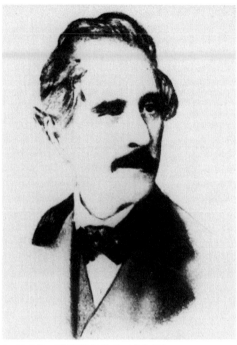

Figure 1.1: *Charles Stent (1845–1901), an English dentist who lent his name to a tooth mould (bottom) and perhaps to endoluminal scaffolding devices.*

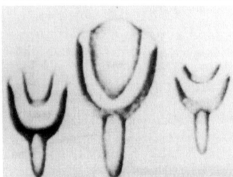

non-heparinized dogs. The work established the potential for the use of such a device in the non-surgical treatment of vascular disease, and was the catalyst for experimentation with a variety of innovative devices.

Not long after the preliminary reports on the use of nitinol coils, Maass and colleagues[7] reported the results of implantation of expanding steel spiral springs in the aortae and vena cavae of dogs and calves. With the application of torque, the springs decreased in diameter, to allow distal delivery. On release of the tension the springs expanded to their predetermined dimensions (figure 1.4). Although the spirals remained stable and did not cause perforation, thrombosis,

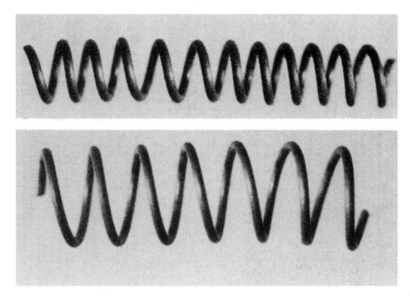

Figure 1.2: *Nitinol coil wire stent. Top: compacted for transcatheter placement. Bottom: same coil after heat-induced (60 °C) reversion to initial, anatomically indicated configuration. (From Dotter CT, Buschmann PAC, McKinney MK, Rösch J. Transluminal expandable nitinol coil stent grafting: preliminary report. Radiology 1983; **147:** 259–60.)*

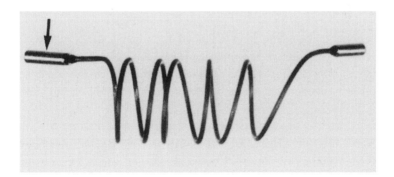

Figure 1.3: *Loosely wound nitinol coil graft. Arrow indicates a threaded adapter which can be attached to a modified guidewire. The coil was straightened in ice water and passed via a catheter into the aorta. The coil reformed when heated to body temperature and could be positioned using the attached guidewire. (From Cragg A, Lund G, Rysavy J, Casteneda F, Casteneda-Zuniga W, Amplatz K. Nonsurgical placement of arterial endoprostheses: a new technique using nitinol wire. Radiology 1983; **147:** 261–63.)*

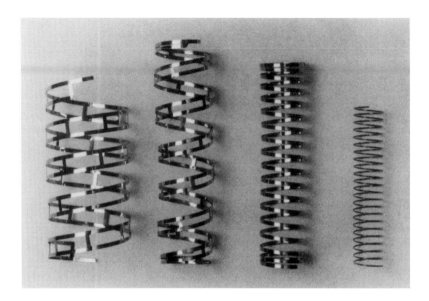

Figure 1.4: *Various types of implanted spiral springs. The devices were made of corrosion resistant heat-treated spring steel alloy. Application of torque to the spiral springs in the direction of the coils increased the number of coils and reduced the diameter of the spiral. (From Maass D, Zollikofer CL, Largiadèr F, Senning A. Radiological follow-up of transluminally inserted vascular endoprostheses: an experimental study using expanding spirals. Radiology 1984; 152: 659–63.)*

or stenosis of the treated vessel, a large diameter applicator was needed for introduction and placement, and this limited target lumen access. In 1985, the initial results of the implantation of spring-loaded self-expanding stents in dogs were described by Gianturco and colleagues[8] (figure 1.5). That research showed the importance of oversizing the stent in relation to the size of the target vessel to prevent migration of the prostheses.

The idea of a balloon-mounted stent for simultaneous dilatation and stent delivery was introduced by Palmaz and colleagues.[9] In 1985, they described preliminary results of the implantation of a balloon expandable stainless-steel wire mesh in canine peripheral arteries. The device was made from 150 μm and 200 μm diameter continuous woven stainless-steel wire. The cross-points of the wire mesh were soldered with silver to give the device a relatively high resistance to radial collapse (figure 1.6). The following year, Palmaz published data on a larger group of 18 balloon expandable stent implantations in canine femoral, renal, mesenteric, and carotid arteries.[10] These early results foretold problems that would plague intravascular stent implantation over the following decade.

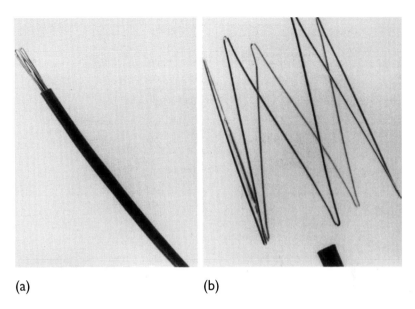

(a)   (b)

Figure 1.5: Zigzag expanding stainless steel stent. (a) Collapsed stent beginning to exit 12 F Teflon sheath. (b) Stent fully expanded after being pushed from the sheath. (From Wright KC, Wallace S, Charnsangavej C, Carrasco CH, Gianturco C. Percutaneous endovascular stents: an experimental evaluation. Radiology 1985; **156**: 69–72.)

Four thrombotic occlusions occurred in the first group of treated animals, which showed that adequate antithrombotic and antiplatelet therapy was needed at the time of stent deployment. Palmaz's group recognized that heparin therapy did not prevent late occlusion of stented segments with low flow, and that the best results were obtained in those without flow restriction. These are now axioms of contemporary stenting. Their observation of an overall patency rate of 77% at 35 weeks was surprisingly similar to the findings of subsequent stent trials.

With the refinement of equipment, smaller vessels could be accessed, and application of stent technology to the coronary system became possible. In 1987, Rousseau and colleagues[11] tested a flexible, self-expanding stainless-steel mesh stent that was restrained with a protective sheath. Forty-seven devices were implanted in 28 dogs, 21 of these devices in coronary arteries. No anticoagulant or antiplatelet agents were used, and partial or total thrombotic occlusion was seen in eight (35%) animals. Thrombus formation occurred at points of rapid reduction of vessel diameter, when the end of the prosthesis impinged upon a side branch of a major vessel and when there was a high ratio of unconstrained (maximal expansion) to implant device diameter. Endothelialization and incorporation of the stent into the vessel wall by neo-intimalization occurred by

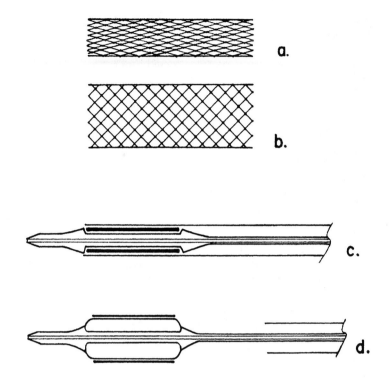

Figure 1.6: *Schematic profile of the balloon expandable wire mesh stent of Palmaz and colleagues in the collapsed (a), and expanded (b) state. The mounted stent was protected from being dislodged off the balloon by oversized leading and trailing retainers (c) and balloon inflation expanded the graft (d). (From Palmaz JC, Sibbit RR, Reuter SR, Tio FO, Rice WJ. Expandable intraluminal graft: a preliminary study. Radiology 1985; **156:** 73–77.)*

the third week after implantation. This was consistent with previously reported results of stainless-steel stents.[8,9]

The feasibility of the implantation of balloon expandable stents into canine coronary arteries was also shown in 1987. Roubin and colleagues[12] described implantation of a balloon mounted interdigitating flexible coil stent with a novel design in 39 animals (figure 1.7). Schatz and colleagues[13] reported their results of the percutaneous implantation of a non-articulated modified Palmaz-type stent in the coronary circulation of 20 dogs. The stent was cut with staggered, parallel, rectangular slots from a stainless-steel tube, and was more streamlined than the wire-mesh Palmaz stent (figure 1.8). No thrombotic events were observed in these animals. The publication of these two studies in the cardiovascular literature rather than in a radiological journal showed that coronary stenting had become separated from the field of vascular radiology.

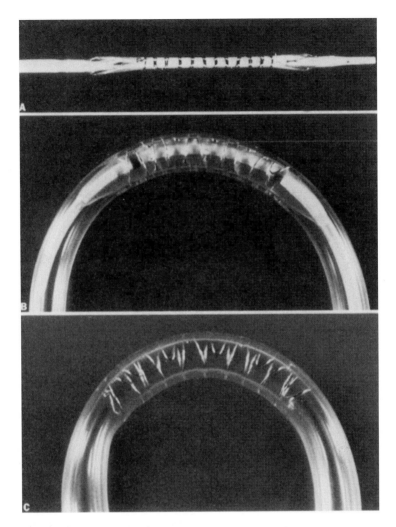

Figure 1.7: *(a) Coil stent coil wrapped firmly on standard PTCA balloon catheter. (b) Stent fully expanded by inflated balloon catheter demonstrated in transparent flexible tubing. (c) Fully expanded stent after removal of deflated balloon catheter. (From Roubin GS, Robinson KA, King III SB, et al. Early and late results of intracoronary arterial stenting after coronary angioplasty in dogs. Circulation 1987; **76**: 891–97.)*

The early experience of Rousseau's group with the implantation of the self-expanding stent in coronary arteries was the impetus for the implantation of a stent in an atheromatous human coronary artery. The first human implantation was done by Jacques Puel (Toulouse, France) in 1986,[14] followed shortly by Ulrich Sigwart (Lausanne, Switzerland). Subsequently, Sigwart, and colleagues[15]

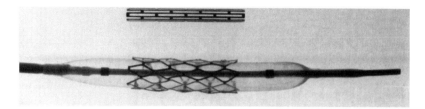

Figure 1.8: *Balloon expandable intravascular stent. Collapsed, the stent fits over any standard coronary angioplasty catheter. Inflation of the balloon results in expansion of each rectangular slot into a diamond configuration. (From Schatz RA, Palmaz JC, Tio FO, Garcia F, Garcia O, Reuter SR. Balloon-expandable intracoronary stents in the adult dog. Circulation 1987;* **76:** *450–57.)*

reported the results of the implantation of 24 self-expanding mesh stents (Medinvent SA, Lausanne, figure 1.9) in the coronary arteries of 19 patients. Three conditions were considered indications for stent insertion:

- restenosis of a segment previously treated with angioplasty;
- stenosis of aortocoronary-bypass grafts;
- acute coronary occlusion secondary to intimal dissection following balloon angioplasty.

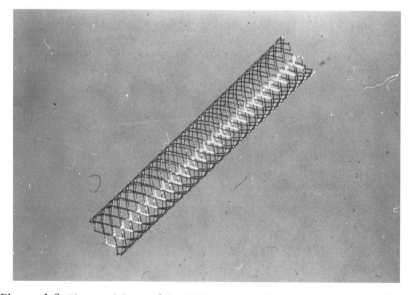

Figure 1.9: *The initial design of the Wallstent used in the early clinical studies. The first stents were made from a stainless-steel alloy with a self-expanding mesh design.*

Two complications related to stent thrombosis occurred (11%) and there were no cases of restenosis within the stented segment 9 weeks to 9 months after implantation. As a consequence of the encouraging results of this landmark study, the US Food and Drug Administration (FDA) gave their approval for phase I trials in the United States. The trials used the balloon expandable Gianturco–Roubin™ and Palmaz–Schatz™ intracoronary stents.

By early 1988, 117 self-expanding intravascular stents, of a type subsequently called the Wallstent™, had been implanted in native coronary arteries (n = 94) or in aortocoronary-bypass grafts (n = 23) of 105 patients.[16] Stents were placed for dilation of a restenosis, acute vessel occlusion after angioplasty, chronic occlusion after angioplasty, and as an adjunct to primary angioplasty. The results of intermediate term follow-up of this first series were sobering. Four patients died before repeat angiography, there was complete stent occlusion of 27 stents in 25 (24%) patients, and a long-term restenosis rate of 14% in those stents that remained patent.[16] The overall mortality rate at 1 year was 7.6%. The results also fuelled the controversy that surrounded the choice of a suitable anticoagulation regimen to minimize postprocedural complications and haemorrhagic side effects. Together with the comments of a daunting editorial that accompanied the manuscript[17] these results diminished the initial optimism for the future of these new devices.

The potential benefit of intracoronary stenting for the treatment of acute and threatened closure complicating percutaneous transluminal coronary angioplasty was demonstrated by Roubin and colleagues.[18] They reported on their experience during 1987–89 using the balloon-expandable Gianturco–Roubin™ stent, which was designed specifically for the control of dissection and acute closure. Stents were successfully deployed in all of the 115 patients studied, and optimum results were obtained in 93% of the patients. Despite the emergent nature of the procedures, the number of complications was low, with 4.2% of cases requiring CABG, an overall myocardial infarction rate of 16%, a subacute thrombosis rate of 7.6%, and an in-hospital mortality rate of 1.7%. These results suggested that stenting for acute or threatened closure limited the need for emergency CABG and reduced the incidence of myocardial infarction. The high incidence of restenosis (41%), similar to rates seen in acute closure successfully managed by balloon dilatation alone, indicated that the stent gave no benefit to late outcome when used for the treatment of acute closure.

More favorable were the results of a multicentre registry of elective stent placement in native coronary vessels (1987–89), presented in 1991 by Schatz and colleagues.[19] Their study compared the implantation of balloon expandable intracoronary stents of two different configurations; the prototypical rigid Palmaz-type stent, and an articulated Palmaz–Schatz™ stent fashioned with a bridging strut between two shorter stainless-steel slotted tubes (figure 1.10). In this study 21% of patients had total occlusion, and 69% had a previously

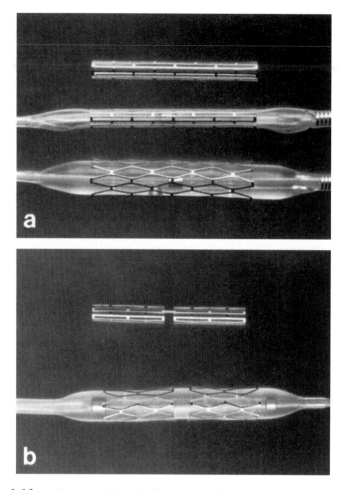

Figure 1.10: *(a) Prototype Palmaz balloon expandable rigid intracoronary stent. (b) Articulated Palmaz-Schatz stent.*

successful coronary angioplasty with clinical and angiographic restenosis. Successful delivery of 299 stents was accomplished in 230 lesions in 213 (93%) patients. Failed delivery occurred with 22 stents, 11 of which were successfully withdrawn, three partially deployed, and eight embolized systemically after failed withdrawal. Two anticoagulation regimens were used. The first 17 stented patients were given procedural dextran and heparin, and discharged on aspirin and dipyridamole only. No episodes of abrupt closure were seen in these patients. Thereafter, as more patients were treated a significant number of thrombotic episodes occurred. Warfarin was added to the postprocedural

10

regimen after the first 35 patients were treated. In the 174 patients stented thereafter, warfarin was administered and continued for 1–3 months. This procedural change brought a dramatic reduction in the incidence of occlusive thrombosis (0.6%). This low incidence of subacute thrombosis could not be confirmed in a retrospective analysis reported by Haude and colleagues[20] in the same year, which used the same device. In the latter study, a subacute thrombosis rate of 14% was reported, although the studies were not directly comparable in terms of selection of patients. Restenosis rates determined at follow-up angiography were 36% in the registry series of Schatz,[21] and 27% in the work of Haude and colleagues.[20] A higher restenosis rate was seen in those lesions treated with multiple stents[21,22] and in those with a history of restenosis in the stented segment.[21]

The first trial to focus specifically on stent implantation for the treatment of restenosis after angioplasty was published in 1992.[22] In this article, de Jaegere and colleagues[22] described their experience with the Medtronic Wiktor™ stent, a unique coil-like prosthesis made of a single loose interdigitating tantalum wire. Stents were successfully implanted in 59 patients. Thrombotic stent occlusion occurred in 10% of the treated patients, all of whom subsequently suffered a myocardial infarction. The restenosis rate, defined as a change in diameter stenosis of greater than 50% at follow-up, was 29%.

Taken together, these early observational trials highlighted problems with the use of stents. Subacute stent thrombosis was clearly a problem despite the very aggressive anticoagulation regimens used in several of the studies. Rigorous anticoagulation resulted in a longer hospital stay, and in bleeding complications that were difficult to control and occasionally serious. Restenosis of the stented segment was also a problem, with restenosis rates comparable to those seen with angioplasty alone. Nonetheless, these technical obstacles to stent deployment helped to define ideal stent characteristics (table 1.1).

Several fundamental questions were raised by these and other small observational trials. Were the disparate results from the various stent registries related to the clinical circumstances that dictated stent implantation, or were they due to properties inherent in the particular device? Was there a clinical situation for which stenting could provide the solution? After these early trials, the utility of stenting for the treatment of obstructive coronary artery disease remained to be proven.

These pioneer investigators were convinced that coronary stenting could become a standard therapeutic modality in interventional cardiology, through improved periprocedural management of patients, better selection of patients, and clearly defined clinical indications. Their convictions led to the initiation of two major important randomized trials comparing balloon angioplasty with elective Palmaz–Schatz coronary stenting. The European BENESTENT[23] and the North American STRESS[24] studies both began recruitment of patients in 1991. In

11

Table 1.1 Desirable stent characteristics
Flexible
Trackable
Low unconstrained profile
Radio-opaque
Thromboresistant
Biocompatible
Reliably expandable
High radial strength
Circumferential coverage
Low surface area
Hydrodynamic compatibility

both studies, patients were randomized to conventional balloon angioplasty or to implantation of a Palmaz–Schatz stent in a primary lesion of a native coronary artery with a length of less than 15 mm and a diameter stenosis of 50% (BENESTENT) or 70% (STRESS). A total of 516 patients (257 balloon, 259 stent) all of whom had stable angina, were recruited in the BENESTENT study: 407 patients (202 balloon, 205 stent), of whom 47% had unstable angina symptoms, were randomized in the STRESS study. The incidence of restenosis, according to the 50% diameter stenosis criterion, was significantly lower after stent implantation (BENESTENT 22%, STRESS 32%) than after balloon dilatation alone (BENESTENT 32%, $p = 0.02$, STRESS 42%, $p = 0.046$). Importantly, this difference was associated with a more favourable long-term clinical outcome in patients who received a stent. The 7-month event-free survival in the BENESTENT trial was 79.9% after stenting and 70.4% after balloon angioplasty ($p < 0.05$). In the STRESS study, the comparable figures were 80.5% and 76.0% respectively (difference not significant). The benefits of stent implantation compared with balloon angioplasty were largely due to a reduced need for reintervention in the stent group. The observed benefit came at a cost, however, with stented patients experiencing increased vascular and bleeding complications, and needing a longer hospital stay. One-year follow-up results of the BENESTENT trial showed a continued benefit for stented patients, with a 1-year event-free survival of 76.8% compared with 68.5% in the balloon angioplasty patients.[25] These two landmark trials conclusively showed that the elective placement of intracoronary stents significantly reduced the incidence of angiographic restenosis in patients with discrete, de-novo lesions in large target vessels. Paradoxically, the BENESTENT and STRESS trials were accepted by clinicians as being positive overall, despite a subacute occlusion rate of 3.7% (which was higher than with balloon angioplasty alone), longer hospitalization times, and more vascular and bleeding complications.

With the publication of the BENESTENT and STRESS trial results and the resultant acceptance of coronary stenting as a promising alternative to angioplasty, attention was then given to improving technical aspects of stent implantation, optimizing adjunctive therapy, and minimizing complication rates. Thrombosis within the self-expanding stainless-steel Medinvent stent, as seen in the early animal experiments,[9] prompted the use of intracoronary urokinase along with heparin, aspirin, dipyridamole, and coumadin in the first human coronary implants.[15] Despite this very aggressive anticoagulation regimen, thrombosis remained a problem. The addition of dextran and sulphinpyrazone[16] increased the number of anticoagulation agents to seven, which led to inevitable bleeding and vascular complications, and a prolonged hospital stay. The high early occlusion rates with these devices[16,17] suggested that stents were highly thrombogenic foreign bodies, and this discouraged investigators from using coronary stents as a primary treatment for coronary artery stenosis. However, Antonio Colombo and his group[26–28] focused attention on the modalities of stent deployment, and questioned the dogma of the intrinsic thrombogenic nature of the stents. The major contribution of these investigators was to assume that the normalization of the rheology inside the stent, as well as its inflow and outflow, would render the anticoagulation treatment superfluous. Intravascular ultrasound imaging had a pivotal role in revealing that most of the angiographically satisfactory stent implantations were far from optimum.[26,27] Incomplete stent apposition, persistence of residual luminal narrowing because of incomplete or asymmetrical stent expansion, and the presence of significant disease of the proximal and distal reference segments could not be easily detected with angiography, and required intravascular ultrasound for visualization. With the use of additional high-pressure non-compliant balloon angioplasty to expand the stent fully, and with stent deployment guided by intravascular ultrasound, Colombo and colleagues progressively decreased the postintervention anticoagulation regimen, and finally stopped it altogether. The procedure had a very low closure rate and a similarly low incidence of vascular complications.[28] Using a strategy of stent deployment largely influenced by the Colombo approach, a multicentre French trial[29] initiated in 1992 examined the feasibility of stenting without postprocedural vitamin-K antagonists and without mandatory ultrasound. With

13

combined aspirin–ticlopidine antiplatelet therapy and subcutaneous low molecule weight heparin treatment, these researchers observed a significant reduction in the rate of subacute thrombosis. These results have been validated in a larger multicentre European prospective observational trial.[30] Neumann and colleagues[31] observed that platelet markers rather than the coagulation parameters indicated the risk of stent thrombosis. This finding supports the use of antiplatelet rather than anticoagulant postprocedural management. The benefits of combined antiplatelet therapy compared with anticoagulant treatment after coronary stenting were confirmed by the pivotal prospective randomized Intracoronary Stenting and Antithrombotic Regimen (ISAR) trial[32] which showed that aspirin plus ticlopidine therapy reduced haemorrhagic and vascular complications, and the incidence of cardiac events.

Today, full antiplatelet therapy, without additional subcutaneous heparin and without ultrasound guidance, has become routine clinical practice. Using this approach, acute and subacute closure rates have become acceptably low, although the search for a better antiplatelet agent continues, and the problem of restenosis remains. All currently available stents are made of metal, and induce significant intimal hyperplasia. New approaches are being tested in order to solve the problem of restenosis, including coatings for metallic stents, stents made of biological materials, biodegradable stents, drug-eluting stents, and radioactive stents. With continued developments and refinements, coronary stenting will remain an integral part of interventional cardiology.

References

1. Dotter CT, Judkins MP. Transluminal treatment of arteriosclerotic obstruction. *Circulation* 1964; **30:** 654–70.

2. Dotter CT. Transluminally-placed coilspring endarterial tube grafts: long term patency in canine popliteal artery. *Invest Radiol* 1969; **4:** 329–32.

3. Ruygrok PN, Serruys PW. Intracoronary stenting: from concept to custom. *Circulation* 1996; **94:** 882–90.

4. Mulliken JB, Goldwyn RM. Impressions of Charles Stent. *Plastic and Reconstructive Surgery* 1978; **62:** 173–76.

5. Dotter CT, Buschmann PAC, McKinney MK, Rösch J. Transluminal expandable nitinol coil stent grafting: preliminary report. *Radiology* 1983; **147:** 259–60.

6. Cragg A, Lund G, Rysavy J, Casteneda F, Casteneda-Zuniga W, Amplatz K. Nonsurgical placement of arterial endoprostheses: a new technique using nitinol wire. *Radiology* 1983; **147:** 261–63.

7. Maass D, Zollikofer CL, Largiadèr F, Senning A. Radiological follow-up of

transluminally inserted vascular endoprostheses: an experimental study using expanding spirals. *Radiology* 1984; **152:** 659–63.

8. Wright KC, Wallace S, Charnsangavej C, Carrasco CH, Gianturco C. Percutaneous endovascular stents: an experimental evaluation. *Radiology* 1985; **156:** 69–72.

9. Palmaz JC, Sibbit RR, Reuter SR, Tio FO, Rice WJ. Expandable intraluminal graft: a preliminary study. *Radiology* 1985; **156:** 73–77.

10. Palmaz JC, Sibbit RR, Tio FO, Reuter SR, Peters JE, Garcia F. Expandable intraluminal vascular graft: a feasibility study. *Surgery* 1986; **99:** 199–205.

11. Rousseau H, Puel J, Joffre F et al. Self-expanding endovascular prosthesis: an experimental study. *Radiology* 1987; **164:** 709–14.

12. Roubin GS, Robinson KA, King SB III et al. Early and late results of intracoronary arterial stenting after coronary angioplasty in dogs. *Circulation* 1987; **76:** 891–97.

13. Schatz RA, Palmaz JC, Tio FO, Garcia F, Garcio O, Reuter SR. Balloon-expandable intracoronary stents in the adult dog. *Circulation* 1987; **76:** 450–57.

14. Puel J, Joffre F, Rousseau H, Guermonprez B, Lancelin B, Morice MC. Endo-prothèses coronariennes auto-expansives dans le prévention des resténoses après angioplastie transluminale. *Arch Mal Coeur* 1987; **8:** 1311–12.

15. Sigwart U, Puel J, Mirkovitch V, Joffre F, Kappenberger L. Intravascular stents to prevent occlusion and restenosis after transluminal angioplasty. *N Engl J Med* 1987; **316:** 701–06.

16. Serruys PW, Strauss BH, Beatt KJ et al. Angiographic follow-up after placement of a self-expanding coronary artery stent. *N Engl J Med* 1991; **324:** 13–17.

17. Block PC. Coronary-artery stents and other endoluminal devices. *N Engl J Med* 1991; **324:** 52–53.

18. Roubin GS, Cannon AD, Agrawal SK et al. Intracoronary stenting for acute and threatened closure complicating percutaneous transluminal coronary angioplasty. *Circulation* 1992; **85:** 916–27.

19. Schatz RA, Baim DS, Leon M et al. Clinical experience with the Palmaz–Schatz coronary stent. Initial results of a multicenter study. *Circulation* 1991; **83:** 148–61.

20. Haude M, Erbel R, Straub U, Dietz U, Meyer J. Short and long term results after intracoronary stenting in human coronary arteries: monocentre experience with the balloon-expandable Palmaz–Schatz stent. *Br Heart J* 1991; **66:** 337–45.

21. Ellis SG, Savage M, Fischman D et al. Restenosis after placement of Palmaz-Schatz stents in native coronary arteries: initial results of a multicenter experience. *Circulation* 1992; **86:** 1836–44.

22. de Jaegere PP, Serruys PW, Bertrand M et al. Wiktor stent implantation in patients with restenosis following balloon angioplasty of a native coronary artery. *Am J Cardiol* 1992; **69:** 598–602.

23. Serruys PW, de Jaegere P, Kiemeneij F et al, for the Benestent Study Group. A comparison of balloon-expandable-stent implantation with balloon angioplasty in patients with coronary artery disease. *N Engl J Med* 1994; **331:** 489–95.

24. Fischman DL, Leon MB, Baim DS et al, for the Stent Restenosis Study investigators. A randomized comparison of coronary-stent placement and balloon angioplasty in the treatment of coronary artery disease. *N Engl J Med* 1994; **331:** 496–501.

25. Macaya C, Serruys PW, Ruygrok P et al. Continued benefit of coronary stenting versus balloon angioplasty: one year clinical follow-up of Benestent trial. *J Am Coll Cardiol* 1996; **27:** 255–61.

26. Goldberg SL, Colombo A, Nakamura S, Almagor Y, Maiello L, Tobis J. Benefit of intracoronary ultrasound in the deployment of Palmaz–Schatz stents. *J Am Coll Cardiol* 1994; **24:** 996–1003.

27. Nakamura S, Colombo A, Gaglione S et al. Intracoronary ultrasound observations during stent implantation. *Circulation* 1994; **89:** 2026–34.

28. Colombo A, Hall P, Nakamura S et al. Intracoronary stenting without anticoagulation accomplished with intravascular ultrasound guidance. *Circulation* 1995; **91:** 1676–88.

29. Morice MC, Zemour G, Beneviste E et al. Intracoronary stenting without coumadin: one month results of a French multicenter study. *Cathet Cardiovasc Diagn* 1995; **35:** 1–7.

30. Morice M.-C. Preliminary results of the MUST trial. *J Invas Cardiol* 1996; **8** (suppl E): 8E–9E.

31. Neumann FJ, Gawaz M, Ott I, May A, Mössmer G, Schömig A. Prospective evaluation of hemostatic predictors of subacute stent thrombosis after coronary Palmaz-Schatz stenting. *J Am Coll Cardiol* 1996; **27:** 15–21.

32. Schömig A, Neumann FJ, Kastrati A et al. A randomized comparison of antiplatelet and anticoagulant therapy after the placement of coronary-artery stents. *N Engl J Med* 1996; **334:** 1084–89.

16

2. STENTS CURRENTLY AVAILABLE

At present there are only five stents approved by the FDA for routine clinical use in the USA. In 1993, the FDA granted approval of the Gianturco–Roubin™ stent for use in the treatment of acute or threatened vessel closure during coronary interventions. In the following year, approval of the Palmaz–Schatz™ stent was given for the treatment of discrete (less than 15 mm in length), de-novo lesions in the native circulation in symptomatic patients (lesion characteristics defined in the BENESTENT and STRESS trials). In 1997, the MULTI-LINK™ stent was approved for use for similar indications, followed by the AVE GFX™ and the NIR™ stents in 1998. In clinical practice however, the use of coronary stents has extended beyond these indications, and as the variety and sophistication of stenting devices improves, new applications are being tested.

Stents that are presently available have five basic design types; tubular, coil, ring, multi-design and mesh (table 2.1). None of these designs incorporates all of the characteristics of the ideal stent, and each has its own particular advantages and disadvantages. The feature common to tubular stents is that they are all laser cut from a continuous cylinder of stainless steel or nitinol. Coil stents are manufactured from a single strand of metal wire wound into a particular pattern, and ring devices are repeating modules of short coils. Both of these designs give a stent that is highly flexible, and both share the disadvantage of uneven expansion at the site of resistance. Therefore, completely performed percutaneous transluminal coronary angioplasty (PTCA) or debulking procedures, with a resultant smooth lumen, are required for the use of these stents. The early generation coil and ring stents were less resistant to external radial forces than the early tubular devices, which may have led to greater recoil of the stented site. Of the newer, more sophisticated designs, however, the best-performing coil stents have crush-resistance properties equal to those of the best-performing tubular stent.[1] Coverage of the lesion site is better with the tubular design, in which the stent is cut from a continuous metal tube. However, the relative inflexibility of most tubular stents makes advancement of the device through tortuous vessels difficult (poor trackability). By nature of the design, the self-expanding mesh stents shorten considerably and often unpredictably in the treated segment, making precise placement difficult even when used by expert operators. With mesh stents, side-branch accessibility is difficult.

Currently, there are more than 55 standard and customized stent types

Table 2.1 Currently available multipurpose stents

Stent type	Composition	Radio-opacity of stent	Radio-opaque markers	Surface area (%) [4 mm expanded]	Expansion mechanism
Coil					
Freedom, Freedom Force	316L stainless steel	Moderate	On balloon	15, 17	Balloon delivery
Wiktor-GX*, –i*	Tantalum	High	On balloon	8, 9	Balloon delivery
Crossflex	316L stainless steel	Moderate	On balloon	22	Balloon delivery
Angiostent	90% Platinum/10% Iridium	High	On balloon and sheath	9	Balloon delivery
GR II	316L stainless steel	High	On stent	16	Balloon delivery
Tubular					
V-Flex, V-Flex Plus	stainless steel	Moderate	On balloon	13, 14	Balloon delivery
Radius	Nitinol	Moderate	On sheath	20	Self-expanding
divYsio	Phoshphorylcholine coated 316L stainless steel	Moderate	None	14	Balloon delivery
beStent (BES, BEL)	316L stainless steel	Moderate	On stent	16, 15	Balloon delivery
IRIS II, Spiral Force, Zebra	316L stainless steel	Moderate	On balloon	16, 12, 15	Balloon delivery
TENSUM, TENAX	a-SiC:H coated tantalum, a-SiC:H coated stainless steel	High Moderate	None On stent	13 13	Balloon delivery Balloon delivery
Palmaz–Schatz* (PS153, Spiral, Crown)	316L stainless steel	Moderate	On balloon	20	Balloon delivery
Paragon	Nitinol	Moderate	None	20	Balloon delivery
JOSTENT Plus*, JOSTENT Flex*	316L stainless steel	Moderate	None	16	Balloon delivery
Balloon Expandable (BX)	316L stainless steel	Moderate	None	16	Balloon delivery
PURA-A, -VARIO	316L stainless steel	Moderate	None	14	Balloon delivery
R Stent	316L stainless steel	Moderate	None	15	Balloon delivery

Table 2.1 continued

InFlow; InFlow-Gold	316L stainless steel	Moderate	On balloon	12	Balloon delivery
Parallel-Serial-Jang	316L stainless steel	Moderate	On balloon	14	Balloon delivery
LP-Stent	316L stainless steel	Moderate	On balloon	15	Balloon delivery
Seaquence	316L stainless steel	Moderate	On balloon	15	Balloon delivery
CIA	316L stainless steel	Moderate	None	<20	Balloon delivery
Diamond AS, Diamond Flex AS	Diamond-like carbon coated 316L stainless steel	Moderate	On balloon	16, 13	Balloon delivery
Terumo	316L stainless steel	Moderate	On balloon	18	Balloon delivery
Synthesis	316L stainless steel	Moderate	On balloon	13	Balloon delivery
PRO-STENT	Heparin-coated 316L stainless steel	Moderate	On balloon	12	Balloon delivery
Medtronic Self-Expanding	Nitinol	Low	On delivery system	13	Self-expanding
Coroflex	316L stainless steel	Low	On balloon	12	Balloon delivery
CrossFlex LC	316L stainless steel	Moderate	On balloon	15	Balloon delivery
MULTI-LINK, MULTI-LINK DUET	316L stainless steel	Moderate	On balloon	15, 14	Balloon delivery
Ring					
AVE Micro II, GFX	316L stainless steel	Moderate	On balloon	8, 20	Balloon delivery
BARD XT	316L stainless steel	High (spine only)	None	13	Balloon delivery
Multi-design					
Navius	Full hard stainless steel	Low	On balloon	38	Balloon delivery
NIR	316L stainless steel	Moderate	On balloon	16	Balloon delivery
Mesh					
Wallstent	Cobalt alloy with platinum core	Moderate	On catheter	14	Self-expanding

* Available with heparin coating.

available for use in the coronary system, manufactured by more than 30 different companies. Most of these devices are second or third generation, with designs that are evolving as stent technology advances.

Mesh stents

Magic Wallstent™ (Schneider [Europe] GmbH [Bülach, Switzerland])

The Wallstent was the first stent to undergo clinical evaluation, and this began a new era in interventional cardiology. The initial evaluation of what was eventually to become the Wallstent began with Rousseau and co-workers[2] who tested a flexible, self-expanding stainless-steel mesh stent that was restrained with a protective sheath. Despite partial or total thrombotic occlusions in 35% of the treated arteries, this early experience provided the impetus for the implantation of a stent in an atheromatous human coronary artery. Clinical evaluation of the Wallstent began in 1986, with the first human implantations done by Jacques Puel (Toulouse, France),[3] followed shortly after by Ulrich Sigwart (Lausanne, Switzerland) and Patrick Serruys (Rotterdam, The Netherlands). The results of the implantation of 24 self-expanding mesh stents (Medinvent SA, Lausanne, Switzerland) in the coronary arteries of 19 patients were reported in 1987.[4] In that year, two additional centres in Lille (France) and London (UK) joined the collaboration, followed in 1989 by Geneva (Switzerland). The European Wallstent experience was an open-ended feasibility study for the possible uses of a coronary stent. At the outset, there was no study protocol to be followed, and each investigator selected the type of lesion to be stented and the anticoagulation regimen. As with all new procedures, operators had to struggle with steep learning curves and develop clinical indications and contraindications from their experience. In May 1988, the five European centres testing the Wallstent agreed to set up a core laboratory in Rotterdam for quantitative angiographic analysis, to assess the results objectively.[5,6] This core laboratory set the standards for the evaluation of new intracoronary treatments that are currently employed.

By the early part of 1988, 117 Wallstents™ had been implanted (94 in native coronary arteries, 23 in aortocoronary-bypass grafts) in 105 patients.[5] Stents were placed for dilation of a restenosis, acute vessel occlusion after angioplasty, chronic occlusion after angioplasty, and as an adjunct to primary angioplasty. The results of intermediate term follow-up of this first series were sobering, with four patient deaths before repeat angiography, complete stent occlusion of 27 stents in 25 (24%) patients, and a long-term restenosis rate of 14% in those that remained patent.[5] A high rate of stent thrombosis emphasized the controversy that surrounded the choice of a suitable anticoagulation regimen to minimize

20

postprocedural complications and haemorrhagic side-effects. In response to published reports of high occlusion rates, the coronary Wallstent was withdrawn from the market in the autumn of 1990, soon after the acquisition of the stent by Schneider (Europe). With better periprocedural anticoagulation regimens and increased operator experience, it became apparent that the high early thrombosis rates in the early trials were not likely to be a result of properties intrinsic to the stent itself, but rather could be attributed to the early learning curve of implantation expertise and errors in periprocedural management. The device was reintroduced in 1994.

The coronary Wallstent has undergone several design modifications since its first release by Medinvent SA (Lausanne, Switzerland). The original stainless-steel Wallstent has been replaced by a device made of strands of a non-ferromagnetic cobalt-based alloy with a platinum core. The wire is arranged into a self-expanding mesh that relies on the elastic range of metal deformation to expand (figure 2.1). The composition and design afford the stent excellent longitudinal flexibility and good radio-opacity. In the expanded state, the metallic surface area of the early devices was roughly 20% of the stented surface. With modification of the wire braid angle, the surface area of later devices was reduced to 14%. Shortly before being withdrawn from the market in 1990, a polymer-coated stent was introduced in an attempt to alleviate the problem of acute thrombosis. The coating was not applied on reintroduction of the devices in 1994.

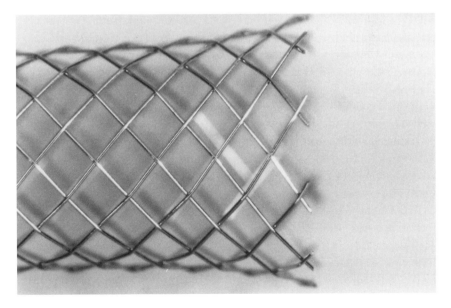

Figure 2.1: *The end of a deployed Wallstent.*

In first-generation devices, the Wallstent was compressed and thus elongated on the delivery system, constrained by a doubled-over membrane system (rolling membrane system). The space between the inner and outer layers of the membrane was filled with contrast medium for lubrication and to enhance fluoroscopic visualization. Retraction of the membrane allowed the stent to be released gradually into the lumen of the coronary artery. With the introduction of the newer Magic Wallstent a few of the disadvantages of the previous design were addressed. With the older device, once the distal end of the stent was released from the protective membrane, the stent could no longer be repositioned. The newer Magic Wallstent has a similar design to the original Wallstent, but the delivery mechanism has been redesigned with a retractable sheath that enables a partially deployed stent (up to 50%) to be recovered with the sheath and repositioned. This improved system allows precise placement of the stent.

Three radio-opaque markers are present on the delivery catheter. These markers are intended to indicate the distal extremity of the stent mounted on the delivery catheter and the approximate length of the implanted stent (indicated by the distance between the middle marker and a proximal marker). Retraction of the membrane progressively releases the stent, which tends to return to its original diameter, thereby anchoring itself against the arterial wall. On expansion, the stent shortens by about 15–20%. Its unconstrained length varies between 15 and 50 mm, and its diameter in the fully expanded state ranges from 3.5 to 6.0 mm.

In general, the Wallstent is placed after dilation of the lesion with a standard balloon angioplasty catheter. In most instances an additional dilation is recommended after stent implantation (the 'Swiss Kiss') to accelerate early expansion of the stent, and in some cases to dissipate clots within the stent. However, this particular stent, due to its self-expanding property, can be implanted without requiring adjunct balloon angioplasty. This is particularly useful in old, diffusely diseased, friable bypass grafts at high risk of embolization with angioplasty. Several centres have advocated the Wallstent as the device of choice for this indication.[7-9] The stent should also be sized so that its unconstrained diameter is 10–20% larger than the reference diameter, which will ensure the presence of a residual radial force. Proper sizing, however, has resulted in continued expansion of the stent after deployment, which can be observed at long-term follow-up.[10] As a result, lumen decrease due to neointimal formation is partially balanced by the self-expanding properties of the Wallstent. This chronic barotrauma does not seem to cause exaggerated neointimal formation. Registry results of the use of the Magic Wallstent in native vessels and bypass grafts are available.[11,12]

Tubular stents

Palmaz–Schatz Stents (PS-153™, Spiral™, Improved Spiral™, Crown™ and Mini-Crown™ [Cordis Corp, a Johnson and Johnson Interventional Systems Co, Warren NJ, USA])

The original Palmaz–Schatz prototype, first described in 1985, consisted of a continuous strand of stainless-steel wire, hand-woven into a mesh on a grooved mandrel.[13] The cross-points of the mesh were silver-soldered to give resistance to radial collapse. The stent was then crimped onto a delivery balloon, and was kept in place by leading and trailing oversized retainers. In early studies, Palmaz and colleagues[13] implanted 11 of these stents of 6–10 mm in diameter into canine common carotid, superior mesenteric, iliac, and renal arteries. Except for three stents for which procedural heparin was used, no anticoagulation therapy was given. After 8 weeks follow-up only one occlusive thrombus in a non-heparinized animal was found. Successful implantation into the coronary circulation of dogs was reported not long afterwards, with the placement of 20 stents which were followed-up for up to 18 months.[14] Aspirin and dipyridamole were given before the procedure, and heparin and low molecular weight dextran were given during the procedure. Aspirin and dipyridamole were then continued for 3 months. All stents remained patent for the duration of the study. The canine model, however, is an unsatisfactory model on which to base conclusions concerning thrombotic potential, in that it has heightened intrinsic plasminogen activator activity and thus has a lessened propensity for thrombosis compared with other models.

In 1986, Palmaz and colleagues reported a further refinement of the prototype stent which they referred to as the BEIG (balloon expandable intraluminal graft).[15] The BEIG was a stainless-steel tube 15 mm long with eight rows of staggered offset slots each 3.5 mm long, similar in design to the current PS-153 stent. This stent was manufactured from a solid tube with the slots etched by electromagnetic discharge. Upon balloon expansion, the rectangular slots assumed a diamond shape with a maximum metal-free area of 80–85%. The inflexibility of this stent made it very difficult to deliver, and its use was restricted almost exclusively to downgoing right coronary artery anatomy. This limitation was addressed first by shortening the stent to 7.0 mm (figure 2.2a) and positioning two or more independent segments on a balloon, and later by connecting two segments with a 1 mm bridge that prevented telescoping and migration of the components at the expense of flexibility (PS-153 series). This stent is currently available mounted on sheathed delivery system (PAS) or unmounted as a "stent-alone" device. The limitations of this device include:

- fixed stent length of 15 mm;
- a "bare area" of 1 mm at the articulation site;

23

- low radio-opacity;
- restricted flexibility;
- high profile and low pressure, compliant balloon of the mounted device.

Despite these limitations, the Palmaz–Schatz PS-153 series stents have undergone the most scrutiny and are the most widely used stents, with more than 1,000,000 patients receiving Palmaz–Schatz stents worldwide. The landmark BENESTENT[16] and STRESS[17] trials used this stent, and the BENESTENT II trial examined the use of heparin-coated Palmaz–Schatz stents in a randomized fashion.[18]

To overcome some of the design weaknesses of the first-generation device, several modifications have been made to the articulated Palmaz–Schatz stent and the delivery system. The result is the Balloon Expandable Spiral Coronary Palmaz–Schatz Stent. This stent is cut with 12 rows and six spiral bridges at the articulation point to eliminate the "bare area" and has twice the radial force of the PS-153 series because of an increase in the thickness of the struts. This stent is better suited for calcified or fibrotic lesions that require added radial force to minimize the degree of residual stenosis. The stent is limited in its longitudinal flexibility, however, and is therefore not suited for the treatment of long tortuous lesions. The stent is available as stent-alone, and mounted on the PAS Delivery System.

The Improved Spiral Coronary Stent incorporates changes with the aim of improving the longitudinal flexibility of the device (figure 2.2b). The wall thickness has been reduced, and the stent is cut with 10 rows and five spiral bridges. The Improved Spiral Coronary Stent is being sold on a high pressure, sheathless, PowerGrip™ rapid exchange delivery system.[19] This delivery system has been designed with a high pressure, non-compliant balloon to eliminate the need for an additional balloon to postdilate the stent after deployment. It has a rapid exchange system with good pushability, trackability, and guidewire movement. The system is compatible with a 6 F guiding catheter to allow use from femoral, brachial, or radial approaches.

The newest stent design from Johnson and Johnson Interventional Systems Co is the Palmaz–Schatz Crown design (figure 2.2c). This design affords increased longitudinal flexibility over the other series without designated articulation points. Longitudinal flexibility in the undeployed state is given by a sinusoidal pattern of slots rather than the previous parallel configuration. In all other respects, the stent possesses similar properties to the PS-153 series and the Improved Spiral Stent in terms of radial force, percent open area, and recoil tendency. With the sinusoidal walls of the diamond shaped cells, passage of a catheter and dilation of "jailed" side branches through these cells is much easier than with other versions of the Palmaz–Schatz stents. This stent is available on the PowerGrip™ delivery system.

24

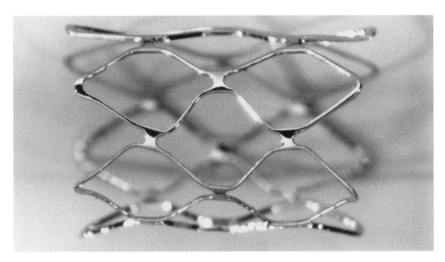

a)

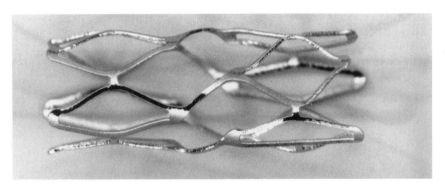

b)

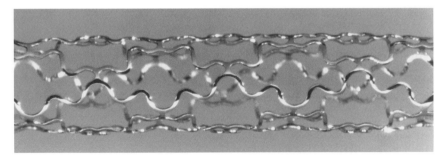

c)

Figure 2.2: (a) An expanded Palmaz–Schatz non-articulated 7 mm long stent; (b) an expanded Improved Spiral Coronary Palmaz–Schatz stent; (c) an expanded Mini-Crown Palmaz–Schatz stent showing the repeating sine wave design.

A more flexible version of the Crown stent, the Mini-Crown, has been developed by reducing the number of rows, the strut thickness, and the strut width, whilst maintaining the sinusoidal wave strut design. Because of the decreased number of rows, optimal expansion ranges from 2.25 to 3.25 mm, thus allowing stent placement in vessels as small as 2 mm. The Mini-Crown stent is available on a new delivery platform, the Dynasty™ Delivery System. This delivery balloon has a very low profile, a high-rated burst pressure of 18 atmospheres, a high-friction surface, favourable rewrapping characteristics, and a 6 F delivery in both over-the-wire and monorail configurations.

The Palmaz–Schatz stents have been further modified by covalently bonding heparin to the stent using the propriety Carmeda process, to render the stent non-thrombogenic. Both the PS-153 series and the Spiral series have been heparin coated and tested. The PS-153 heparin-coated stents have been tested in the BENESTENT II Pilot Study[20] and the BENESTENT II Randomized Trial.[18,21] Of the 616 patients receiving the heparin-coated stent in these two groups of patients, only one patient suffered subacute occlusion, yielding an overall subacute thrombosis rate of less than 0.2%.

Radioactive Palmaz–Schatz PS-153 series stents are also available. These devices are made radioactive by ion implantation of the pure β emitter ^{32}P implanted beneath the stent surface. Clinical trials of the radioactive stent have been done.

ACS MULTI-LINK™, ACS MULTI-LINK RX DUET™ (Guidant/Advanced Cardiovascular Systems [Santa Clara, CA, USA])

The ACS MULTI-LINK stent is a stainless-steel balloon expandable tubular stent, cut to form a series of nested rings interconnected with small bridging struts (figure 2.3a). The perimeter length of the individual cells allows easy side branch access and the cells can be dilated up to 3.6 mm in diameter. The first-generation devices were covered with a protective sleeve to prevent stent dislodgement before proper positioning of the device. The sheath was withdrawn by activation of a manipulator handle. Second-generation devices do not include this protective sheath. Positioned between the delivery balloon and the stent is a layer of elastomeric material, which is designed to ensure radial concentric stent deployment and to prevent uneven stent expansion, a problem with most balloon expandable devices.

Clinical use of this device began in Europe in 1993[22] and led to two small European registry trials, WEST I[23-25] and WEST II[26] (Western European Stent Trial), which were done in 1995–96. The stent was released for commercial use in Europe in 1995. WEST I studied 102 patients on an anticoagulation protocol

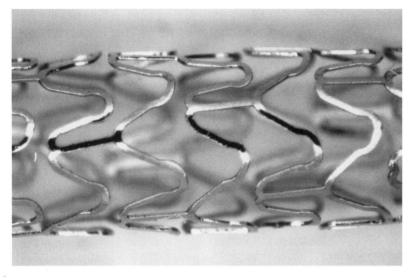

a)

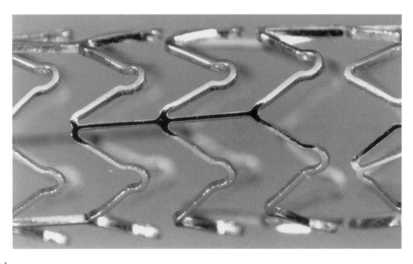

b)

Figure 2.3: (a) An expanded MULTI-LINK stent; (b) an expanded MULTI-LINK RX DUET stent showing the triangular repeating unit with a rounded apex and the difference in articulation compared with the earlier generation MULTI-LINK stent.

of ASA plus coumadin, and WEST II studied 165 patients on an antiplatelet regimen of ASA plus ticlopidine. The major adverse cardiac event rate at 30 days was reported as 5.9% in WEST I, and 1.8% in WEST II. The first US implants of the MULTI-LINK stent were done in 1995,[27,28] and several North American

27

registry trials[29,30] were done in parallel to the large multicentre randomized ASCENT equivalency trial, which compared a 15-mm sheathed MULTI-LINK stent to the Palmaz–Schatz stent in focal de-novo lesions.[31]

The ACS stent is available on four different delivery systems, a rapid exchange delivery system (RX MULTI-LINK™), a rapid exchange high pressure delivery system (RX MULTI-LINK™ HP), an over-the-wire delivery system (MULTI-LINK™), and an over-the-wire high-pressure delivery system (MULTI-LINK™ HP). The favourable early clinical results and registry data collected with the use of this stent,[22–30,32–41] and the proven equivalence with the Palmaz–Schatz stent,[31] led to FDA approval for the use of this device in October 1997.

The newest ACS stent, the ACS MULTI-LINK RX DUET stent, is the next generation of MULTI-LINK stent (figure 2.3b). The modifications made to create the ACS MULTI-LINK RX DUET stent involve the pattern, strut thickness, and articulation frequency. The rounded repeating unit of the MULTI-LINK has been replaced with a triangular unit with a rounded apex. In addition, to augment its radio-opacity and radial strength, the strut thickness has been increased. To maintain flexibility, the number of articulations between the repeating units has been decreased. On the earlier MULTI-LINK design there are three articulations per ring, but the ACS MULTI-LINK RX DUET stent has an alternating pattern of two or three articulations per ring. These modifications were made to produce a stent which will be available both loose (ACS MULTI-LINK SOLO) and premounted (ACS MULTI-LINK RX DUET), with performance characteristics similar or superior to the original MULTI-LINK design.

Radius™ (SciMED Life Systems [Maple Grove MN, USA])

The SciMED Radius stent has a multiple zigzag segment design, and is cut from a single cylinder of nitinol metal (figure 2.4). The stent is delivered by wire pull-

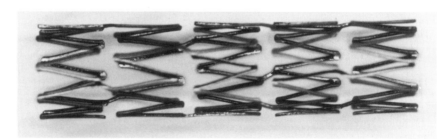

Figure 2.4: A deployed Radius stent.

back of the restraining sheath, and does not shorten after full stent expansion. There is no mechanical recoil of this stent, but as the stent does not expand beyond its nominal size, proper sizing is very important. In clinical application, implantation of the Radius stent is associated with a low injury score[42] and, with modest oversizing, the stent continues to expand after implantation, which has a favourable influence on the luminal diameter measured at follow-up.[43] With human implantations, it has also been shown that the nitinol Radius stent induces less platelet aggregation than the stainless-steel Palmaz–Schatz and GR-II stents.[44] This finding may be due to the type of metal used, the unique architecture of the Radius stent, or both. A disadvantage of the Radius stent design is the limitation to side branch access. Favourable results of animal testing[45] has led to the initiation of clinical registry series,[46] and to an equivalency trial comparing the Radius with the Palmaz–Schatz stent (SCORES; Stent COmparative REStenosis trial).[47,48]

beStent™ (Medtronic Instent [Minneapolis MN, USA])

The beStent is a stainless-steel, second generation, balloon expandable tubular stent. The wires are arranged in a serpentine design with no welding points, and upon expansion the stent assumes a mesh-like appearance (figure 2.5).[49,50] The unique design of this stent, with its rotational junctions, ensures relative low stress concentration. As the stent expands, the orthogonal cross junctions rotate,

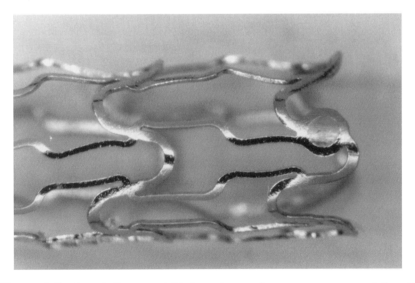

Figure 2.5: The end of an expanded beStent showing the rotating junctions and the gold end-marker.

and the serpentine struts straighten in both longitudinal and radial directions. This mechanism ensures zero shortening during stent expansion, and orthogonal concentration of forces in the radial direction, which provides superior strength. The stent has two radio-opaque terminal gold markers for visibility of the stent ends, which allow for precise positioning. The stent is supplied both bare (in three lengths) and mounted on a delivery balloon (Artist™) in a 15 mm length. The beStent is available in two versions, the beStent small (BES) for use in vessels with a diameter range of 2.5–3.00 mm, and the beStent large (BEL) for vessels with a diameter range of 3.0–5.5 mm. Registry trials are currently underway.[51–57]

TENSUM™ and TENAX™ (Biotronik [Berlin, Germany])

The TENSUM Biotronik stent is a silicon-carbide coated, balloon expandable, tantalum tubular stent configured with two articulations (figure 2.6a). The stent is supplied as a bare device, not mounted on a delivery balloon. The stent material provides high radio-opacity that allows precise positioning of this stent. Disadvantages of this stent are similar to those of the Palmaz–Schatz stent. The connecting bridge may serve as a site for intimal hyperplasia and increased restenosis. The design also results in "stent jail" and lack of access of entrapped side branches. Feasibility and registry data are currently being collected, and randomized trials are planned.[58,59]

The second generation TENAX stent has been designed to address some of the disadvantages of the TENSUM design. Like the TENSUM stent, the TENAX stent is a balloon expandable tubular stent, but the TENAX stent has been redesigned as a series of repeating rings connected with small bridges, and is configured from 316L stainless steel (figure 2.6b). Tantalum radio-opaque marker rings at both ends of the stent allow for better visualization and precise positioning in tortuous arteries. Like the TENSUM stent, the TENAX stent surface is coated with a semiconducting ceramic coating, amorphous silicon carbide (a-SiC:H),[60] applied by a modified plasma-enhanced chemical vapour deposition (PECVD) process.[61] It is thought that the semiconducting material inhibits electrochemical thrombogenic interactions by preventing the transfer of electrons from blood proteins to the stent, thus reducing the polymerization of proteins and activation of circulating platelets.[61]

IRIS II™, Spiral Force™, Zebra™ (Uni-cath Inc [Saddle Brook, NJ, USA])

The IRIS II is a second-generation balloon expandable stainless steel tubular stent. It is designed with unique alternating "C" flex joints that allow for a great deal of flexibility and radial force (figure 2.7a). The unique design, with flex joints and

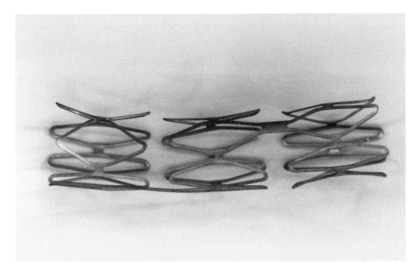

a)

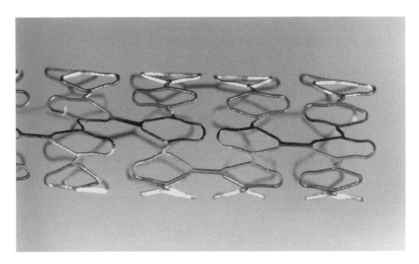

b)

Figure 2.6: (a) An expanded TENSUM stent; (b) an expanded TENAX stent.

diagonal struts, allows the stent to crimp securely and open uniformly upon expansion, yet maintains straight struts to provide scaffolding with maximum radial force. The flex joints also allow the stent to conform to bends in the coronary artery, by closing the segment in the tight portion while opening the joint in the wider portion of the curve. The stent is available as a bare stent, or

31

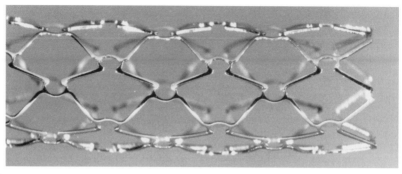

a)

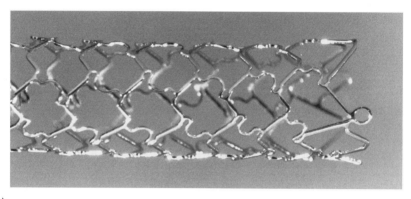

b)

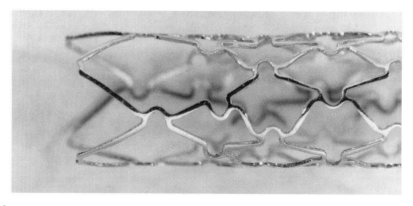

c)

Figure 2.7: *(a) An expanded IRIS II stent showing the "C" flex joints; (b) an expanded Spiral Force stent; (c) an expanded Zebra stent showing the larger cells and less metal content at the the extremes of the stent.*

mounted on a delivery balloon catheter. The mounted device is unique in that the stent is secured onto the balloon and therefore shifting during complex deliveries is prevented. The stent can be released only upon balloon expansion.

The Spiral Force stent is a third-generation, balloon expandable stainless-steel stent (figure 2.7b). The struts in this design are spiral cut, with "C" flex joints similar to the IRIS II stent. Like the IRIS II stent, the Spiral Force stent is available both mounted and bare.

The Zebra stent is the latest generation Uni-cath stent (figure 2.7c). Like the IRIS and Spiral Force stents, it is also a balloon expandable, stainless-steel tubular device. The Zebra stent is configured with inverted "C" joints with diagonal struts. A unique feature of this stent is that the last two circumferential rows of cells at the ends of the stent are larger than those in the central region. The Zebra stent therefore provides more metal coverage in the central 75% of the stent, where it is needed, and less metal coverage at the ends. It is currently available in a single length of 17 mm, with a diameter expansion range of 2.5–4.0 mm.

divYsio™ (Biocompatibles Ltd [Surrey, UK])

The divYsio stents are stainless-steel tubular devices with two configurations. They are based on a similar design, and both have a surface coating of a chemical analogue of naturally occurring phosphorylcholine. Phosphorylcholine is the predominant lipid head group of membrane phospholipids. It is a zwitterionic compound (both positive and negative charge in the same molecule and thus no net charge) and as such will not adsorb proteins. In preclinical studies in vitro, passage of blood containing indium-labelled platelets through an uncoated stainless-steel tube resulted in an exponential increase of platelet adhesion to the metal surface over time, with ensuing total occlusion of the tube by a platelet plug 1 hour after the start of perfusion. Phosphorylcholine coated stents, in contrast, showed a minimum amount of platelet adhesion, and the tubes remained patent after 2 hours of perfusion.[67] Early animal experiments showed that the coating was not associated with excessive tissue reaction[62-66] or with increased neointima formation.[67,68] It is hoped that the phosphorylcholine coating will improve the haemocompatibility of the stent and reduce the incidence of acute and subacute thrombosis in clinical situations, perhaps permitting a reduction in the periprocedural and postprocedural antithrombotic and antiplatelet regimens and consequently reducing vascular and bleeding complications.

The divYsio stent is available in two configurations (figures 2.8a, and 2.8b). Although the basic design of the two models is similar, the slots are cut differently, which results in an open and closed cell configuration. The ends of the stent are rounded to minimize the risk of balloon and vessel damage.

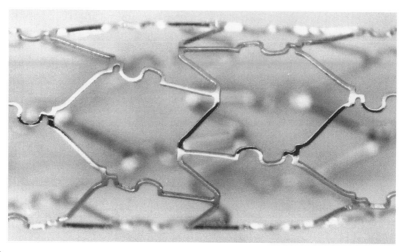

a)

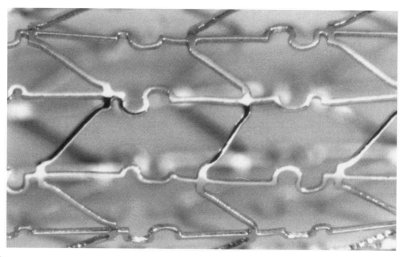

b)

Figure 2.8: (a) An Expanded divYsio stent with an open cell design; (b) an expanded divYsio stent with a closed cell design.

JOSTENT™ Plus, JOSTENT™ Flex (Jomed International AB [Drottninggatan, Sweden])

The JOSTENT Plus and Flex stents are second generation JOSTENTs. Both are stainless-steel, balloon expandable, tubular stents, but each was designed to suit particular applications. The JOSTENT Plus is based upon a multicellular geometry, includes a stronger strut for improved radial strength, and

34

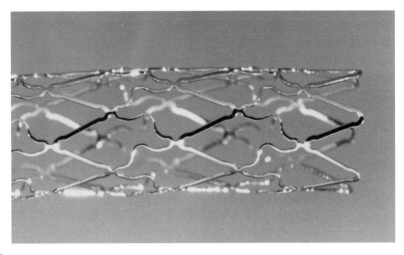

a)

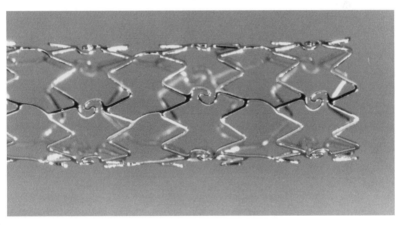

b)

Figure 2.9: (a) The end of an expanded JOSTENT plus; (b) the end of an expanded JOSTENT flex.

incorporates a "loop design" to enhance flexibility (figure 2.9a). This new design provides increased individual cell area and allows the stent to be implanted in vessels up to 6 mm in diameter. The JOSTENT Flex was created specifically for lesions that are difficult to reach (figure 2.9b), and was designed to combine flexibility with high radial strength. The cells are connected with unique spiral bridges. The JOSTENT Flex can be implanted in vessels of up to 5 mm in diameter.

35

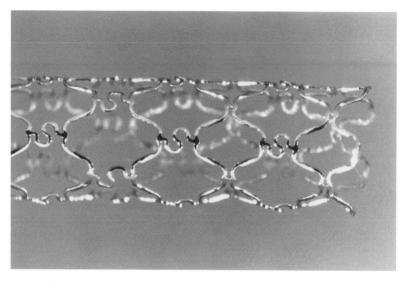

Figure 2.10: *The end of an expanded BX stent showing the unique "H" and "S" struts.*

Balloon Expandable (BX)™ (IsoStent Inc [San Carlos, CA, USA])

The IsoStent BX is a third-generation, balloon expandable, stainless-steel, tubular stent. The configuration combines a unique pattern of two different cell types, both with negative angle struts, with each cell interconnected by either straight "H" or undulating "S" links (figure 2.10). The "H" links provide radial strength, particularly at the stent ends, and "S" links improve longitudinal flexibility. Three of the centrally located "S" cells can be balloon-expanded to 2.5 mm diameter for side branch access. A ^{32}P β-particle-emitting IsoStent BX has also been developed.

PURA-A™, PURA-VARIO™, PURA-VARIO-AS™, PURA-VARIO-AL™ (Devon Medical [Hamburg, Germany])

The first-generation stainless-steel, balloon expandable PURA-A stents were developed in 1995. They are tubular devices with a "Y" shaped geometry of the longitudinal connecting branch points. This design allows the stent to be crimped to very small outer diameters on low-profile balloon catheters. The low profile of the crimped stent and its high radial force make it a good choice for use in calcified lesions. The PURA-A stent is available as a single segment 7 mm long for the treatment of short lesions, and in both articulated (with a single 1 mm articulation bridge) and non-articulated versions for use in longer lesions. The

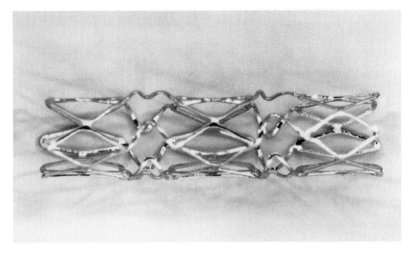

a)

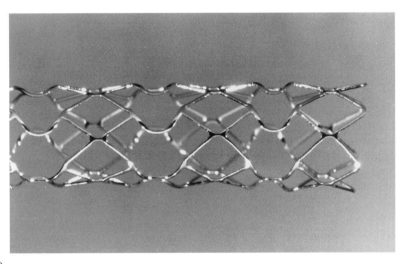

b)

Figure 2.11: *(a) An expanded PURA-VARIO stent; (b) the end of a PURA-VARIO-AS stent showing shortened segment and articulation length compared with the PURA-VARIO device.*

original design of the PURA-A stent has been modified to create the PURA-VARIO family of devices. Like the first-generation device, they are also balloon expandable, stainless-steel, tubular stents (figure 2.11a). PURA-VARIO stents are configured with 4 mm segments connected with specially designed, radially arranged articulating curved bridges. Each segment is comprised of six

37

radially arranged cells. The 2 mm long curved articulations give the device high flexibility and, uniquely, allow the stent to be "customized" prior to crimping and implantation. By pushing the segments together, the metallic coverage of the vessel wall can be increased. By pulling the segments apart, a wider opening can be created to facilitate sidebranch access. The PURA-VARIO stents are not suitable for crimping on low profile PTCA balloons, as the stent may perforate the balloon. In the newer generation PURA-VARIO-AS and -AL stents the strut width has been decreased, which results in a lower profile device compared with the previous generation PURA-VARIO. Like the PURA-VARIO stents, the newer PURA-VARIO-AS device ("S" is for small) also has six cells arranged circumferentially around each segment, with six connecting articulations between each segment. However, in the PURA-VARIO-AS stent, the length of each segment and the span of the articulating bridges have been shortened significantly (figure 2.11b). The -AS stent was designed for use in vessels 3.5 mm in diameter or less. For use in vessels of 3.5 mm or more, the PURA-VARIO-AL device ("L" indicating large), with eight circumferentially arranged cells and eight articulations, has been introduced. Since the PURA-VARIO-AS and -AL stents have an intricate design, side branch access is difficult, and the thinness of the struts results in low radio-opacity. These stents are available both premounted and bare. There is much experience of the use of the PURA family of devices in Europe.[69,70]

Paragon™ (Vascular Therapies, a division of United States Surgical Corporation [Norwalk, CT, USA])

The Paragon stent is a third-generation balloon expandable device (figure 2.12a). The stent has a tubular design cut from a cylinder of martensitic nitinol metal. Nitinol is a unique alloy with thermal-elastic shape-memory properties. It exists either in a martensite or austenite crystal phase.[71] Phase transition is effected by heating the metal above a characteristic temperature determined by the composition of the alloy. At body temperature, the alloy contains a higher martensitic fraction, which gives it a deformable structure. Unlike stainless-steel self-expanding stents and balloon expandable stents, the material properties of the nitinol do not allow the stent to expand beyond its nominal size. Proper sizing is therefore important, and a stent to vessel wall ratio 1.1 to 1.2 is recommended. Also important is the difference in angiographic appearance of a properly deployed nitinol stent compared with that of a thin-walled stainless steel stent. Nitinol has a radio-opacity very similar to that of standard angiographic contrast medium. The angiographic appearance of a sub-optimally deployed stainless-steel stent shows a narrowing in the column of contrast, or a "step-down". This is a result of the relative radio-lucency of stainless-steel compared with contrast. Proper deployment results in a smooth contour to the contrast

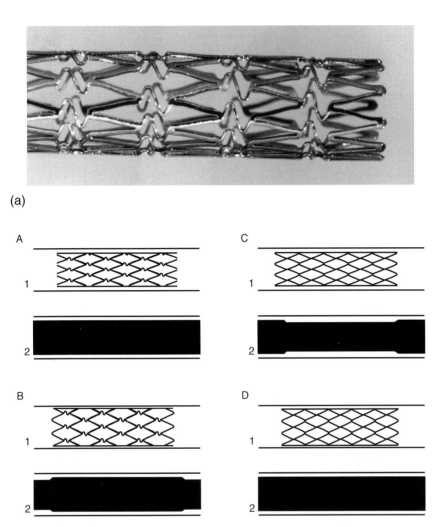

(a)

(b)

Figure 2.12: (a) *The end of an unexpanded Paragon stent.* (b) *angiographic evaluation of the implantation of the nitinol Paragon stent compared with a stainless-steel device. A. A consequence of the sub-optimal implantation of a Paragon stent may be that the stent will not have complete coverage of the arterial wall (1). In this situation, angiography will reveal a smooth linear contrast column (2). This is because the stent and contrast have a similar radio-opacity. B. Correct deployment of Paragon and the stent reveals a "step-up / step down" appearance with angiography. C. The angiographic appearance of a sub-optimally deployed stainless-steel stent is different than that of a nitinol stent. In this instance the lower radio-opacity of the metallic struts gives a "step-down / step-up" appearance to the contrast column (2). D. In contrast to the appearance of a properly deployed Paragon stent, a properly deployed stainless-steel stent will yield a contrast column with a smooth linear contour on angiography.*

column and indicates that the stent is embedded in the vessel wall. Because of the similar radio-opacity between the nitinol Paragon stent and contrast, a smooth contour of the contrast column suggests sub-optimal deployment. Optimal deployment, with the struts embedded in the vessel wall provides a "step-up/step-down" angiographic image (figure 2.12b). The first-generation devices (Act-One™) were composed of two segments connected with a single 0.5 mm articulation bridge. Each segment was comprised of a single cell. Implantation of these first-generation devices in animals began in 1994, and the first clinical experience with this device occurred in 1995. The latest generation Paragon stent has a sinusoidal geometry and no longer has the central articulation point. It is available in lengths of 9, 16, 26 and 36 mm. Several clinical trials of this device are currently underway, including an equivalency trial with the Palmaz–Schatz stent (PAS Trial).

V-Flex™, V-Flex Plus™ (Global Therapeutics Inc [Broomfield, CO, USA])

The V-Flex and V-Flex Plus stents are stainless-steel tubular stents, designed with crown segments linked by alternating "V" bridges or tie bars. The modular design affords a high degree of flexibility and trackability to these devices. The V-Flex stent has six "crowns" on each repeating module, and each module is connected with three tie bars or V bridges (figure 2.13a). The spaces between the segments allow access to side branches, and this stent is well suited for use in bifurcation lesions. The V-Flex Plus stent is configured with segments consisting of eight crowns, and has closer spacing between the modules to give this design improved vessel coverage and radial strength (figure 2.13b). Clinical trials of this stent are underway.[72]

R Stent™(Orbus/Spectranetics [Fort Lauderdale FL, USA])

The R stent is a balloon expandable tubular stainless-steel stent with a helical spiral configuration. The stent was designed for particular use in long and diffuse lesions. The stent has a modular design, segmented into five zones with three different configurations (figure 2.14). Each helical module or zone serves to orient the structure during deployment. The end zones have squared ends and are configured in a double helix lattice. Between the centre zone and the end zones are transition zones which, in combination with the squared end zones, retard premature expansion of the ends and foreshortening of the stent during deployment. The centre zone consists of a dual helix lattice which affords trackability and flexibility to the device. The cells of the end zones are attached with "S" connections, and the transition and central module attachments have

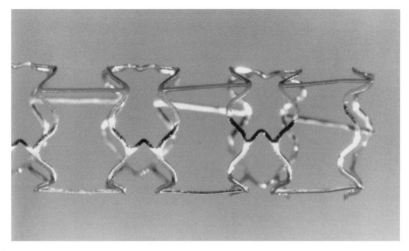

a)

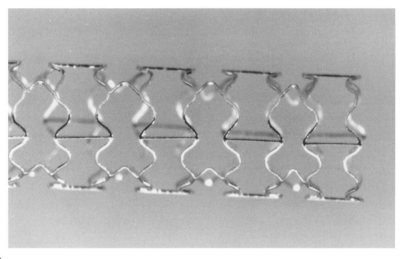

b)

Figure 2.13: (a) An expanded V-Flex stent; (b) an expanded V-Flex Plus stent.

more flexible "X" connections. The "S" connections require more force to open than the "X" connections, which results in the distribution of the balloon expansion forces inward and allows uniform stent deployment. Another unique feature of this design is the oblique orientation of the strut loops. When flexed, the stent struts do not overlap on the lesser curvature. Several other stent designs suffer from this "fish-scaling" effect, and in these devices the protruding strut can

41

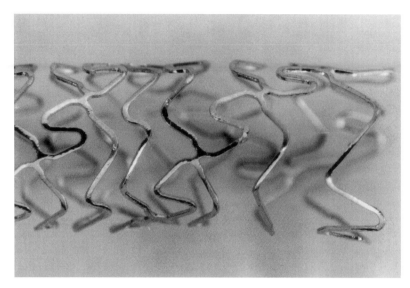

Figure 2.14: *The end of an expanded R stent showing the three zones with different configurations.*

catch on calcium in the vessel wall during positioning. Also of note is the potential for side branch access with the R stent. The cells of the R stent can expand to 4.3 mm in diameter: this is much greater than other slotted-tube devices and allows side branch access. The R stent is currently available bare and premounted.

Parallel-Serial-Jang™ (PSJ-3) (InVentCa Technologies [Redlands, CA, USA])

The PSJ-3 stent is a balloon expandable stainless-steel tubular stent (figure 2.15). The stent has a continuous chain-mesh strut pattern. The rigidity of the expanded device is provided by the interlocking rhomboidal stent geometry. The blind loops of the stent are interlinked by serial connector struts. Reinforced expansion struts at the ends of the PSJ-3 stent provide extra focal radial strength to those regions most vulnerable to strut deformity and loose scaffolding after deployment in the vessel lumen. These reinforced areas also produce tighter focal crimping at both ends of the stent.

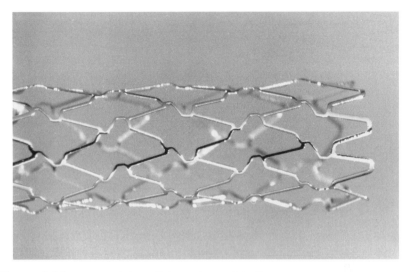

Figure 2.15: *An expanded Parallel-Serial-Jang (PSJ-3) stent.*

InFlow-Stent™, InFlow-Gold-Stent™ (InFlow Dynamics AG [Munich, Germany])

The InFlow stent is a balloon expandable stainless-steel tubular device (figure 2.16a). The stent design has interconnected sinusoidal waves, with six waves around the circumference. The struts of the InFlow stent are oval in cross-section. In addition to bare stainless steel, the InFlow stent is available with a 5 μm thick gold coating (figure 2.16b). Gold is resistant to corrosion and has been shown less thrombogenic than stainless steel in an in-vitro human stasis model.[73,74] Gold has the added advantage of antibacterial properties, and may have antiproliferative effects.[75] The gold-coated InFlow stents have been made radioactive by neutron bombardment to produce the β particle emitter [198]Au. A dose-dependent reduction in neointimal hyperplasia was seen with implantation of stents with activities of 0.2–20 Gray (Gy) in a swine coronary model.[76] The first human implants of the Inflow and Inflow-Gold stents were done in 1996, and there is a large amount of clinical experience with these devices.[77,78]

LP-Stent™ (Interventional Technologies Inc (IVT) [San Diego CA, USA])

The IVT LP-Stent system is a balloon expandable stainless-steel tubular coronary stent with a rapid exchange deployment catheter (figure 2.17a). The struts of the

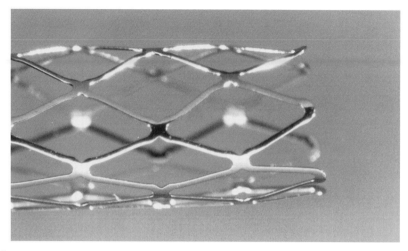

a)

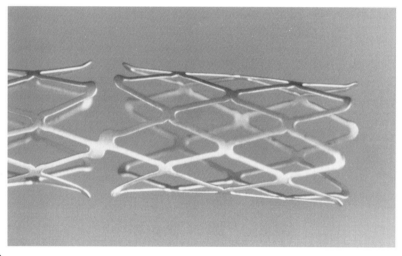

b)

Figure 2.16: (a) The end of an InFlow-Stent; (b) the end of an InFlow-Gold stent.

LP-Stent are pentagonal in cross-section, and configured in a continuous loop design. The lesser angles of the pentagonal struts are radially directed, with the flat portion of the strut apposed to the balloon. A consequence of this orientation is that on deployment the stent struts penetrate the atherosclerotic or restenotic tissue. As a result, the delivered stent struts present no obstruction to blood flow, which improves the hydrodynamic compatibility of this device (figure

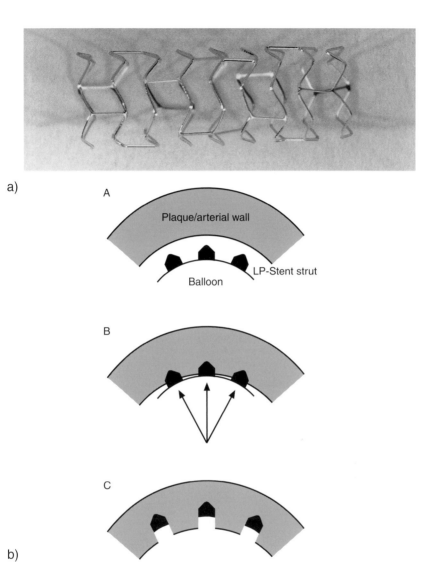

a)

b)

Figure 2.17: *(a) An expanded LP stent. (b) deployment of the LP-Stent. (A) The design of the strut improves the penetration capabilities of the stent and lowers the pressure requirements. (B) The flat strut bottom ensures efficient balloon pressure transmission. (C) The delivered stent struts do not obstruct flow.*

2.17b). The unique shape and configuration of the struts allows for full deployment of the stent at pressures at or below 8 atmospheres. It is thought that the low pressure deployment will enhance long-term vessel patency by reducing pressure-induced barotrauma.

45

The stent is designed with repeating, looped rings. Each repeating unit is joined to its neighbour with two connecting bridges. The connecting bridges are asymmetrically placed, to give a staggered spine that confers high flexibility to the device. The stent is premounted on a rapid-exchange balloon angioplasty system. It is available in diameters of 3.0 and 3.5 mm, and in lengths of 12, 18, and 24 mm.

Seaquence™ (Nycomed Amersham Medical Systems [Paris, France])

The Seaquence stent is a balloon expandable stainless-steel, tubular stent. It is designed as a series of linked rings with a repeating "S" shape, which on expansion yields five circumferential cells (figure 2.18). The lack of obstructing struts in each of the cells allows for easy side branch access. Each ring segment is connected to its neighbour by a single asymmetrically placed bridge, which provides a staggered backbone to improve the flexibility of the device. The principal innovation of the Seaquence stent is the uniform deployment afforded by its unique struts, which are cut to be of variable width. This permits implantation without jutting or twisting of the stent during expansion, results in an improved distribution of mechanical stress, and ensures uniform circumferential coverage of the arterial wall. The Seaquence stent is available premounted on a balloon dilatation catheter in four lengths (8, 18, 28, 38 mm) and in four diameters (2.5, 3.0, 3.5, 4.0 mm). All are 6F-compatible.

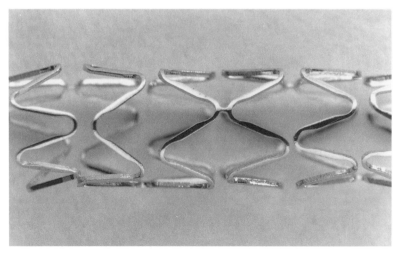

Figure 2.18: An expanded Seaquence stent showing variable width of the stent struts.

CIA (Coronary Improved Architecture) (Stent Tech [Saint Nom La Bretèche, France])

The CIA stent is a stainless-steel, balloon expandable, tubular stent. It has repeating segments each with eight crowns, each of which is linked to its neighbour by eight "S" shaped bridges (figure 2.19). The struts are 0.1 mm thick (0.004 in), and the metallic surface coverage of the vessel wall is less than 20%. The design of this device provides high flexibility and high radial strength, and the relatively large diameter of the cells of the expanded device allows for vessel side branch access. The stent is available bare in lengths of 10, 14, and 20 mm, with an expansion range of 2.5–6.0 mm.

Diamond AS™, Diamond Flex AS™ (Phytis Comércio Internacional LDA [Funchal, Portugal])

The Diamond AS and Diamond AS Flex stents are balloon expandable, tubular, stainless-steel devices coated with a unique diamond-like carbon (DLC) coating (figure 2.20). DLC is an amorphous form of carbon which, when applied to the surface of stainless-steel stents by a chemical vapour deposition method (plasma technology), improves their haemocompatibility[71] and may improve their biocompatibility. In vitro analyses have shown that stents coated with DLC cause less platelet activation[79,80] and are less thrombogenic than their stainless-steel counterparts.[80] The release of cytotoxic heavy metal ions is also greatly reduced in the coated devices.[79]

The repeating unit of the Diamond AS and Diamond Flex AS stents is a sinusoidal ring. The rings of the Diamond AS stent are joined out of phase, which results in open cells on expansion. The repeating units of the Diamond Flex AS stent are connected with bridges of two alternating lengths. This design affords the stent a high degree of flexibility. The Diamond AS stent is available in lengths

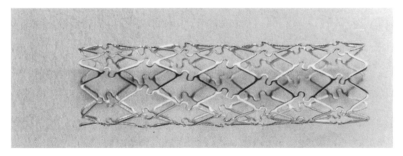

Figure 2.19: *An expanded CIA stent*

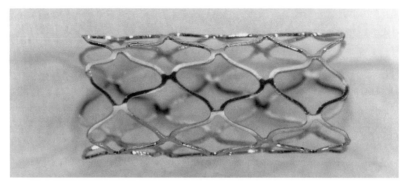

a)

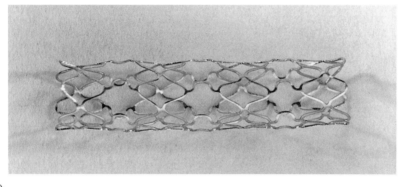

b)

Figure 2.20: (a) An expanded Diamond AS stent; (b) an expanded Diamond Flex AS stent

of 9 mm and 16 mm, and the Diamond Flex AS stent is supplied in lengths of 16 mm and 25 mm. The strut thickness of the Diamond AS stent is 0.06 mm (0.0024 in) and that of the Diamond Flex AS stent is 0.08 mm (0.0032 in, 16 mm stent) and 0.10 mm (0.004 in, 25 mm stent). The expansion range of the Diamond AS stents is between 2.5 and 5.0 mm, and that of the Diamond Flex AS stent is between 2.5 and 6.0 mm. The stents are supplied balloon mounted and are compatible with 6F guiding catheters. Clinical data on the implantation of these stents is currently being collected.

PRO-STENT™ (Medical Concepts Company [Bangalore, India])

The PRO-STENT is a balloon expandable heparin-coated stainless-steel stent (figure 2.21). It has a modular, multi-cellular, tubular design. Each repeating module of the stent is 5 mm in length, and modules are joined with four connecting bridges. The PRO-STENT is available in three lengths; 10, 15, and 20 mm. The 10 mm stent is comprised of two connected modules, and the 15 and 20 mm stents have three and four modules, respectively. The strut thickness of the PRO-STENT is 0.15 mm (0.006 in). It is available both bare and premounted on a low compliance rapid-exchange balloon catheter. The expansion range for the PRO-STENT is between 2.5 and 4.0 mm.

Terumo™ (Terumo Deutschland GmbH [Frankfurt am Main, Germany])

The Terumo stent, developed in Japan, is a balloon expandable, stainless-steel, tubular stent (figure 2.22). The repeating unit of the stent is four radially

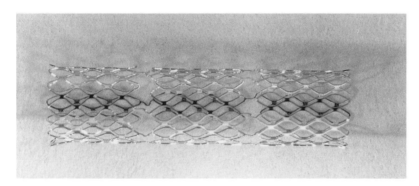

Figure 2.21: *An expanded PRO-STENT*

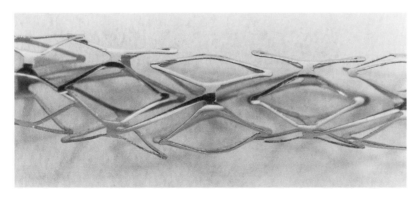

Figure 2.22: *An expanded Terumo Stent*

49

arranged diamonds joined by a single connecting bridge. The thickness of the struts is 0.08 mm (0.0031 in). The Terumo stent is available premounted in lengths of 20, 30, and 40 mm, and in diameters of 2.5, 3.0, and 3.5 mm. Favourable results of a single-centre registry trial of the Terumo stent have been reported.[81]

Synthesis™ (CardioVascular Dynamics Inc (CVD) [Irvine CA, USA])

The Synthesis stent is a balloon expandable, stainless-steel, tubular stent (figure 2.23). It is constructed with serpentine rings linked together with two connecting bridges. The connecting bridges alternate between straight and oblique along the length of the stent. The struts of the Synthesis stent are 0.08 mm (0.0032 in) thick. These design features give the Synthesis stent a high degree of trackability and radial strength. The Synthesis stent is available bare in lengths of 17 and 28 mm, and premounted on the Star™ delivery system in a 17 mm length only.

The Synthesis Star System™ is a truly unique concept. The Synthesis stent is mounted on a multicompliant, multidiameter balloon. At nominal pressure, the balloon expands evenly and starts to focalize. As pressure increases, the focalization becomes more distinct, and radial dilating forces are concentrated within the stent segment. By directing the force, stent expansion is maximized whilst damage to the adjoining inflow and outflow regions is minimized. This "focal stenting" concept has been successfully employed in several controlled series. In the MUSCAT (MUSic using CAT) trial, Palmaz–Schatz stents were implanted using a CAT™ focal angioplasty balloon (CVD).[82] The key observation of this trial was the ability to both predilate and high-pressure postdilate the stents with a single balloon, thereby reducing the number of balloons used per

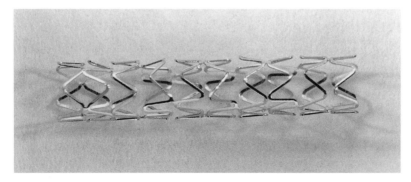

Figure 2.23: *An expanded synthesis stent*

case. The relatively small number of patients (47) prevented any conclusions regarding the potential clinical benefits of this approach. The OSTI-II (Optimal Stent Implantation II) trial has been designed to give more information on the potential benefits of focal stenting.[83] In this multicentre study, two groups of patients are being studied. In vessels greater than 3 mm in diameter, standard angioplasty balloons sized 1:1 are used to high-pressure postdilate Palmaz–Schatz stents until a successful angiographic result is achieved. Intravascular ultrasound (IVUS) followed by focal balloon dilatation is done to improve the final results. In the second group of patients, vessels with angiographic lumen reference diameters of less than 3 mm are stented using the focal stenting concept. Preliminary results of the OSTI-II trial show that with focal stenting a larger lumen diameter is obtained, which may improve long-term results.[84,85]

The single-centre randomized SIPS (Strategy of Intracoronary ultrasound guided PTCA and Stenting) trial was designed to test the hypothesis that a combination of intracoronary ultrasound (ICUS) guidance and focal angioplasty could provide a cost-effective approach to improved interventional results compared with routine angiographically guided intervention with conventional unidiameter balloons.[86,87] In all, 269 patients were randomized, but stent use was not regulated and occurred in 52% of each group of patients. The primary angiographic endpoints of this trial were the acute minimal luminal diameter (MLD) and the MLD at follow-up; the clinical endpoints were the occurrence of major cardiac events (death, myocardial infarction, repeat revascularization) at 6 months' follow-up. Results of the SIPS trial show that procedural ICUS guidance leads to an improved net gain in MLD (1.25 ± 0.95 mm for ICUS guidance *vs*

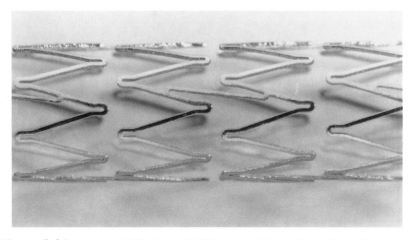

Figure 2.24: An expanded Medtronic Self-Expanding Nitinol Stent. The midpoint attachment of the connecting bridges is shown

0.78 ± 0.89 mm for angiographic guidance, p = 0.01) and a trend towards lower target lesion revascularization procedures and restenosis rates.[88]

Medtronic Self-Expanding Nitinol Stent (Medtronic Instent [Minneapolis MN, USA])

The Medtronic Nitinol Stent is a self-expanding nitinol tubular device with a "Christmas tree" mesh design (figure 2.24). It is supplied on SOE (single operator exchange) delivery catheter protected by an overtube which radially constrains the stent prior to deployment. Upon retraction of the overtube, the stent is self-expanded in situ to the required vessel diameter. The stent is available in diameters of 3.0–4.5 mm and in lengths of 8, 15, 25, and 36 mm. Registry studies are currently underway.

Coroflex™ (B. Braun Melsungen AG, [Berlin, Germany])

The Coroflex stent is a pre-mounted, balloon expandable, stainless-steel, tubular stent (figure 2.25). The stent is designed with sinusoidal ring elements connected with flexible bridges. The connecting bridges are mid-point attached to the ring elements which results in low shortening during expansion. The geometry, length and diameter of the bridges give the device high flexibility. The strut thickness is 0.080 mm (0.0032 in). The Coroflex stent is available in lengths of 9, 16 and 24 mm, and in diameters of 2.5–4.0 mm.

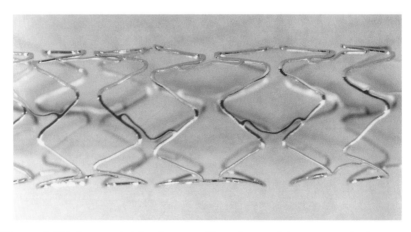

Figure 2.25: An expanded Coroflex stent. The midpoint of the connecting bridges is shown

CrossFlex LC™ (Cordis Corp., a Johnson and Johnson Interventional Systems Co. [Warren NJ, USA])

The CrossFlex LC (laser cut) is a balloon expandable stainless-steel tubular stent (figure 2.26). The helical coil design of the CrossFlex LC stent is similar to that of its predecessor, the CrossFlex coil stent. Unlike the coil CrossFlex stent, the CrossFlex LC stent has staggered connecting bridges along the length of the stent. These design changes were made with the hope of creating a device with the flexibility of a coil stent and the radial strength of a tubular device. The stent is available in diameters of 3.0 to 4.0 mm and in expanded lengths of 18 and 27 mm.

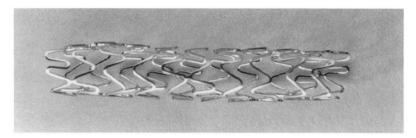

Figure 2.26: *An expanded CrossFlex LC stent*

Coil stents

GR II™ (Cook Inc [Bloomington IN, USA])

In 1985, the initial results of the percutaneous implantation of spring loaded self-expanding Z-type stents in dogs was described by Cesare Gianturco and colleagues.[89] They appreciated the importance of oversizing the stent in relation to the size of the target vessel to prevent migration of the prostheses. However, the inflexibility of this early device, difficulties in its precise placement, and its apparent thrombogenicity in the canine coronary circulation, led to the abandonment of its development and a reconsideration of a balloon expandable stent which had been initially investigated by Gianturco and associates at MD Anderson Hospital in Houston, Texas, in 1981. In collaboration with Gary Roubin, the design of the original device was modified to an incomplete serpentine coil structure, and the first-generation stainless-steel Gianturco–Roubin Flex-Stent was released. It was first placed in human subjects in 1987, and was the first intracoronary stent approved by the FDA (1993) for clinical use in the USA. The first-generation stent was made from a single continuous strand of 0.15 mm (0.006 in) stainless-steel wire. The wire was folded to form a series of loops that were then mounted around a compliant balloon catheter to form a cylinder of interdigitating loops.

In the initial phase I clinical evaluation in humans, the Flex-Stent was used for the treatment of acute closure in patients as a bridge to emergency bypass surgery.[90] The encouraging results of these initial implantations prompted a phase II multicentre registry evaluation, which assessed the clinical outcome and angiographic result at 6 months follow-up after placement of the stent in cases of acute or threatened closure following angioplasty. Between September 1988, and September 1992, 973 patients were included in this series. The initial results were reported in 1992 and included 115 patients.[91] In the study, threatened closure was defined by the presence of two or more of:

- a residual stenosis of more than 50%;
- TIMI grade 2 flow;
- a significant dissection;
- ECG or clinical evidence of ischaemia.

Despite the emergent nature of the procedures, the number of complications was low, with 4.2% of cases requiring CABG, an overall myocardial infarction rate of 16%, a subacute thrombosis rate of 7.6%, and an in-hospital mortality rate of 1.7%. A later report from one of the centres participating in the multicentre registry included 288 patients who received the Flex-Stent. Of these patients, 240 were treated for acute or threatened closure.[92] Predictors of stent thrombosis included angiographic evidence of persistent dissection after stenting, a stent size of less than 2.5 mm, and the presence of a filling defect after stent placement. The use of a 20 mm stent, compared with the shorter 12 mm stent, and the use of multiple stents, were also associated with an increased risk of stent thrombosis.

Since the phase II trial was not randomized, it is not clear from the results whether there was any clinical benefit from Flex-Stent placement in the setting of acute or threatened closure compared with prolonged inflation with an autoperfusion catheter. A case control study[93] that examined the effects of stent placement on clinical outcome in the setting of threatened or acute closure compared 61 patients treated with the Flex-Stent to historical controls who were treated before the availability of stents. Although there was a benefit of stenting on the initial angiographic appearance, there was no reduction in mortality or in the occurrence of myocardial infarction between the two groups. There were, however, fewer emergency bypass procedures done in the stented patients.

In 1995, a randomized trial reported by Rodriguez and colleagues[94] suggested that the elective placement of the Flex-Stent gave a reduction in the incidence of angiographic restenosis compared with conventional balloon angioplasty. The study included 66 patients who, on angiography 24 hours after successful PTCA,

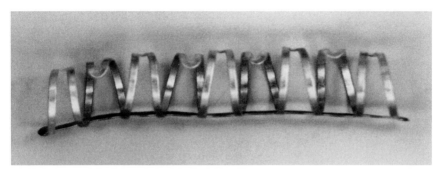

Figure 2.27: *A GR II stent showing flat wire coil design.*

showed "early loss" with angiographic characteristics suggestive of a higher risk of developing restenosis (lesions with >0.3 mm loss in Minimum luminal diameter (MLD) and/or >10% increase in diameter stenosis[95]). These patients were randomized to receive no further intervention or implantation of a Flex-Stent. Follow-up angiography was done at 3.6 ($\pm$1) months after PTCA, and with a binary definition of restenosis (>50% diameter narrowing) the restenosis rate was 21% in the stent group and 76% in the control group (p < 0.001).

The first human implant of the second-generation GR II stent was done in France in May 1995. The GR II stent has the same basic design as the Flex-Stent, but the stent coils are flattened to give the device a lower profile, allowing the smaller stents to be placed through a 6F guiding catheter. There are gold radio-opaque markers at each end of the stent, and a longitudinal spine (figure 2.27). The GR II stent is mounted on a low profile, moderately non-compliant balloon, unlike the first generation device which was supplied on a highly compliant balloon making high-pressure deployment inappropriate. The GR II stent has been shown effective for the treatment of de-novo[96,97] and restenotic lesions, small vessel,[98–100] bifurcation,[101,102] and long lesions,[101] and in the treatment of acute/threatened closure[103–105] and in acute coronary syndromes.[106–109]

Wiktor (-GX™ and -i™) (Medtronic Interventional Vascular [Kerkrade, Netherlands])

The Wiktor-GX stent, originally designed by Dominik Wiktor, is a balloon expandable prosthesis made of a single loose interdigitating tantalum wire formed into a sinusoidal wave and configured as a helical coil. It is mounted on a single operator exchange low-compliance balloon angioplasty catheter. Tantalum wire was chosen over stainless steel because it is more radio-opaque and less elastic,

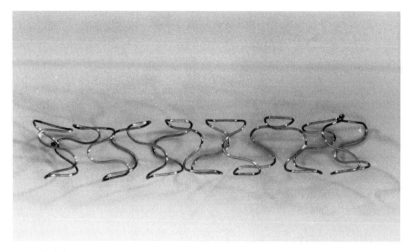

Figure 2.28: *A Wiktor-i stent showing coil design and secured wire end.*

and in-vitro observations suggested that its greater electronegative charge gave greater thromboresistance to the stent.[110,111]

The first human implantation of the Wiktor stent was done in 1989,[112] and the first clinical series was reported in 1991.[113] There is considerable clinical experience[114] with this device and several advantages of the stent design have been recognized. During stent expansion, each wave of the wire stent opens individually, which results in minimal shortening. The coil configuration gives pronounced flexibility and trackability, to allow placement in tortuous coronary arteries. The open design avoids the disadvantage of overlap of important side branches, which subsequently limits blood flow and future access to that vessel ("stent jail"[115,116]) – a problem with mesh and tubular stents. The single-wire design also allows simple extraction of the stent by grasping any portion of the stent with a snare and pulling back to unwrap the helical coil. Observational studies have shown that the Wiktor stent is effective for use in restenotic lesions[117] and in bailout situations.[117,118] Several randomized trials are currently underway to clarify the specific indications for the use of this stent.

The newer Wiktor-i stent is of similar design to the -GX series stents but with a more dense wave pattern (figure 2.28). An increased wire density and resultant wall coverage (7% for a 4.0 mm diameter -GX stent compared with 8.8% for a similarly sized -i series device) gives enhanced vessel support, improved scaffolding properties, and a lower risk of prolapse of fragile plaque material. Results from animal studies comparing the Wiktor-GX and -i stents have been published,[119,120] and there are some data to show that the Wiktor-i series stent induced less neointimal proliferation compared with the standard Wiktor-GX stent.[119]

Both the Wiktor-GX and -i stents are available with biologically active heparin covalently bonded to their surfaces – the Wiktor-GX Hepamed and Wiktor-i Hepamed coated coronary stents.[121] The coating is conformable, and stretches with the stent upon expansion. This property ensures that blood and tissue elements interact only with the coating and not with metal. Studies in vitro indicate that the heparin coating gives the stent improved thromboresistance, with decreased platelet adhesion and thrombin generation on the stent surface. The clinical benefits of the Hepamed-coated Wiktor stents have yet to be determined.

CrossFlex™ (Cordis Corp, a Johnson and Johnson Interventional Systems Co [Warren NJ, USA])

The Cordis CrossFlex stent is a balloon expandable stent comprised of stainless-steel wire configured into sinusoidal wavelets and wound into a helical coil. Much of the experience with this stent was obtained by the use of a previous generation device with a similar configuration but made of tantalum (figure 2.29).[122–128] Although data are limited, the short-term and medium-term results with the use of the stainless-steel device appear promising.[129,130] The open design and the flexibility of the CrossFlex stent suggest that it may have advantages for use at

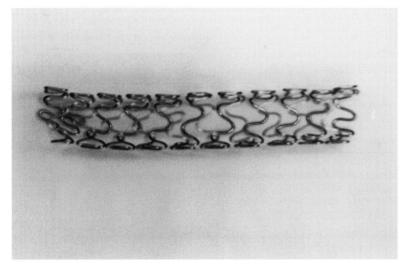

Figure 2.29: A tantalum CrossFlex stent showing the helically wound wire design.

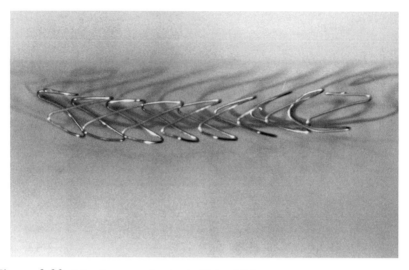

Figure 2.30: A Freedom stent showing its "fishscale" design.

branch points and in distal or tortuous segments. Side branch access is very good, and this stent may be used for bifurcation "Y" stenting for one or both vessels.

Freedom™ and Freedom Force™ (Global Therapeutics Inc [Broomfield, CO, USA])

The Freedom and Freedom Force stents are balloon expandable, single wire, stainless-steel coil stents arranged in a "fishscale" design (figure 2.30). They are available premounted on a delivery balloon or as a bare stent. The Freedom Force version has thicker stent struts for greater radial strength. The advantages of this stent design are its flexibility and the variety of available sizes, which allow the stenting of very long lesions with a single stent. This avoids the problems of overlapping stents, which may increase the risk of subacute thrombosis and late restenosis. The first human implant of the Freedom stent was done in Europe in 1994, and since that time there has been considerable experience with this stent in Europe.[131–135] Registry data are being collected and randomized clinical trials are underway.[136–140]

AngioStent™ (Angiodynamics [Glens Falls NY, USA])

The AngioStent is a balloon expandable stent made of a single platinum–iridium alloy wire, sinusoidal in form, wrapped helically, and connected end-to-end by a

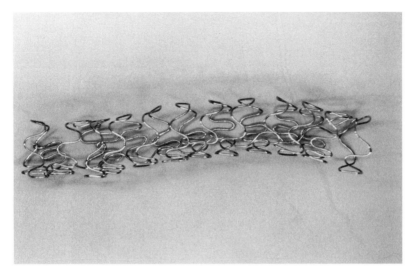

Figure 2.31: *An expanded Angiostent showing the helically wound wire design.*

second longitudinal wire (figure 2.31). The stents are supplied premounted on semicompliant balloons, both as rapid exchange and over-the-wire systems. A protective sheath covers the stent in the over-the-wire design. The AngioStent possesses the advantages of flexibility and side branch accessibility seen with other coil devices. However, as with some other coil devices, it has the disadvantage of uneven expansion in angioplastied lesions without a smooth profile. The radio-opacity of this device is high. The first human coronary artery implantation was done in 1995 in Jordan, and clinical trials with this stent began shortly afterwards. A large amount of registry data is currently available.

Ring stents

AVE Micro Stent II™ and GFX™ (Applied Vascular Engineering Inc [Santa Rosa, CA, USA])

The impetus behind the design for the AVE Micro Stent came from the concept that in order to reduce the risk of subacute stent thrombosis, the implantation of a minimal amount of metal was desirable. The result was the balloon expandable first-generation Micro Stent PL, which consisted of unconnected stainless-steel segments each with a length of 4 mm.[141] Each discrete module had a zigzag configuration with four waves or "crowns". They were supplied on a semicompliant delivery system as four or six segments.

59

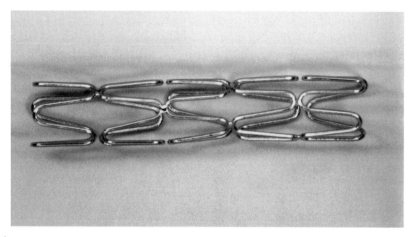

a)

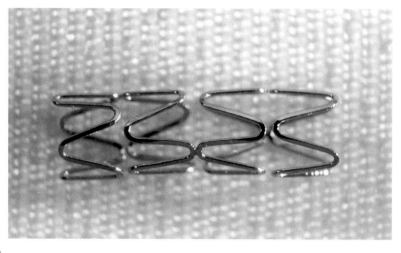

b)

Figure 2.32: *(a) A Micro Stent II; (b) the GFX stent showing sinusoidal ring design.*

In the second-generation Micro Stent, the individual 4 mm four-crown modules were welded together, either at all junctions (fully connected) or at half of the junctions (half connected). The length of the stent was determined by the number of individual segments that were welded together. This design gave the stent an exceptional degree of longitudinal flexibility, and it could be passed through a 6F guiding catheter. Animal data[142] and clinical observational data are available for the use of this stent.[143–146]

60

The design of the AVE Micro Stent II is a modification of the second-generation device (figure 2.32a). In the Micro Stent II, the individual segment length has been reduced to 3 mm. The effect of this revision is an increase in the radial strength of the stent. In addition to its flexibility, an advantage of the Micro Stent design is its low profile on the delivery balloon, which allows the stent to traverse proximally deployed stents. Observational studies had suggested that implantation of the second generation Micro Stent was associated with higher restenosis rates and higher rates of intervention when compared with matched lesions treated with the Palmaz–Schatz stent.[147–149] Encouraging medium-term results have been reported with the use of the Micro Stent II.[150] The randomized SMART trial (Study of AVE-Micro stent Ability to limit Restenosis Trial) of the Micro Stent II has shown that the use of this stent may yield better midterm results than with the Palmaz–Schatz stent.

In the fourth-generation GFX stent the design of the individual segments was again modified (figure 2.32b). The individual segment length was further shortened to 2 mm and the number of crowns per segment was increased to six. The geometry of the device was also changed to a more rounded configuration. The segments are fully connected at all junctions using laser fusion technology. These changes in design were made with the intent of generating a stent with the radial strength of a tubular stent and the flexibility of a coil. Preliminary clinical results show that the design changes in the GFX stent have resulted in a device with favourable properties.[151–153] For use in small vessels, the GFX 2.5 was released. In this design, the number of crowns was decreased to four.

Bard XT™ (CR Bard Inc [Billerica, MA, USA])

The Bard XT coronary stent was designed by Enzo Borghi from Bologna, Italy, and was first used in the coronary circulation in 1995. It is a balloon expandable stainless-steel stent made of discrete zigzag modules mounted on a flexible spine (figure 2.33). The attachment points of the zigzag modules to the spine have relatively high radio-opacity, which facilitates placement of the stent. During deployment there is no stent shortening. The design affords reasonable flexibility to the device, although long tortuous lesions may impose some restriction on trackability. The modular configuration allows for differential expansion of each segment, allowing the stent to conform to tapering vessels. In lesions at points of vessel bifurcation, the side branch remains easily accessible with the Bard XT stent. The bare stent is available on a special mounting tool. International observational and registry data are being compiled, and an equivalency trial comparing the XT stent to the Palmaz–Schatz stent is currently underway (EXTRA Trial).[154–156]

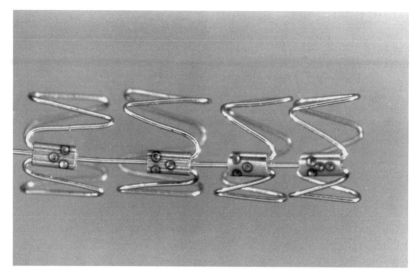

Figure 2.33: *The end of a Bard XT stent showing the zig zag modules and spine. The three indentations on the connecting piece are the weld points.*

Multidesign stents

Navius™ (Navius Corporation [San Diego, CA, USA])

The Navius stent is a balloon expandable device with a very unique ratcheting mechanism. It is constructed from 0.025 mm (0.001 in) full hard stainless steel, which is chemically milled to a pattern of multiple radial bands attached to twin backbones (figure 2.34). The stent is deployed by balloon inflation that initiates a series of "lock-outs" on the radial bands, to give a range of predictable locked stent diameters depending on balloon deployment pressure. By virtue of the fact that the Navius stent is manufactured from 316L full hard stainless steel, it can be made several times thinner than other devices made from annealed material. It is thought that by putting a thinner stent in the coronary vessel there will be less shear stress developed at the step-up between the vessel wall and the stent struts, and therefore the activation of platelets will be diminished. As a consequence, the incidence of subacute thrombosis, and the signal for neointimal proliferation and restenosis, will be reduced. There is some experimental evidence to support this speculation.[157,158] Another benefit of the full hard stainless-steel design of this stent is that the stent does not have to be forced into the vessel wall by high-pressure inflation in order to mould the metal to the vessel surface. Rather, the mechanism of multiple lock-out positions achieved with balloon pressures from 4

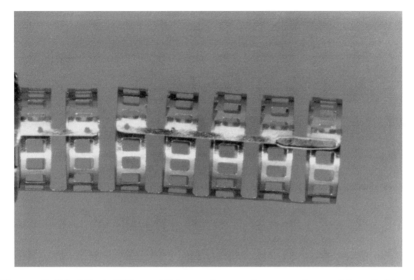

Figure 2.34: *A "locked" Navius ZR1 stent showing the unique design of the radial bands and locking mechanism.*

to 14 atmospheres allows precise sizing of the stent to the arterial wall during deployment. Lower-pressure deployment limits the degree of vessel injury, potentially reducing the degree of subsequent neointimal proliferation.[159] The radial strength of this device ensures no recoil, and therefore maintains the MLD achieved at the stenting procedure. The design of the Navius stent also gives the stent a high degree of flexibility postdeployment, minimizing the mechanical strain associated with straightening of tortuous vessels. Because of its unique ratcheting design, accurate sizing of the Navius stent is more important than with other stent designs. A small Navius stent cannot be grown to fit a large vessel simply by introducing a larger PTCA balloon. Compared with other stents, the metallic surface area of the Navius stent is quite high, which may affect long-term outcome. Clinical experience with this stent is being obtained.[160]

NIR™ and NIROYAL™ (Medinol/SciMed Life Systems [Maple Grove, MN, USA])

NIR stents comprise three families of balloon expandable stainless-steel devices (figure 2.35a). They are all laser-cut from a metal sheet, rolled, and welded. The configuration of the repeating unit or "cell" of each family is identical (figure 2.35b). What distinguishes each family is the number of circumferentially arranged cells. NIR stents are available in 5, 7, and 9 cell constructions: the digit

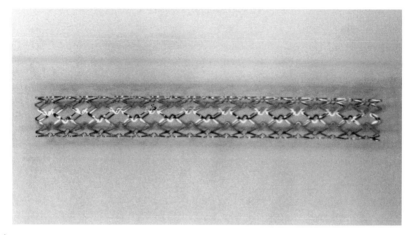

a)

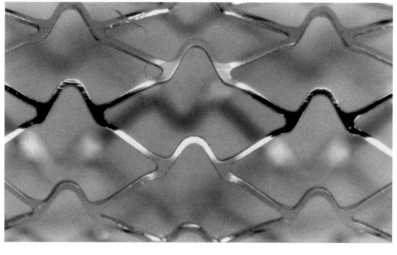

b)

Figure 2.35: *(a) A NIR stent; (b) photograph showing details of the repeating cell configuration of the NIR stent.*

denotes the number of closed cells in the circumference of the stent. The length of the stent is determined by the number of longitudinally arranged cells in each stent. Each of the uniform cells of the NIR stent is capable of extending or foreshortening, which allows for differential elongation of areas of the stent and permits navigation of tortuous segments. This feature also ensures that the rigid

64

expanded stent does not straighten the vessel or create a sharp kink at the interface between the stented and non-stented segment. Another feature that increases the trackability of the stent is that the stent has no "free internal loops" or ends not connected longitudinally to their neighbours, which in some other stent designs can flare out and latch on plaque surfaces upon insertion. The relatively small cells decrease the chance for tissue prolapse and plaque protrusion into vessel lumen. The small cells and short struts give a high radial resistance and reduce wall trauma since the local stress on the wall caused by the individual struts is decreased.

Each of the NIR stent families spans a range of expanded diameters. For each family, a size range is specified. The lower limit of this range is defined by the diameter at which the stent has less than 20% metal area coverage, and the upper limit is the diameter at which the cells are fully opened. At the maximum recommended diameter the metal area coverage is less than 12% and the stent gives maximum radial strength. Clinical observational and registry data have been published for the NIR stent,[161–166] and results of a multicentre randomized trial comparing the NIR stent with the Palmaz–Schatz stent will soon be available (NIRVANA Trial).[167,168] A gold plated NIR stent is also available (NIROYAL), which is more radio-opaque and may be less thrombogenic than its stainless-steel predecessor.

The NIR Conformer™ incorporates a novel design idea. The terminal rows of cells at the extreme ends of the stent are smaller than the cells of the main body of the stent. As a consequence, these rows have a slightly greater resistance to expansion than the cells of the main body of the stent. The result of this subtle design modification is that the balloon expansion forces are directed inward, and there is no flaring of the ends of the stent on balloon expansion, which may reduce the prevalence of traumatic vessel dissection upon implantation of these devices.

Custom designed stents

With recent improvements in deployment techniques for intracoronary stents, and with increased operator experience, lesions previously judged not amenable to percutaneous treatment are now being treated with intracoronary stent implantation. Industry has responded to the demand by producing a myriad of customized stents for very particular applications.

Bifurcation lesions

Several new stent designs are available which are constructed specifically for use in bifurcation lesions. The JOSTEN B (Jomed International AB [Drottninggatan,

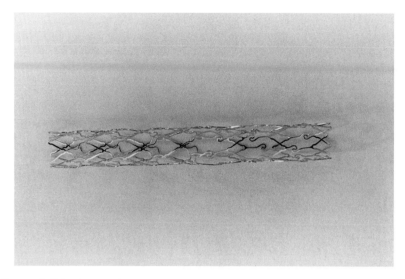

Figure 2.36: *The end of the JOSTENT B showing the larger cells at one extreme of the stent.*

Sweden]) is one such device.[182] The JOSTENT B is a stainless-steel, balloon expandable, tubular stent composed of expanding closed cells. The configuration and size of the cells at one end of the JOSTENT B is similar to the second generation JOSTENT Plus stent. At the other end of the stent, the cells are larger with a JOSTENT Flex configuration (figure 2.36). On full expansion, the larger cells have a diameter of 3.5 mm, allowing easy access to the other arm of the vessel bifurcation.

Devon Medical (Hamburg, Germany) also supplies a unique pair of stents to be used for bifurcation lesions. The stents are balloon expandable and laser-cut from a stainless-steel tube. One stent has two segments connected with a single bridge. This stent can be folded at the articulation point and crimped over two balloons, which can then be introduced to implant two stents at the two arms of the bifurcation, with the connecting bridge positioned over the bifurcation point. The second stent is cut with an oblique edge at one end of the stent. This oblique single stent can be placed in the main vessel aligned with one arm of the bifurcation segment. The distal end of the oblique stent is cut with larger cells, allowing free access to the joining vessel.

CR Bard Inc (Billerica MA, USA) has developed a true bifurcation stent which is currently in clinical trial. The Bard XT Carina Bifurcate stent is shaped like a "Y" and mounted on two balloons (figure 2.37). The main body of the stent is a single coil through which the two balloons pass. The balloons diverge at the crux

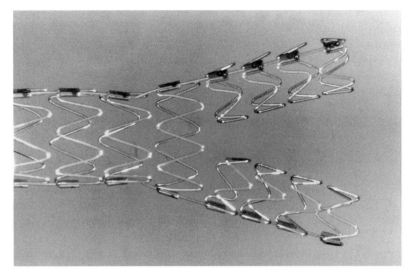

Figure 2.37: *The Bard Carina Bifurcate Stent, a true bifurcated device.*

of the "Y" to pass separately through the two arms. The stent can accommodate angles of up to 120°. The first human implants of this stent have been done.

Side branch

Stents specifically designed for use in the treatment of lesions at the site of significant side branches are also available. Medinol/SciMed Life Systems (Maple Grove MN, USA) supplies the NIRSide, which has the same basic design as the standard family of NIR stents. The stent is cut from a sheet of stainless steel, rolled, and welded to form a tube. However, the cells in the middle of the stent are larger than those at the ends. When properly positioned, the number of obstructing struts over the entrance to the side branch is minimized and side branch access is facilitated. The design concept of the JOSTENT S (Jomed International AB [Drottninggatan, Sweden]) is similar to that of the NIRSide stent. The JOSTENT S is a balloon expandable stainless-steel tubular device.[183] It is configured with segments similar to the JOSTENT Plus stent. The segments flank a row of larger cells connected with spiral bridges (figure 2.38). The larger cells of the JOSTENT S have a diameter of 3.5 mm on full expansion, which allows for easy access to the side branch vessel through the implanted stent. The design of the Devon Medical Side-Arm stent (Hamburg, Germany) is slightly different than the NIRSide and the JOSTENT S. The Devon Side-Arm stent is

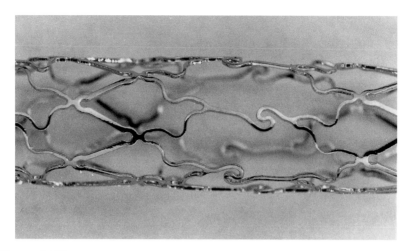

Figure 2.38: *The JOSTENT S showing the region of the stent with larger cells.*

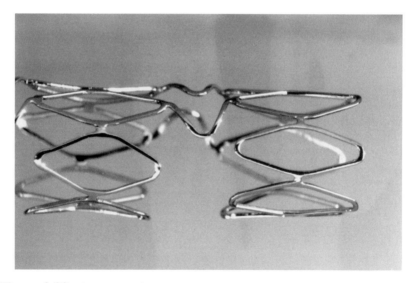

Figure 2.39: *The Devon Side-Arm Stent showing the region with omitted struts.*

based on the PURA-VARIO design. Customization for use in lesions with side branches involves the omission of a single connecting bridge to provide side branch access (figure 2.39).

Ostial lesions

Devon Medical (Hamburg, Germany) produces a stent designed exclusively for use in ostial lesions (figure 2.40). The base design for the stent is the PURA-VARIO A. At one end of the stent, however, the terminal row of cells is slightly longer and the struts slightly thicker. This not only increases the radial force of this portion of the stent, but also increases its radio-opacity, which allows precise positioning.

Aneurysms or perforations
The JOSTENT Coronary Stent Graft (Jomed International AB [Drottninggatan, Sweden]) is a unique integration of graft material into a coronary stent[184] (figure 2.41). This device is constructed using a sandwich technique whereby an ultra-thin layer of expandable PTFE, specially developed for integration into a stent graft system, is placed between two stents with reduced strut thickness. The design of the metallic portion of the Coronary Stent Graft is identical to that of the JOSTENT Flex, and the profile is only slightly larger than a standard coronary stent. The Stent Graft is also offered coated with the Corline Heparin Surface, which has the potential to reduce the risk of thrombosis after stent implantation.

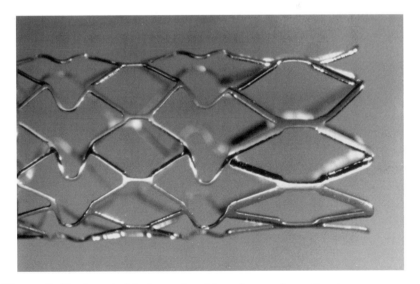

Figure 2.40: The end of the Devon Osteal Stent showing the reinforced struts at one extreme of the stent.

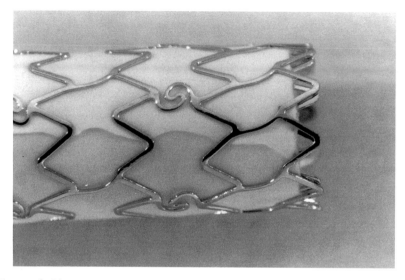

Figure 2.41: *The end of a JOSTENT Coronary Stent Graft showing the expandable PTFE material sandwiched between two thin-strut metal stents.*

Is there a difference?

With this plethora of intracoronary stenting devices, it must be asked whether stent design dictates the injury imposed at implantation, and whether the choice of a particular stent makes a difference with respect to clinical outcome. There is both experimental and clinical evidence suggesting that a difference does indeed exist between different stents. Animal studies have shown that the degree of deep injury caused by stent struts at the time of implantation dictates the amount of stenosis.[169–174] Altering a stent's configuration to cause less strut-related deep injury, while achieving the same gain in lumen diameter, has been shown to reduce neointimal thickening when implanted in peripheral[169] and coronary[175] arteries of animals. However, it has also been shown that features of stent design, such as the amount of coverage of the vessel wall by metal, can dictate the vascular response independent of the extent of wall injury.[176] In addition, recent experimental findings indicate that an inflammatory reaction plays as important a part as strut-related arterial injury in neointimal formation after coronary stenting.[177,178] Thus, the clinical observation that stent design may affect the relation between acute gain and late lumen loss, indicative of neointimal proliferation,[179] may be explained by the amount of wall injury caused by the struts of a particular design, or independent properties of deep wall injury such as vessel wall coverage and the amount of inflammation a design causes. Even design characteristics such as regular spacing between stent struts has been shown to reduce vessel wall reaction.[176,180] In a clinical study comparing stents with two different designs, Goy and colleagues[181] reported that only the stent with the slotted tubular design gave benefit over balloon dilatation alone in the observed restenosis rates when compared with a coil stent. A similar finding was reported by Fernández-Ortiz et al who compared the tubular Palmaz–Schatz stent to the coil Gianturco–Roubin stent. In their study, 50 consecutive patients were matched according to vessel size, location of the target lesion and dissection type among patients who underwent coronary stenting to treat an acute dissection following coronary angioplasty.[182] Despite similar acute angiographic results, late loss in luminal diameter was significantly higher in the lesions treated with the coil stent. This translated into a significantly higher restenosis rate in those patients treated with a coil stent (40%) compared with those treated with the tubular stent (16%, p<0.05). Large randomized trials are currently underway comparing various stent designs "head to head" to answer the question whether design can affect clinical outcome. With the large number of stents currently available, it is questionable what practical purpose will be served by comparing all the available stents with the "standard" Palmaz–Schatz stent or with each other. Furthermore, is similar performance at 6-months follow-up angiography adequate to show equivalency? Other issues that must be considered when evaluating a stent, aside from equivalency to an arbitrary standard, are ease of use, versatility, and cost.

With these continued developments and refinements, it is possible that stenting will lead the coup over angioplasty and surgery for coronary artery revascularization.

References

1. Grégoire J, Smith DG, Ragheb A et al. Stent collapse resistance to external pressure: comparison between coil and slotted tube stent designs. *J Am Coll Cardiol* 1998; **31** (suppl): 414A.

2. Rousseau H, Puel J, Joffre F et al. Self-expanding endovascular prosthesis: an experimental study. *Radiology* 1987; **164:** 709–14.

3. Puel J, Joffre F, Rousseau H, Guermonprez B, Lancelin B, Morice MC. Endo-prothèses coronariennes auto-expansives dans le prévention des resténoses après angioplastie transluminale. *Arch Mal Coeur* 1987; **8:** 1311–12.

4. Sigwart U, Puel J, Mirkovitch V, Joffre F, Kappenberger L. Intravascular stents to

prevent occlusion and restenosis after transluminal angioplasty. *N Engl J Med* 1987; **316:** 701–06.

5. Serruys PW, Strauss BH, Beatt KJ et al. Angiographic follow-up after placement of a self-expanding coronary artery stent. *N Engl J Med* 1991; **324:** 13–17.

6. Strauss BH, Serruys PW, Bertrand ME et al. Qualitative angiographic follow-up of the coronary Wallstent in native vessel and bypass grafts (European experience: March 1986–March 1990). *Am J Cardiol* 1992; **69:** 475–81.

7. Kelly P.A., Kurbaan AS, Clague JR, Sigwart U. Total endovascular reconstruction of occluded saphenous vein grafts using coronary or peripheral Wallstents. *J Invas Cardiol* 1997; **9:** 513–17.

8. Joseph T, Fajadet J, Jordan C et al. Reconstruction of old diffusely degenerated saphenous vein grafts with less-shortening Wallstents [abstract]. *Circulation* 1997; **96** (suppl): I-275.

9. Pieper MJ, Heyndrickx G, Meier B et al. Wallstent implantation as first choice for venous graft angioplasty: the Wellstent-CABG-Study [abstract]. *J Am Coll Cardiol* 1998; **31** (suppl): 216A.

10. König A, Regar E, Henneke K-H et al. Interaction of the Wallstent with the coronary artery during a longterm follow-up: morphological assessment by serial intravascular ultrasound with a motorized pullback system [abstract]. *J Am Coll Cardiol* 1998; **31** (suppl): 494A.

11. Foley DP, Heyndrickx G, Macaya C et al, on behalf of the Wellstent Native Investigators. Implantation of the self-expanding less-shortening Wallstent for primary, coronary artery lesions: final results of the Wellstent Native study [abstract]. *Eur Heart J* 1997; **18** (suppl): 156.

12. Foley DP, Wijns W, Suryapranata H et al. Bypass graft angioplasty using the self-expanding less shortening Wallstent – results of the Wallstent CABG study [abstract]. *Eur Heart J* 1997; **18** (suppl): 157.

13. Palmaz JC, Sibbit RR, Reuter SR, Tio FOR, Rice WJ. Expandable intraluminal graft: a preliminary study. *Radiology* 1985; **156:** 73–77.

14. Palmaz JC, Sibbit RR, Tio FOR, Reuter SR, Peters JE, Garcia F. Expandable intraluminal vascular graft: a feasibility study. *Surgery* 1986; **99:** 199–205.

15. Palmaz JC, Windelar SA, Garcia F, Tio FOR, Sibbit RR, Reuter SR. Atherosclerotic rabbit aortas: expandable intraluminal grafting. *Radiology* 1986; **160:** 723–26.

16. Serruys PW, de Jaegere P, Kiemeneij F et al, for the Benestent Study Group. A comparison of balloon-expandable-stent implantation with balloon angioplasty in patients with coronary artery disease. *N Engl J Med* 1994; **331:** 489–95.

17. Fischman DL, Leon MB, Baim DS et al, for the Stent Restenosis Study investigators. A randomized comparison of coronary-stent placement and balloon

angioplasty in the treatment of coronary artery disease. *N Engl J Med* 1994; **331:** 496–501.

18. Serruys PW, van Hout B, Bonnier H et al, for the Benestent Study Group. Effectiveness, costs and cost-effectiveness of a strategy of elective heparin-coated stenting compared to balloon angioplasty in selected patients with coronary artery disease: the BENESTENT II study. *Lancet* 1998; in press.

19. di Mario C, Reimers B, Reinhardt R, Ferraro M, Moussa I, Colombo A. New stent delivery balloon: a technical note. *Cathet Cardiovasc Diagn* 1997; **42:** 452–56.

20. Serruys PW, Emanuelsson H, van der Giessen W et al, on behalf of the BENESTENT II Study Group. Heparin coated Palmaz–Schatz stents on human coronary arteries: early outcome of the BENESTENT II pilot study. *Circulation* 1996; **93:** 412–22.

21. Garcia E, Serruys PW, Dawkins K et al. BENESTENT-II trial: final results of visit II & III: a 7 month follow-up [abstract]. *Eur Heart J* 1997; **18** (suppl): 350.

22. Priestly KA, Clague JR , Buller NP, Sigwart U. First clinical experience with a new flexible low profile metallic stent and delivery system. *Eur Heart J* 1996; **17:** 438–44.

23. Dawkins KD, Emanuelsson HU, van der Giessen WJ et al. Preliminary results of a European multicentre feasibility and safety registry on an innovative stent: the "W.E.S.T." study [abstract]. *Circulation* 1995; **92** (suppl I): I-280.

24. van der Giessen W, Emanuelsson H, Dawkins K et al. Six month clinical outcome and angiographic follow up of the WEST study [abstract]. *Eur Heart J* 1996; **17** (suppl): 990.

25. Emanuelsson H, Serruys PW, van der Giessen WJ et al, on behalf of the WEST Study Group. Clinical and angiographic results with the Multi-Link™ coronary stent system – the West European Stent Trial (WEST). *J Invas Cardiol* 1997; **9:** 561–68.

26. Serruys PW, van der Giessen W, Garcia E et al, for the WEST-2 Investigators. Clinical and angiographic results with the Multi-Link stent implanted under intravascular ultrasound guidance (WEST-2 Study). *J Invas Cardiol* 1998; **10** (suppl B): 20B–27B.

27. Wong P, Wong CM, Chang CH et al. Early clinical experience with the Multi-Link Coronary stent. *Cathet Cardiovasc Diagn* 1996; **39:** 413–19.

28. Chevalier B, Royer T, Glatt B et al. Early clinical experience with the Multi-Link coronary stent [abstract]. *Circulation* 1996; **94** (suppl I): I-1198.

29. Carrozza JP, Zhang Y, Robertson LK, Chauhan M. Acute 30-day and late clinical outcome in the prior restenosis registry of the ACS Multi-Link coronary stent system [abstract]. *Circulation* 1997; **96** (suppl): I-654.

30. Linnemeier TJ. The Rx Multi-Link™ stent parallel registries to the ASCENT Trial. *J Invas Cardiol* 1998; **10** (suppl B): 55B–56B.

31. Baim DS. ASCENT Trial – evaluation of the ACS Multi-Link stent. *J Invas Cardiol* 1998; **10** (suppl B): 53B–54B.

32. Clague JR, Kurbaan AS, Kelly PA et al. The new ACS Multilink coronary stent: a single centre experience in 103 consecutive patients with and without oral anticoagulation. *J Intervent Cardiol* 1997; **10**: 183–91.

33. Anzai H, Nakamura S, Nishida T et al. Comparison of radial force of Palmaz–Schatz stent, Multi-Link stent, and Act-One stent by intravascular ultrasound [abstract]. *Eur Heart J* 1996; **17** (suppl): 2862.

34. Waigand J, Uhlich F, Gulba DC, Gross M, Dietz R, Volhard F. Intracoronary stenting with the Multi-Link stent – single centre experience [abstract]. *Circulation* 1996; **94** (suppl I): I-506.

35. Carrozza JP, Yock PG, Linnemeier TJ et al. Serial expansion of the ACS Multi-Link stent after 8, 12 and 16 atmospheres: a QCA and IVUS pilot study [abstract]. *Circulation* 1996; **94** (suppl I): I-509.

36. Hermiller JB, Baim DS, Linnemeier TJ et al. Clinical results with the ACS Multi-Link stent in the US pilot phase [abstract]. *Circulation* 1996; **94** (suppl I): I-505.

37. Honda Y, Yock CA, Hermiller JB, Fitzgerald PJ, Yock PG, for the MULTI-LINK™ Investigators. Longitudinal redistribution of plaque is an important mechanism for luminal expansion in stenting [abstract]. *J Am Coll Cardiol* 1997; **29** (suppl A): 218A.

38. Hamasaki N, Nakano Y, Nosaka H et al. Initial experience with the ACS Multi-Link stent: serial angiographic follow-up and comparison with Palmaz–Schatz stent in matched lesions. *J Invas Cardiol* 1998; **10**: 76–82.

39. Carrozza JP, Hermiller JB, Linnemeier TJ et al. Quantitative coronary angiographic and intravascular ultrasound assessment of a new nonarticulated stent: report from the Advanced Cardiovascular Systems MultiLink Stent pilot study. *J Am Coll Cardiol* 1998; **31**: 50–56.

40. Moreno R, Delcán JL, Abeytua M et al. Multi-Link stenting in acute myocardial infarction. *J Invas Cardiol* 1998; **10**: 213–17.

41. Seth A, Chandra P, Chugh SK et al. Immediate results and angiographic follow up of intracoronary stenting with the ACS™ MULTILINK stent [abstract]. *J Invas Cardiol* 1997; **9** (suppl C): 20C.

42. Kobayashi Y, Mukai S, Brown CL III et al. Geometric expansion in a self-expandable stent and a balloon-expandable stent: interim results from the IVUS substudy of the SCORES trial [abstract]. *Circulation* 1998; **96** (suppl): I-584.

43. Kobayashi Y, Teirstein PS, Bailey SR et al. Self-expandable stent versus balloon-

expandable stent: a serial volumetric analysis by intravascular ultrasound [abstract]. *J Am Coll Cardiol* 1998; **31** (suppl): 396A.

44. Isshiki T, Eto K, Ochiai M et al. Nitinol Radius stent induces less platelet aggregation than stainless steel Palmaz–Schatz/Gianturco–Rubin II stents [abstract]. *J Am Coll Cardiol* 1998; **31** (suppl): 312A.

45. Carter AJ, Scott D, Laird JR et al. Progressive vascular remodeling and reduced neointimal formation after placement of a thermoelastic self-expanding nitinol stent in an experimental model. *Cathet Cardiovasc Diagn* 1998; **44:** 193–201.

46. van der Giessen WJ, Grollier G, Hoorntje JC, Heyndrickx G, Morel MM, Serruys PW. The ESSEX Study: first clinical experience with the self-expanding, nitinol Radius stent [abstract]. *Eur Heart J* 1997; **18** (suppl): 158.

47. Goldberg S, Schwartz RS, Mann TJ III et al. Comparison of a novel self-expanding Nitinol stent (RADIUS™) with a balloon expandable (Palmaz–Schatz™) stent: initial results of a randomized trial (SCORES) [abstract]. *Circulation* 1997; **96** (suppl): I-654.

48. Han RO, Schwartz RS, Mann JT et al. Comparative efficacy of self expanding and balloon expandable stents for the reduction of restenosis [abstract]. *J Am Coll Cardiol* 1998; **31** (suppl): 314A.

49. Beyar R, Roguin A. Newer stents: materials and designs. *J Invas Cardiol* 1997; **9:** 363–71.

50. Roguin A, Beyar R. BeStent – the serpentine balloon expandable stent: review of mechanical properties and clinical experience. *Artificial Organs* 1998; **22:** 243–49.

51. Bartorelli AL, Trabattoni D, de Cesare N et al. Treatment of non-BENESTENT-STRESS type coronary lesions with a new balloon-expandable stent (beStent) [abstract]. *J Invas Cardiol* 1997; **9** (suppl C): 5C.

52. Bartorelli AL, Trabattoni D, de Cesare N et al. A new serpentine balloon-expandable stent (beStent) for the treatment of real life coronary lesions: immediate and follow-up results [abstract]. *Eur Heart J* 1997; **18** (suppl): 384.

53. Beyar R, Roguin A, Hamburger J et al, on behalf of the beStent investigators. Longer lesion coverage is associated with an increase in six months clinical events: results from a multicentre evaluation of the serpentine balloon-expandable stent (beStent™) [abstract]. *Eur Heart J* 1997; **18** (suppl): 158.

54. Beyar R, Hamburger J, Saaiman A et al, for the beStent Investigators. A multi-center pilot study of a serpentine balloon-expandable stent (beStent™): acute angiographic and clinical results [abstract]. *J Am Coll Cardiol* 1997; **29** (suppl A): 494A.

55. Beyar R, Roguin A, Hamburger J et al, for the beStent investigators. Longer lesion coverage is associated with an increase in six months clinical events: results from a multicenter evaluation of the serpentine balloon-expandable stent (beStent™) [abstract]. *Am J Cardiol* 1997; **80** (suppl 7A): 32S.

56. Beyar R, Roguin A, Hamburger J et al. Multi-center pilot study of a serpentine balloon-expandable stent (beStent™): acute angiographic and clinical results. *J Interven Cardiol* 1997; **10**: 277–86.

57. Roguin A, Grenadier E, Peled B, Markiewicz W, Beyar R. Acute and 30-day results of the serpentine balloon expandable stent implantation in simple and complex coronary arterial narrowings. *Am J Cardiol* 1997; **80**: 1155–62.

58. Hanenkamp CEE, Bonnier HJRM, Michels RH et al. Feasibility study with an amorphous hydrogenated siliciumcarbide coated tantalum stent in daily practice [abstract]. *Am J Cardiol* 1997; **80** (suppl 7A): 30S.

59. Heublein B, Pethig K, Elsayed A-M. Silicon carbide coating – a semiconducting hybrid design of coronary stents – a feasibility study. *J Invas Cardiol* 1998; **10**: 255–62.

60. Hanenkamp CEE, Koolen JJ, Pijls NHJ, van Gelder BM, Bonnier HJRM. A new flexible amorphous hydrogenated siliciumcarbide, aSiCH, coated stainless steel slotted tube coronary stent [abstract]. *Am J Cardiol* 1997; **80** (suppl 7A): 30S.

61. Amon M, Bolz A, Schaldach M. Improvement of stenting therapy with a silicon carbide coated tantalum stent. *J Materials Science: Materials in Medicine* 1996; **7**: 273–78.

62. Chronos NAF, Robinson KA, Kelly AB et al. Thromboresistant phosphorylcholine coatings for coronary stents [abstract]. *Circulation* 1995; **92** (suppl I): I-685.

63. Malik N, Gunn J, Shepard L, Newman CMH, Crossman DC, Cumberland DC. Phosphorylcholine-coated stents in porcine coronary arteries: angiographic and morphometric assessment. *Eur J Cardiol* 1997; **18** (suppl): 152.

64. Bonan R, Paiement P, Tanguay JF et al. Recoil evaluation of a new stent with phosphorylcholine coating in porcine coronary arteries. *Eur J Cardiol* 1997; **18** (suppl): 153.

65. Gunn J, Malik N, Holt C et al. The BioDivYsio® stent: morphometric superiority to the Palmaz–Schatz stent in the porcine coronary model [abstract]. *Am J Cardiol* 1997; **80** (suppl 7A): 29S.

66. Beusekom HMM, Whelan DM, Krabbendam SC et al. Biocompatibility of phosphorylcholine coated stents in a porcine coronary model [abstract]. *Circulation* 1998; **96** (suppl): I-289.

67. Kuiper KJ, Robinson KA, Chronos NAF, Nordrehaug JE. Implantation of metal phosphorylcholine coated stents in rabbit iliac and porcine coronary arteries [abstract]. *Circulation* 1997; **96** (suppl): I-289.

68. Malik N, Gunn J, Newman C, Crossman DC, Cumberland DC. Phosphorylcholine coated stents: angiographic and morphometric assessment in porcine coronary arteries [abstract]. *J Am Coll Cardiol* 1998; **31** (suppl): 414A.

69. Machraoui A, Germing A, von Dryander S, Grewe P, Jäger D, Lemke B. Clinical

and angiographic results of coronary stenting using PURA stents [abstract]. *Am J Cardiol* 1997; **80** (suppl 7A): 32S.

70. Reimers B, Moussa I, Kobayashi Y et al. Immediate results with the newly designed PURA-VARIO coronary stent [abstract]. *Am J Cardiol* 1997; **80** (suppl 7A): 38S.

71. Shetky LM. Shape-memory alloys. *Sci Am* 1979; **241:** 74–83.

72. De Scheerder I, Dens J, Desmet W, Coussement P, Piessens J. First clinical experience with a new tubular coronary stent (Dart™): clinical and angiographic results [abstract]. *Am J Cardiol* 1997; **80** (suppl 7A): 39S.

73. Herrmann R, Schmidmaier G, Alt E et al. Comparison of the thrombogenicity of steel and gold-surface coronary stents with a biodegradable, drug releasing coating in a human stasis model [abstract]. *Eur Heart J* 1997; **18** (suppl): 152.

74. Herrmann RA, Rybnikar A, Resch A et al. Thrombogenicity of stainless steel coronary stents with a completely gold coated surface [abstract]. *J Am Coll Cardiol* 1998; **31** (suppl): 413A.

75. Hehrlein C, Zimmerman M, Metz J, Ensinger W, Kübler W. Influence of surface texture and charge on the biocompatibility of endovascular stents. *Coron Artery Dis* 1995; **6:** 581–86.

76. Alt E, Herrmann RA, Rybnikar A et al. Reduction of neointimal proliferation after implantation of a beta particle emitting gold Au 198 coated stent. *J Am Coll Cardiol* 1998; **31** (suppl): 350A.

77. Alt E, Pasquantonio J, Fliedner T et al. Effect of endovascular stent design on experimental restenosis [abstract]. *J Am Coll Cardiol* 1997; **29** (suppl A): 242A.

78. Alt E, Elezi S, Zitzmann E, Hausleiter J, Rybnikar A, Schömig A. The new Inflow stent: clinical and angiographic results [abstract]. *J Am Coll Cardiol* 1997; 29 (suppl A): 416A.

79. Gutensohn K, Fenner T, Padmanaban K et al. Diamond-like carbon coating of intracoronary stents reduces platelet activation and the release of metal atoms [abstract]. *Infusionther Transfusionmed* 1997; **24:** 299.

80. Beythien C, Gutensohn K, Kühnl P, Hamm CW, Alt E, Terres W. Influence of "diamond-like" and gold coating on platelet activation: a flow cytometry analysis in a pulsed floating model [abstract]. *J Am Coll Cardiol* 1998; **31** (suppl): 413A.

81. Yokoi H, Nakagawa Y, Tamura T et al. Preliminary experiences with the Terumo coronary stent [abstract]. *J Am Coll Cardiol* 1998; **31** (suppl): 314A.

82. Mudra H, Werner F, Reger E et al. One balloon approach for optimized Palmaz–Schatz stent implantation: the MUSCAT trial. *Cathet Cardiovasc Diagn* 1997; **42:** 130–36.

83. Hodgson JMcB. Focal angioplasty: theory and clinical application. *Cathet Cardiovasc Diagn* 1997; **42:** 445–51.

84. Stone GW, Kiesz S, Bailey S et al. Improved procedural results of coronary stenting with focal balloon "overexpansion" – final core lab analysis from the prospective, multicenter OSTI-2A trial [abstract]. *J Am Coll Cardiol* 1998; **31** (suppl): 16A.

85. Stone GW, Kiesz RS, Oshima K et al. Improved procedural results of coronary stenting with focal balloon "overexpansion:" the OSTI-2A trial [abstract]. *Circulation* 1997; 96 (suppl): I-402.

86. Hodgson JMcB, Frey AW, Roskamm H. Net gain after six month angiographic follow-up is greater when IVUS is used to guide initial interventions: chronic SIPS trial results [abstract]. *Am J Cardiol* 1997; **80** (suppl 7A): 17S.

87. Hodgson JMcB, Frey AW, Müller C, Roskamm H. Comparison of acute procedure cost and equipment utilization with strategies of ICUS guided vs angiographic guided PTCA and stenting: preliminary results of the Strategy of ICUS-guided PTCA and Stenting (SIPS) study [abstract]. *Circulation* 1996; **94** (suppl): I-235.

88. Frey AW, Roskamm H, Hodgson JMcB. Ivus-guided stenting: does acute angiography predict long term outcome? Insights from the strategy of Ivus-guided PTCA and stenting (SIPS) trial [abstract]. *Circulation* 1997; **96** (suppl): I-222.

89. Wright KC, Wallace S, Charnsangavej C, Carrasco CH, Gianturco C. Percutaneous endovascular stents: an experimental evaluation. *Radiology* 1985; **156:** 69–72.

90. Berger PB. The Cook Inc Gianturco–Roubin Flex-Stent. *J Interven Cardiol* 1996; **9:** 145–52.

91. Roubin GS, Cannon AD, Agrawal SK et al. Intracoronary stenting for acute and threatened closure complicating percutaneous transluminal coronary angioplasty. *Circulation* 1992; **85:** 916–27.

92. Agrawal SK, Ho DSW, Lie MW et al. Predictors of thrombolytic complications after placement of the flexible coil stent. *Am J Cardiol* 1994; **73:** 1216–19.

93. Lincoff AM, Topol EJ, Chapekis AT et al. Intracoronary stenting compared with conventional therapy for abrupt vessel closure complicating coronary angioplasty: a matched case-control study. *J Am Coll Cardiol* 1993; **21:** 866–75.

94. Rodriguez AE, Santaera O, Larribau M et al. Coronary stenting decreases restenosis in lesions with early loss in luminal diameter 24 hours after successful PTCA. *Circulation* 1995; **91:** 1397–402.

95. Rodriguez AE, Santaera O, Larribau M, Sosa MI, Palacios IF. Early decreases in minimal luminal diameter predicts late restenosis after successful coronary angioplasty. *Am J Cardiol* 1993; **71:** 1391–95.

96. Dean LS, O'Shaughnessy CD, Moore PB et al, on behalf of the GR II™ Clinical Investigators. Elective stenting of de novo lesions: randomized, multicentre trial comparing two stent designs [abstract]. *Eur Heart J* 1997; **18** (suppl): 349.

97. Multicenter GRII™ Investigator Group, Leon M. A multicenter randomized trial comparing the second generation Gianturco-Roubin (GRII™) and the Palmaz–Schatz coronary stents [abstract]. *J Am Coll Cardiol* 1997; **29** (suppl A): 170A.

98. Zidar JP, O'Shaughnessy CD, Dean LS et al, for the GR II™ Clinical Investigators. Elective second generation stenting in small diameter vessels: a multicentre trial [abstract]. *Eur Heart J* 1997; **18** (suppl): 156.

99. Dean LS, Zidar JP, Voorhees WD et al. Stenting in small vessels: a re-evaluation using the GRII intracoronary stent in a multicenter registry study [abstract]. *J Am Coll Cardiol* 1997; **29** (suppl A): 396A.

100. Zidar JP, O'Shaughnessy CD, Dean LS et al. Elective GR II® stenting in small vessels: multicenter results [abstract]. *J Am Coll Cardiol* 1998; **31** (suppl): 274A.

101. Dean LS. Improved treatment for difficult lesions: using the GR II™ coronary stent for bailout, bifurcations, and long lesions: data presented at the Endovascular Therapy Course, Paris, France, May 21, 1997.

102. Colombo A. Use of a second-generation flexible stent in small vessels and bifurcation lesions: data presented at the XVIIth Congress of the European Society of Cardiology, Birmingham, UK, August 25, 1996.

103. Garratt K, O'Shaughnessy CD, Leon MB et al, on behalf of the GR II™ Clinical Investigators. Improved early outcomes after coronary stent placement for abrupt or threatened closure: results of a multicenter trial using second generation stents [abstract]. *Eur Heart J* 1997; **18** (suppl): 388.

104. O'Shaughnessy CD, Popma JJ, Dean LS et al. The new Gianturco-Roubin coronary stent is an improved therapy for abrupt and threatened closure syndrome. [abstract]. *J Am Coll Cardiol* 1997; **29** (suppl A): 416A–17A.

105. Leon MB, Fry ETA, O'Shaughnessy CD et al. Preliminary multicenter experiences with the new GR-II stent for abrupt and threatened closure syndrome [abstract]. *Circulation* 1996; **94** (suppl): I-207.

106. Rodriguez A, Fernández M, Bernardi V et al, on behalf of the GRAMI Investigators. Coronary stents improved hospital results during coronary angioplasty in acute myocardial infarction: preliminary results of a randomized controlled study (GRAMI trial) [abstract]. *J Am Coll Cardiol* 1997; **29** (suppl A): 221A.

107. Rodriguez A, Bernardi V, Fernández M et al, on behalf of the GRAMI Investigators. Coronary stents improved hospital outcome in patients undergoing angioplasty in acute myocardial infarction: results of a randomized multicenter study (GRAMI trial) [abstract]. *Eur Heart J* 1997; **18** (suppl): 586.

108. Antoniucci D, Santoro GM, Bolognese L et al. Stenting in acute myocardial infarction: preliminary results of the FRESCO study (Florence Randomized

Elective Stenting in Acute Coronary Occlusions) [abstract]. *Eur Heart J* 1997; **18** (suppl): 586.

109. Antoniucci D, Santoro GM, Bolognese L et al. Elective stenting in acute myocardial infarction: preliminary results of the Florence randomized elective stenting in acute coronary occlusions (FRESCO) study [abstract]. *J Am Coll Cardiol* 1997; **29** (suppl A): 456A.

110. Baier R. Initial events in interaction of blood with a foreign surface. *J Biomed Mat Res* 1969; **3:** 191–206.

111. De Palma VE, Baier RE. Investigation of three-surface properties of several metals and their relation to blood biocompatibility. *J Biomed Mat Res* 1972; **6:** 37–75.

112. de Jaegere PP, Serruys PW, Bertrand M et al. Wiktor stent implantation in patients with restenosis following balloon angioplasty of a native coronary artery. *Am J Cardiol* 1992; **69:** 598–602.

113. Buchwald A, Unterberg C, Werner G, Voth E, Kreuzer H, Wiegand V. Initial clinical results with the Wiktor stent: a new balloon expandable coronary stent. *Clin Cardiol* 1991; **14:** 374–79.

114. Buchwald AB, Werner GS, Möller K, Unterberg C. Expansion of Wiktor stents by oversizing versus high-pressure dilatation: a randomized, intracoronary ultrasound-controlled study. *Am Heart J* 1997; **133:** 190–96.

115. Corcos T, Guérin Y, Garcia-Cantu E et al. Bail-out of stent jail: stent delivery through stent struts. *J Invas Cardiol* 1996; **8:** 113–16.

116. Nakamura S, Hall P, Maiello L, Colombo A. Techniques for Palmaz–Schatz stent deployment in lesions with a large side branch. *Cathet Cardiovasc Diagn* 1995; **34:** 353–61.

117. Buchwald A, Unterbert C, Werner GS, Wiegand V. Acute coronary occlusion after angioplasty management by a new balloon-expandable stent [abstract]. *Eur Heart J* 1990; **11** (suppl): 370.

118. Bertrand OF, Legrand V, Bilodeau L, Martinez CA, Kulbertus HE. Emergency coronary stenting with Wiktor stents – immediate and late results. *J Invas Cardiol* 1997; **9:** 2–9.

119. Buchwald AB, Stevens J, Zilz R et al. Influence of increased wave density of coil stents on the proliferative response in a minipig coronary stent-angioplasty model [abstract]. *Eur Heart J* 1997; **18** (suppl): 152.

120. Wang K, Verbeken E, Zhou XR, De Scheerder IK. Experimental evaluation of a new single wire tantalum coil coronary stent (Wiktor-i™). *J Invas Cardiol* 1998; **10:** 64–69.

121. Vrolix MC, Grolier G, Legrand V et al. Heparin-coated wire coil (Wiktor) for elective stent placement – the MENTOR Trial [abstract]. *Eur Heart J* 1997; **18** (suppl): 152.

122. Penn IM, Barbeau G, Brown RIG et al. Initial human implants with a flexible radio-opaque tantalum stent [abstract]. *J Am Coll Cardiol* 1995; **25**: 288A.

123. Hamasaki N, Nosaka H, Nobuyoshi M. Initial experience of Cordis Stent implantation [abstract]. *J Am Coll Cardiol* 1995; **25**: 239A.

124. Ozaki Y, Keane D, Nobuyoshi M, Hamasaki N, Popma JJ, Serruys PW. Coronary lumen at six-months follow-up of a new radio-opaque Cordis tantalum stent using quantitative angiography and intracoronary ultrasound. *Am J Cardiol* 1995; **76**: 1135–43.

125. Rothman MT, Serruys PW, Horntje JCA, Grollier G, vd Bos AA, Wijns W, on behalf of the EASI Investigators. Easi study: 6 months results of a multicentre evaluation of a short-wave tantalum coil stent [abstract]. *Eur Heart J* 1997; **18** (suppl): 152.

126. Watson PS, Ponde CK, Aroney CN et al. Angiographic follow-up and clinical experience with the flexible tantalum Cordis stent. *Cathet Cardiovasc Diagn* 1998; **43**: 168–73.

127. Park S-J, Park S-W, Hong M-K et al. Late clinical outcomes of Cordis tantalum coronary stenting without anticoagulation. *Am J Cardiol* 1997; **80**: 943–47.

128. Hamasaki N, Nosaka H, Kimura T et al. Initial experience with the Cordis stent: analysis of serial angiographic follow-up. *Cathet Cardiovasc Diagn* 1997; **42**: 166–72.

129. Park S-J, Park S-W, Hong M-K, Cheong S-S, Lee CW, Kim J-J. Intracoronary stainless steel Cordis (CrossFlex) stent implantation: initial results and late outcome [abstract]. *Am J Cardiol* 1997; **80** (suppl 7A): 27S.

130. Feres F, Sousa E, Londero H et al. Early results of the SOLACI Registry of a new coil stent (Cross-flex®) [abstract]. *Am J Cardiol* 1997; **80** (suppl 7A): 28S.

131. De Scheerder I, Wang K, Verbeken E et al. Experimental evaluation of a new single wire stainless steel fishscale coronary stent (Freedom). *J Invas Cardiol* 1996; **8**: 357–62.

132. De Scheerder I, Wang K, Kerdsinchai P et al. Clinical and angiographic experience with coronary stenting using Freedom™ stent. *J Invas Cardiol* 1996; **8**: 418–27.

133. Chevalier B, Glatt B, Royer T. Kissing stenting in bifurcation lesions [abstract]. *Eur Heart J* 1996; **17** (suppl): 218.

134. Chevalier B, Glatt B, Royer T. Coronary artery reconstruction with the Freedom stent [abstract]. *Eur Heart J* 1996; **17** (suppl): 459.

135. Antoniucci D, Valenti R, Santoro M, Bolognese L, Trapani M, Fazzini PF. Preliminary experience with stent-supported coronary angioplasty in long narrowings using the long Freedom Force stent: acute and six-month clinical and angiographic results in a series of 27 consecutive patients. *Cathet Cardiovasc Diagn* 1998; **43**: 163–67.

136. Chevalier B, Montserrat P, Huguet R et al. French Freedom stent registry: short-term results [abstract]. *Eur Heart J* 1996; **17** (suppl): 412.

137. Chevalier B, De Scheerder I, Simon R, Vassanelli C, Royer T, Glatt B. Long bare stent registry [abstract]. *Circulation* 1996; **92** (suppl): I-207.

138. De Scheerder I, Chevalier B, Vassanelli C. European Freedom stent registry [abstract]. *J Am Coll Cardiol* 1997; **29** (suppl A): 495A.

139. Chevalier B, Montserrat P, Huguet R et al. French Freedom stent registry: midterm results [abstract]. *J Am Coll Cardiol* 1997; **29** (suppl A): 495A.

140. De Scheerder I, Chevalier B, Vassanelli C. European Freedom stent registry [abstract]. *Eur Heart J* 1997; **18** (suppl): 156.

141. Webb JG, Popma JJ, Lansky AJ et al. Early and late assessment of the Micro Stent PL coronary stent for restenosis and suboptimal balloon angioplasty. *Am Heart J* 1997; **133**: 369–74.

142. Pomerantsev EV, Kim C, Kernoff RS et al. Coronary AVE Micro Stents: serial quantitative angiography and histology in a canine model. *Cathet Cardiovasc Diagn* 1997; **41**: 213–24.

143. Schalij MJ, Savalle LH, Tresukosol D, Jukema JW, Reiber JHC, Bruschke AVG. Micro Stent I, initial results, and six months follow-up by quantitative coronary angiography. *Cathet Cardiovasc Diagn* 1998; **43**: 19–27.

144. Haase J, Geimer M, Göhring S et al. Results of Micro Stent implantations in coronary lesions of various complexity. *Am J Cardiol* 1997; **80**: 1601–02.

145. Clague JR, Vasudeva A, Ward DE, Pumphrey CW, Redwood DR. The AVE micro coronary stent as a bailout device. *J Invas Cardiol* 1997; **9**: 339–43.

146. Tresukosol D, Schalij MJ, Savalle LH et al. Micro Stent™, quantitative coronary angiography, and procedural results. *Cathet Cardiovasc Diagn* 1996; **38**: 135–43.

147. Rau T, Schofer J, Golestani R, Schlhter M, Mathey DG. Increased restenosis rate associated with the Microstent™ compared to the Palmaz–Schatz stent in matched coronary lesions [abstract]. *Eur Heart J* 1997; **18** (suppl): 157.

148. Agarwal R, Bhargava B, Kaul U et al. Angiographic follow-up after A.V.E. Microstent implantation: lesion matched comparison with Palmaz–Schatz stent [abstract]. *Eur Heart J* 1997; **18** (suppl): 155.

149. Rau T, Schofer J, Mathey DG. Increased restenosis rate associated with the Microstent™ compared to the Palmaz–Schatz stent in matched coronary lesions [abstract]. *Circulation* 1997; **96** (suppl): I-710.

150. Oemrawsingh PV, Tuinenburg JC, Schalij MJ, Jukema WJ, Reiber JHC, Bruschke AVG. Clinical and angiographic outcome of Micro Stent II implantation in native coronary arteries. *Am J Cardiol* 1998; **81**: 152–57.

151. Gerckens U, Cattelaens N, Möller R, Grube E. Clinical application of the new

AVE-Stents (GFX®) in 331 complex coronary stenoses [abstract]. *Eur Heart J* 1997; **18** (suppl): 158.

152. Kiemeneij F, Laarman GJ, Odekerken D, Slagboom T, van der Wieken R. Safety and efficacy of AVE gfx stent implantation via 6 french guiding catheters: results of a pilot study [abstract]. *Am J Cardiol* 1997; **80** (suppl 7A): 29S.

153. Joseph T, Fajadet J, Cassagneau B et al. Initial experience with the new GFX coronary stent [abstract]. *Circulation* 1997; **96** (suppl): I-528.

154. Violini R, Marzocchi A, Antoniucci D et al, on behalf of the Italian Modular Stent Study Group. Multicentre evaluation of a new modular coronary stent [abstract]. *Eur Heart J* 1997; **18** (suppl): 159.

155. Corcos T, Pentousis D, Guérin Y et al. Initial experience with the BARD XT stent [abstract]. *Am J Cardiol* 1997; **80** (suppl 7A): 29S.

156. Sievart H, Rohde S, Ensslen R et al. Initial clinical experience with the new EBI (BARD-XT) flexible coronary stent: acute results and follow-up. *Cathet Cardiovasc Diagn* 1998; **43:** 159–62.

157. Xu XY, Collins MW. Fluid dynamics in stents. In: Sigwart U (ed.), Endoluminal Stenting. London: W.B. Saunders, 1996: 52–59.

158. Brown CH, Leverett LB, Lewis CE. Morphological, biochemical, and functional changes in human platelets subject to shear stress. *J Lab Clin Med* 1975; **86:** 462–71.

159. Schwartz RS, Huber KC, Murphy JG et al. Restenosis and proportional neointimal response to coronary artery injury: results in a porcine model. *J Am Coll Cardiol* 1992; **19:** 267–74.

160. Ischinger TA. The Navius racheting stent: clinical introduction of a novel vascular stent concept. *Am J Cardiol* 1997; **80** (suppl 7A): 225.

161. Almagor Y, Feld S, Kiemeneij F et al, for the FINESS Trial Investigators. First international new intravascular rigid-flex endovascular stent study (FINESS): clinical and angiographic results after elective and urgent stent implantation. *J Am Coll Cardiol* 1997; **30:** 847–54.

162. Almagor Y, Feld S, Kiemeneij F et al. First international new intravascular rigid-flex endovascular stent study: angiographic results and six month clinical follow-up. *Eur Heart J* 1997; **18** (suppl): 156.

163. Di Mario C, Reimers B, Almagor Y et al. Procedural and follow-up results with a new balloon expandable stent in unselected lesions. *Heart* 1998; **79:** 234–41.

164. Zheng H, Corcos T, Favereau X, Pentousis D, Guérin Y, Ouzan J. Preliminary experience with the NIR coronary stent. *Cathet Cardiovasc Diagn* 1998; **43:** 153–58.

165. Lau KW, He Q, Ding ZP, Quek S, Johan A. Early experience with the NIR intracoronary stent. *Am J Cardiol* 1998; **81:** 927–29.

166. Chevalier B, Lefevre T, Meyer P et al. French registry of seven cells NIRstent implantation in ≤2.5 mm coronary arteries [abstract]. *Circulation* 1997; **96** (suppl): I-274.

167. Lansky AJ, Popma JJ, Mehran R et al. Late quantitative angiographic results after NIR stent use: results from the NIRVANA randomized trial and registries [abstract]. *J Am Coll Cardiol* 1998; **31** (suppl): 80A

168. Baim DS. Acute and 30-day clinical results of the NIRVANA Trial [abstract]. *Circulation* 1997; **96** (suppl): I-594.

169. Rogers C, Edelman ER. Endovascular stent design dictates experimental restenosis and thrombosis. *Circulation* 1995; **91:** 2995–3001.

170. Barth KH, Virmani R, Froelich J et al. Paired comparison of vascular wall reactions to Palmaz stents, Streker tantalum stents, and Wallstents in canine iliac and femoral arteries. *Circulation* 1996; **93:** 2161–69.

171. Carter AJ, Laird JR, Farb A, Kufs W, Wortham DC, Virmani R. Morphological characteristics of lesion formation and time course of smooth muscle proliferation in a porcine proliferative restenosis model. *J Am Coll Cardiol* 1994; **24:** 1398–405.

172. Schwartz RS, Huber KC, Murphey JG et al. Restenosis and proportional neointimal response to coronary artery injury: results in a porcine model. *J Am Coll Cardiol* 1991; **19:** 267–74.

173. Schwartz RS, Holmes DH, Topol EJ. The restenosis paradigm revisited: an alternative proposal for cellular mechanisms. *J Am Coll Cardiol* 1992; **20:** 1284–93.

174. Carter AJ, Scott D, Bailey LR, Jones R, Fischell TA. Stent design: in the "ends" it matters [abstract]. *Circulation* 1997; **96** (suppl): I-402.

175. Alt E, Pasquantonio J, Fliedner T et al. Effect of endovascular stent design on experimental restenosis. *J Am Coll Cardiol* 1997; **29** (suppl A): 242A.

176. Garasic JM, Squire JC, Edelman ER, Rogers C. Stent and artery geometry determine intimal thickening independent of deep arterial injury [abstract]. *Circulation* 1997; **96** (suppl): I-402.

177. Kornowski R, Hong MK, Tio FO, Bramwell O, Wu H, Leon MB. In-stent restenosis: contributions of inflammatory responses and arterial injury to neointimal hyperplasia. *J Am Coll Cardiol* 1998; **31:** 224–30.

178. Hofma SH, Whelen DM, van Beusekon HM, Verdouw PD, van der Giessen WJ. Increasing arterial wall injury after long-term implantation of two types of stent in a porcine coronary model. *Eur Heart J* 1998; **19:** 601–09.

179. Escaned J, Goicolea J, Alfonso F et al. Influence of stent design on the relationship between acute gain and late luminal loss [abstract]. *J Am Coll Cardiol* 1998; **31** (suppl): 415A.

180. Gunn J, Malik N, Shepherd L et al. In-stent restenosis: relationship to strut

protrusion and asymmetrical deployment [abstract]. *Eur Heart J* 1997; **18** (suppl): 451.

181. Goy JJ, Eeckhout E, Debbas N, Stauffer JC, Vogt P. Stenting of the right coronary artery for de novo stenosis: a comparison of the Wicktor and the Palmaz–Schatz stents [abstract]. *Circulation* 1995; **92** (suppl I): I-536.

182. Fernández-Ortiz A, Goicolea J, Pérez-Vizcayno MJ et al. Six-month follow-up of successful stenting for acute dissection after coronary angioplasty: Comparison between slotted tube (Palmaz–Schatz) and flexible coil (Gianturco–Roubin) stent designs. *J Interven Cardiol* 1998; **11**: 41–7.

183. Lowe HC. New balloon expandable stent for bifurcation lesions. *Cathet Cardiovasc Diagn* 1997; **42**: 235–36.

184. Gerckens U, Müller R, Cattelaens N, Herchenbach M, Grube E. The new Coronary Stent Graft JoStent®: first clinical experience [abstract]. *J Am Coll Cardiol* 1998; **31** (suppl): 414A.

3. RANDOMIZED CLINICAL TRIALS

Stenting compared with PTCA

Native vessel de-novo stenoses

Completed trials

Early observational trials showed the feasibility and safety of stent implantation in humans. Since stents have been available for elective applications only since 1993, there is a limited number of published randomized trials. The first trials to show conclusively the superiority of coronary stenting over conventional balloon angioplasty in clinical and angiographic outcome were the large prospective randomized trials BENESTENT[1] (BElgium NEtherlands STENT trial) and STRESS[2] (STent REStenosis Study). Both trials compared elective Palmaz–Schatz stent placement with elective balloon angioplasty in patients with single, discrete, de-novo lesions in the native coronary circulation. The BENESTENT study randomized a total of 520 patients and the STRESS study (STRESS I) successfully enrolled 407 patients. A further 189 patients were subsequently enrolled in the STRESS cohort (STRESS II) to make the combined number of 596 patients studied (STRESS I and II). The design and results of these trials are summarized in tables 3.1, 3.2, and 3.3. In both BENESTENT and STRESS, the luminal diameter immediately after the procedure was larger in the patients treated by stent implantation than in those treated with conventional balloon angioplasty. Although the loss in luminal diameter was greater at follow-up, there was a trend towards greater luminal diameter in those patients treated with a stent. Both studies showed that stent implantation significantly reduced the angiographic restenosis rate. In the BENESTENT study, this lower restenosis rate translated into a better 6-month event-free survival, mainly as a result of a 51% reduction in the need for repeat angioplasty. The STRESS study showed only a trend towards an improved long-term clinical outcome. Unfortunately, these favourable results were obtained at the cost of a prolonged hospital stay, and an increased risk of bleeding and vascular complications. One-year follow-up results from STRESS[3] and BENESTENT[4] showed that the clinical benefits observed at 6-months follow-up persisted.

The START (STent versus Angioplasty Restenosis Trial) study was a multicentre Spanish trial that, like the STRESS trial, compared elective

Table 3.1 Design of the BENESTENT and STRESS trials

	BENESTENT study	STRESS study
Study design	Open, multicentre, randomized	Open, multicentre, randomized
Randomization	Telephone service	Sealed envelope
Angiographic endpoint	MLD at FU Restenosis rate (≥50% DS at FU)	MLD at FU Restenosis rate (≥50% DS at FU)
Clinical endpoint	Composite clinical endpoint analysis of the occurrence of death, CVA, AMI, CABG, repeat intervention	Composite clinical endpoint analysis of the occurrence of death, AMI, CABG, bailout stent, repeat intervention
Type of analysis	Intention to treat	Intention to treat
Power calculation	Based on an assumed clinical event rate of 30% in the control group and a reduction of 40% in the stent group, power of 0.80	Based on an assumed restenosis rate of 30% after PTCA and of 15% after stent implantation, power of 0.90
Study population	Stable angina De-novo lesion in coronary artery	Symptomatic ischaemic heart disease De-novo lesion in coronary artery
Patients randomized	520	410
Final study population	516	407
Study period	June 1991–March 1993	January 1991–February 1993
Number of centres	28	20

AMI = acute myocardial infarction; CABG = coronary artery bypass graft; CVA = cerebrovascular accident; DS = diameter stenosis; FU = follow-up; MLD = minimum luminal diameter; PTCA = percutaneous transluminal coronary angioplasty.

Table 3.2 Angiographic results of the BENESTENT, STRESS, and START trials

	BENESTENT Study			STRESS Study			START Study		
	Pre-intervention	Post-intervention	FU	Pre-intervention	Post-intervention	FU	Pre-intervention	Post-intervention	FU
Balloon									
RD (mm)	3.01 ± 0.46	3.09 ± 0.44	3.05 ± 0.49	2.99 ± 0.50	2.99 ± 0.46	2.98 ± 0.49	NR	NR	NR
MLD (mm)	1.08 ± 0.31	2.05 ± 0.33	1.73 ± 0.55	0.75 ± 0.25	1.99 ± 0.47	1.56 ± 0.65	0.80 ± 0.03	2.28 ± 0.5	1.63 ± 0.7
Diameter stenosis (%)	64 ± 10	33 ± 16	43 ± 16	75 ± 8	35 ± 14	49 ± 19	NR	NR	NR
Stent									
RD (mm)	2.99 ± 0.45	3.16 ± 0.43	2.96 ± 0.48	3.03 ± 0.42	3.05 ± 0.40	3.00 ± 0.41	NR	NR	NR
MLD (mm)	1.07 ± 0.33	2.48 ± 0.39	1.82 ± 0.64	0.77 ± 0.27	2.49 ± 0.44	1.74 ± 0.60	0.79 ± 0.3	2.85 ± 0.5	1.96 ± 0.8
Diameter stenosis (%)	64 ± 10	22 ± 8	38 ± 18	75 ± 9	19 ± 11	42 ± 18	NR	NR	NR
Restenosis rate (%) (≥50% DS at FU)									
Balloon			32			42			37
Stent			22			31			22

DS = diameter stenosis; FU = follow-up; MLD = minimum luminal diameter; RD = reference diameter; NR = not reported

Table 3.3 Clinical results of the BENESTENT and STRESS trials

	BENESTENT Study			STRESS Study		
	Balloon (n = 257)	Stent (n = 259)	P	Balloon (n = 202)	Stent (n = 205)	P
Composite clinical endpoint analysis						
In-hospital period	6.2%	6.9%	NR	11.4%	5.9%	NR
At 6 months	29.6%	20.1%	<0.05	23.8%	19.5%	NS
6-month event-free survival	70.4%	79.9%	<0.05	76.2%	80.5%	NS
1-year event-free survival	68.5%	76.8%	<0.05	71.5%*	80.3%*	<0.05
Acute closure/stent thrombosis	2.7%	3.5%	NR	1.5%	3.4%	NS
Bleeding and vascular complications	3.1%	13.5%	<0.05	4.0%	7.3%	NS
Hospital stay (days)	3.1	8.5	<0.05	2.8	5.8	<0.05

NS = nonsignificant; NR = not reported; * combined STRESS I and II data angioplasty and Palmaz–Schatz coronary stenting in patients with symptomatic coronary artery disease and de-novo lesions in the native circulation.[5] A total of 452 patients were included in this trial, and the primary endpoint was restenosis at a 6-months follow-up. As with the results of the BENESTENT and STRESS trials, stenting was associated with a greater initial gain and late loss, and a significantly lower restenosis rate when compared with balloon angioplasty alone.

The BENESTENT II (BElgium NEtherlands STENT trial) was a multicentre randomized trial with a 12-months follow-up.[6–9] The primary objective of the BENESTENT II trial was to assess the long-term effect on cardiac events of the implantation of heparin-coated Palmaz–Schatz stents, in patients with stable or unstable angina and one or more de-novo lesions in the coronary circulation, compared with balloon angioplasty alone. Secondary objectives of this trial included assessments of safety and the effect on restenosis, and consideration of the cost-effectiveness of implantation of a heparin-coated stent in these patients. A total of 824 patients were entered into the trial from around 40 clinical sites. Patients were randomized to treatment with either a heparin-coated stent or with conventional angioplasty. A 1:1 subrandomization was done to assign patients to either clinical and angiographic follow-up or to clinical follow-up only. The subacute thrombosis rate in the patients receiving the heparin-coated stent was less than 0.2%.[6,7] Angiographic follow-up showed a restenosis rate in the stented patients of 17%, compared with a rate of 31% in the balloon angioplasty group (p = 0.001).[6,8] Clinical follow-up showed a 14.3% event rate in the stent-treated group compared with 19.4% in the balloon group. Data concerning the costs of the primary procedure and costs of hospital admission were collected (direct medical costs), and an assessment of indirect costs was obtained with a questionnaire. Cost-effectiveness analysis of the results of the BENESTENT I and II trials suggest that there may be an overall cost benefit for the use of heparin-coated stents in combination with antiplatelet therapy over angioplasty alone.[6,9]

The multicentre Canadian trial TASC-I (Trial of Angioplasty and Stents in Canada) was designed to determine the effects of stenting compared with balloon angioplasty on the late (6-months) restenosis rate.[10] In this trial, 270 patients with de-novo lesions (n = 148) or restenotic (n = 122) lesions in the native coronary circulation that required elective intervention were randomized to either percutaneous transluminal coronary angioplasty (PTCA) or stenting with a Palmaz–Schatz stent. Preliminary Results from this trial showed that the restenosis rate in the patients treated with stents was significantly lower than those treated with angioplasty alone.[10]

Retrospective analysis of the STRESS trial showed that, compared with PTCA, the net gain in luminal diameter was greater in patients who had stents placed in the left anterior descending coronary artery than in those who had stents implanted in other coronary arteries.[11] To verify this observation, a single-centre prospective trial was done in Italy. An advantage of coronary stenting over balloon angioplasty for the treatment of de-novo stenoses in the "high risk" proximal left anterior descending artery location was shown in that study.[12] A total of 120 patients with symptomatic isolated stenosis of the left anterior descending artery were randomly assigned to either stent implantation with a Palmaz–Schatz stent or standard coronary angioplasty. Twelve months event-free survival was significantly better in the stent-treated group than in the angioplasty group (87% *vs* 70% respectively, p = 0.04). Angiographically determined restenosis rates were also significantly improved in stent treated patients (19% after stent implantation and 40% after angioplasty, p = 0.02).

The OCBAS (Optimal Coronary Balloon Angioplasty versus Stent) trial[13] addressed the concept of provisional stenting, that is, the use of balloon angioplasty as the principal strategy for coronary revascularization, with stent implantation only for unsatisfactory results.[14] The trial was designed to assess angiographic restenosis and target lesion revascularization rates of optimal balloon angioplasty compared with those of coronary stenting. The investigators judged an optimal balloon procedure to have a satisfactory acute result and less than 0.3 mm loss in minimum luminal diameter (MLD) after a 30-minute observation period (no early loss). A total of 116 patients were randomized in this trial, 57 to stent and 59 to PTCA. After randomization to the PTCA group, 14% of these patients required crossover to stent due to an early loss in diameter. Final results of this trial showed a greater acute gain in MLD in the stent-treated group (1.6 $\pm$ 0.51 mm balloon *vs* 1.0 $\pm$ 0.3 mm stent, p < 0.03), as expected. However, late loss was greater in the stent group (0.28 $\pm$ 0.44 mm *vs* 0.63 $\pm$ 0.59 mm, p < 0.0001), and as a consequence, the restenosis and target vessel revascularization (TVR) rates were similar in both groups (restenosis rates, 16.6% balloon *vs* 18.8% stent; TVR rates 9.2% balloon *vs* 9.4% stent). These results support the concept that stents should be viewed not as an alternative to, but rather as an adjunct to balloon angioplasty in select lesion subsets consistent with the doctrine of provisional stenting.

The notion of provisional stenting was also tested in a single-centre trial in England.[15] In this trial, 143 unselected patients scheduled for PTCA were enrolled. Of the 143 patients, 50 (35%) required bailout stenting for abrupt or threatened vessel closure. For the remaining patients, the angiographic result was assessed immediately using on-line quantitative coronary angiography (QCA). Sixteen patients had an optimum result (<15% residual stenosis, no visible dissection) after PTCA. The remaining 77 patients were randomized either to no further treatment or to the placement of a Palmaz–Schatz stent. Six months angiographic follow-up was done in 132 of the original 143 patients enrolled. Restenosis ($\geq$50% diameter stenosis) occurred in 17 (45%) of 38 patients with a suboptimum result randomized to PTCA, but in only eight (22%) of 37 patients randomized to stenting (p = 0.05). Patients who had an optimum result had a similar rate of restenosis as the stented patients.

The effectiveness of the Wallstent to reduce the rate of restenosis was tested in the WIN (Wallstent In Native arteries) trial.[16,17] In this trial, 586 eligible patients were randomized to treatment either with implantation of a Wallstent (287) or to conventional balloon angioplasty (299). Patients with both de-novo and restenotic lesions in the native coronary circulation were included in this trial by 26 centres. The objectives were the assessment of clinical and angiographic restenosis as indicated by event-free survival and repeat angiography at 6 months after treatment. The first 8 stented patients were treated with aspirin and coumadin the remaining with aspirin and ticlopidine postimplantation, while patients in the PTCA-only group were treated with aspirin alone. The Wallstent was sized 0.5 to 1.0 mm greater than the on-line maximum reference diameter. 14.4% of the stented patients and 12.2% of the balloon angioplasty patients were treated for restenosis. At six months follow-up, there was no difference in the clinical event rates (death, MI, target lesion revascularization, cerebrovascular accident) between the two groups (28.1% stent *vs* 26.8% balloon). Restenosis rates of the two treatment groups were identical (39% stent *vs* 39% balloon). Thus in this selected population, there was no advantage of elective stenting with the Wallstent compared with balloon angioplasty.

Ongoing trials
There are only a few trials underway comparing stent implantation with conventional angioplasty for de-novo stenoses in the native coronary circulation.

The BOSS (Balloon Optimization *vs* Stent Study) trial was designed to assess whether an optimized PTCA result yields restenosis rates similar to stenting in single discrete de-novo lesions[18] (the concept of provisional stenting). In this trial, a 2:1 randomization of perfusion balloons versus Palmaz–Schatz stenting is being used, and cross-over after PTCA can occur for an inadequate initial result (>30% residual stenosis by QCA) or for recoil assessed visually after 20 minutes. For PTCA, large balloons at low pressures are encouraged (<4 atmospheres), and stent deployment is followed by high-pressure dilatation. Primary endpoints are 6-months angiographically determined restenosis rates, costs, and need for target lesion revascularization. Early analysis of the data suggests that optimum PTCA results in restenosis rates similar to stented lesions.[18]

The primary objective of the ADVANCE (ADditional VAlue of NIR stents for treatment of long Coronary 1Esions) trial is to compare stenting following successful balloon angioplasty to successful balloon angioplasty alone in patients with a single de novo long lesion (treatable by a single balloon longer than 20 mm and shorter than or equal to 40 mm) with respect to major adverse cardiac events at 9 months follow-up. After successful balloon angioplasty, 500 patients are to be randomized to either no further treatment or to implantation of a long NIR stent. Enrolment in this trial is currently underway.

Saphenous vein graft disease

Completed trials

The results of the SAVED trial (SAphenous VEin graft De novo) showed an improved clinical outcome at 6-months' follow-up in patients with vein graft disease treated with stent implantation.[19,20] In this multicentre randomized trial, 220 patients with angina and/or documented ischaemia due to a discrete, non-ostial, de-novo lesion ($\geq$60% on visual estimate) in a vein graft of 3.0–5.0 mm, were randomized to either Palmaz–Schatz stent implantation (110 patients) or convential balloon angioplasty (110 patients). Those with a lesion requiring treatment with more than two stents were excluded. The study endpoints were angiographic restenosis rate ($\geq$50% diameter stenosis at 6 months), the procedural success rate ($\leq$50% diameter stenosis after stenting without complications), and a composite analysis of the clinical endpoints of death, myocardial infarction, repeat surgery, and target lesion revascularization. Results indicate a graft age of roughly 10 years, a lesion length of 10 mm or less, and a mean vessel diameter of 3.19 mm. Postprocedural MLD was 2.81 $\pm$ 0.49 mm in stented vessels compared with 2.16 $\pm$ 0.057 mm with PTCA (p < 0.0001). Procedural success was 95% after stent implantation and 75% after balloon angioplasty. However, stented patients more commonly required blood transfusion (11 stent *vs* 1 PTCA patient, p = 0.003). In the stent group, late loss in MLD at 6 months was greater (1.04 mm stent *vs* 0.68 mm PTCA, p = 0.01), but net gain was greater (0.87 mm stent *vs* 0.52 mm PTCA) than in vessels treated with PTCA. The major cardiac event rate at 6 months was 26% in the stented patients compared with 38% after PTCA (p = 0.05). Thus, in short non-restenotic non-ostial vein graft lesions, these data suggest that stent implantation is the preferred treatment compared with PTCA.

Restenotic lesions

Completed trials

The role of stents to reduce recurrent restenosis compared with balloon angioplasty was evaluated in the REST (stent versus PTCA RESTenosis) trial,[21] a multicentre randomized trial comparing the implantation of a single Palmaz–Schatz stent with conventional angioplasty in patients with restenosis after successful PTCA of a native coronary artery. The primary objectives of this trial were the assessment of the MLD, late loss, and restenosis rate at 6-months follow-up angiography. Secondary objectives included clinical events in and out of hospital. A total of 351 patients were randomized. Significant differences in favour of stent treatment were seen in acute and 6-months follow-up MLD (figure 3.1), in the need for target vessel revascularization during the follow-up period (10% in the stent group *vs* 27% in the PTCA group, p = 0.006) and the

Rest Trial Results

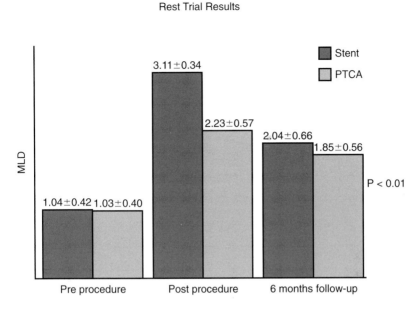

Figure 3.1: Angiographic results of the REST (stent versus PTCA RESTenosis) trial (MLD = minimum luminal diameter).

rate of restenosis (18% stent *vs* 32% PTCA). Patients with "stent-like" post-PTCA results in this trial (≤30% residual diameter stenosis) had a similar requirement for target vessel revascularization to the stented patients, despite a significantly smaller MLD at follow-up.[22]

Total occlusions

Completed trials
Balloon angioplasty of chronically occluded arteries is not only technically demanding, but is also associated with a high incidence of luminal re-narrowing and re-occlusion.[23] The Scandinavian SICCO (Stenting in Chronic Coronary Occlusion) trial randomized 119 patients after initial recanalization of chronic coronary occlusions (duration of occlusion greater than 2 weeks and Thrombolysis in Myocardial Infarction [TIMI] flow grade 0 or 1) to conventional PTCA or Palmaz–Schatz stenting.[24] Restenosis (≥50% diameter stenosis) developed in 32% of patients who were stented compared with 74% of patients with PTCA only (p < 0.001) at 6-months angiographic follow-up.[25] Up to 300 days after randomization, 42.4% of patients in the PTCA group underwent target

vessel revascularization, in contrast to 22.4% of patients in the stented group. A continued clinical benefit was seen at a mean of 2.6 years of follow-up.[26] These results show that the angiographic and clinical long-term outcome after PTCA of chronic coronary occlusions are substantially improved by the insertion of Palmaz–Schatz stents.

A two centre German trial has assessed the benefit of the implantation of the Wiktor stent over balloon angioplasty alone after recanalization of chronic total occlusions (the SPACTO trial).[27] In this trial, 85 patients with chronic total occlusions (duration 25–292 days with TIMI 0 flow) and documented ischemia were randomly assigned to either PTCA alone or Wiktor stent implantation after successful recanalization of the occluded vessel. Seven (8%) patients in the PTCA-only group required crossover to stenting. At 6-months follow-up, the MLD of the stented vessels was significantly larger than that of the PTCA-only group (1.57 $\pm$ 0.59 mm stent vs 1.06 $\pm$ 0.90 mm PTCA, p $=$ 0.01). Consistent with the larger SICCO trial, the restenosis rate was also significantly lower (32% stent vs 64% PTCA, p $=$ 0.01). One patient in the stent group had reocclusion (3%), but eight patients treated with PTCA had reocclusion (24.2%, p$=$0.003). Cumulative cardiac events (death, MI, bypass surgery, repeat PTCA, unstable angina) were also less frequent in the stented group.

A single-centre randomized trial from Japan, in which 60 patients with total occlusions were enrolled, showed a similar favourable acute angiographic outcome in stented patients, with an MLD of 2.29 mm in the stent-treated patients compared with 1.87 in those treated with balloon angioplasty alone (p $<$ 0.001).[28] In this trial, multiple stents were used in 37% of the treated patients, and 39% of the patients in the balloon angioplasty group required crossover to stent treatment, nine (30%) patients for bailout indications, and two patients for reocclusion at 24 hours after initial intervention. This trial failed to show any benefit in the rate of restenosis at follow-up (36% in the stent treated patients vs 33% in balloon treated), which may be a reflection of the high crossover rate.

In the multicentre GISSOC (Grupo Italiano di Studio sullo Stent nelle Occlusioni Coronariche) trial, 110 patients were randomized after successful recanalization of a chronic total occlusion to either balloon angioplasty or implantation of a Palmaz–Schatz stent.[29] The primary endpoint of this trial was the MLD at follow-up angiography. Secondary endpoints included the binary restenosis rate, and the clinical endpoints of death, myocardial infarction, coronary artery bypass surgery, repeat angioplasty, and target vessel revascularization. Clinical follow-up was done at 3, 6, and 9 months after the procedure, and repeat angiography was done at 9 months. Results showed a significantly larger MLD at follow-up in the stent-treated group compared with those treated with balloon angioplasty (1.74 $\pm$ 0.88 mm stent vs 0.85 $\pm$ 0.75 mm balloon, p $<$ 0.001). Stent implantation was also associated with a lower incidence of restenosis (diameter stenosis $\geq$ 50%) at follow-up (32% stent vs 68% balloon, p < 0.001), and a lower rate of reocclusion (8% stent vs 34% balloon, p = 0.003) than balloon angioplasty alone. In addition, stent-treated patients had less recurrent ischaemia (14% stent vs 46% balloon, p = 0.038) and fewer target lesion revascularization procedures (5.3% stent vs 22% balloon, p = 0.038).

Ongoing trials
Three other trials comparing stent implantation to balloon angioplasty alone for chronic total occlusions are underway. Favourable results have been reported in a single centre randomized trial from the UK.[30] Sixty patients with total coronary occlusions were randomized to "stent" or "no stent" after successful balloon angioplasty. Postprocedure angiographic results in these 60 patients showed a significantly larger MLD in stented patients (2.8 mm) compared with those treated with balloon angioplasty (3.3 mm, p < 0.01). Intermediate-term follow-up results (mean 37 weeks) in 40 patients showed a significant benefit in vessel patency, residual percent stenosis, and ejection fraction in stent-treated patients, with no significant difference in the incidence of clinical events. The restenosis rate in the angioplasty-alone treated patients was 30%, compared with 20% in the stent-treated patients. No significant difference between groups was seen, probably due to the small sample size.

The STOP (Stents in Total Occlusion and restenosis Prevention) study is a randomized multicentre Israeli trial being done to assess the benefit of additional coronary stenting using the AVE Micro Stent in chronic (greater than 7 days) occluded coronary arteries.[31] After obtaining optimal PTCA results, patients were randomized either to no further treatment or additional stent implantation. A total of 95 patients have been enrolled in this study. The mean time of coronary occlusion was 45 $\pm$ 20 days. Forty-five patients randomized to the stent arm, received 51 stents (lengths 18–39 mm) with 100% implantation success and no procedure related major complication. Final results of this trial will soon be available.

Six months patient follow-up has recently been completed in the CORSICA (Chronic Occlusion Revascularization with Stent Implantation versus Coronary Angioplasty) trial.[32,33] From November 1995 to July 1997, 142 patients with chronic (greater than 15 days) total occlusions were included in this prospective randomized study. The original intention was to include 170 patients, but the study was stopped after 142 patients were randomized because of the favourable results of the SICCO study. Allocation treatment was done at the end of the balloon PTCA when a stable result was obtained. In both groups, patients received aspirin and ticlopidine for 1 month. In the stent treated group, patients were treated with a single or multiple Palmaz–Schatz stent. At 1 month follow-up, the clinical event rate (death, myocardial infarction, bypass surgery, re-PTCA) was significantly lower in the stent treated group than in the balloon only group (0% stent *vs* 17.1% balloon, p < 0.001). At 6-months follow-up, however, no significant difference in the clinical event rate was seen (22.2% stent *vs* 27.1% balloon, p = 0.5). Similarly, there was no difference in the target vessel revascularization rate at 6 months (22.2% stent *vs* 34.3% balloon, p = 0.1). The angiographic follow-up data will soon be available.

Acute or threatened closure after PTCA

Completed trials
The Canadian TASC II (Trial of Angioplasty and Stents in Canada) was a small scale multicentre trial which included 43 patients randomized to Palmaz–Schatz stent implantation or prolonged autoperfusion balloon angioplasty for failed PTCA (residual stenosis > 50% with ischaemia and dissection or reduction in TIMI flow).[34] A higher clinical success rate (90% stent *vs* 42% balloon) and superior immediate angiographic results were seen in the stented patients. Although small, this trial provided early encouraging results on the efficacy of bailout stent implantation.

Ongoing trials
The GRACE (Gianturco–Roubin stent Acute Closure Evaluation) study randomized patients with true closure (TIMI 0 or 1 flow, or TIMI 2 flow with angina or ECG evidence of ischaemia) and threatened closure (TIMI 2 or 3 flow with >50% residual stenosis or TIMI 3 flow with dissection) to either Gianturco–Roubin stent implantation or prolonged balloon angioplasty.[35] Designed in 1992, this study was hindered by slow recruitment, partly due to an unwillingness on the part of many interventionalists to subject their patients with acute and threatened closure to prolonged and repeated balloon dilatation, because of the availability of stents and the ease of their use. Results of this trial will soon be published.

The STENT-BY trial is a recently completed study from eight German centres that compared immediate Palmaz–Schatz stent implantation to conservative techniques (autoperfusion catheters, high pressure, longer inflation, emergency CABG) for the treatment of abrupt vessel closure (TIMI 0) or symptomatic dissections (TIMI 1 flow + angina + persistent ECG changes refractory to standard intravenous therapy with heparin, nitroglycerin, and calcium channel blockers) during coronary balloon angioplasty.[36] The strict inclusion criteria required that the lesion be less than 15 mm long in a vessel larger than 2.5 mm suitable to receive a single stent. A total of 100 patients were randomized into this trial, and interim analysis of the results of the first 75 patients suggest improved stabilization, fewer complications, and a better short-term and long-term outcome in patients with stent implantation, compared with conservative strategies for the treatment of abrupt closure of symptomatic postintervention dissections.[36]

Stenting in acute myocardial infarction

Completed trials

The GRAMI (GR II in Acute Myocardial Infarction) trial was designed to determine whether implantation of the GR II would improve outcome in patients undergoing percutaneous intervention during acute myocardial infarction.[37–40] A total of 104 patients presenting within 24 hours of the onset of symptoms of an acute myocardial infarction were randomized to either primary PTCA alone or PTCA plus elective stent implantation with the GR II stent. The primary endpoints were comparison of in-hospital major cardiac complications (death, recurrent ischaemia, reinfarction, and emergent coronary bypass), and TIMI 3 flow at discharge, between patients assigned to coronary stenting and patients assigned to balloon angioplasty alone. The secondary endpoints included procedural success, event-free survival, need for target vessel revascularization, and angiographic restenosis at follow-up. The procedural success rate in the stent-treated group was 98%, and that of the PTCA group was 94.2% (no in-laboratory death or emergent coronary bypass surgery, TIMI 2 or 3 flow in the index vessel, and a residual stenosis of ≤30% for coronary angioplasty and <20% for stent). Thirteen patients in the PTCA group required bailout stent implantation. The composite in-hospital outcome of death, CABG, or recurrent ischaemia occurred in 19.2% of the PTCA-treated patients and in only 3.8% of the stented group (p = 0.03). In-hospital target vessel revascularization was required in 13.4% of the balloon group and in 9.6% of the stented lesions (p = not significant). Repeat angiography done immediately before discharge revealed TIMI 3 flow in the infarct-related artery in 98% of the stented patients versus 83% of the angioplasty-only group (p = 0.002). At 1-year clinical follow-up, target vessel revascularization was required in 14% of the stent group, which was not significantly different from the figure of 21% in the angioplasty group. However, event-free survival was significantly better in the stent group than in the coronary angioplasty group (83% stent *vs* 65% PTCA respectively, p = 0.002). Follow-up angiographic data has not yet been presented.

The Japanese PASTA (Primary Angioplasty versus STent in Acute myocardial infarction) trial randomized 136 patients with acute myocardial infarction within 12 hours of symptom onset to balloon angioplasty or Palmaz–Schatz stent implantation.[41,42] The clinical success rate in this trial was 97% in the stented patients and 87% in the balloon-angioplasty-treated patients (p = 0.03). In-hospital clinical events (death, target lesion revascularization) occurred in 6% of the stented patients and in 19% of the balloon-treated patients (p = 0.02).

Target lesion revascularization was required in 18.6% of the stented patients versus 37.6% of the angioplasty group (p = 0.009).

The Zwolle Myocardial Infarction Study (previous acronym ESCOBAR; Emergency Stenting COmpared to conventional Balloon Angioplasty Randomized trial) was a single-centre trial in The Netherlands.[43-45] In this trial, 227 patients with acute myocardial infarction were randomized to either PTCA or primary stent implantation. The clinical endpoints were death, recurrent infarction, subsequent bypass surgery, or repeat angioplasty of the infarct-related vessel at 6 months follow-up. Recurrent infarction occurred in eight (7%) patients after balloon angioplasty and in one (1%) patient after stenting (p = 0.036). Target vessel revascularization was necessary in 19 (17%) and four (4%) patients respectively (p = 0.0016). The cardiac-event-free survival rate at 6 months follow-up in the stent group was significantly higher than in the balloon angioplasty group (95% stent *vs* 80% balloon, p = 0.012).

The FRESCO (Florence Randomized Elective Stenting in Acute Coronary Occlusions) trial was a single-centre trial undertaken in Italy.[46-48] After successful primary PTCA (residual stenosis <30%, reference vessel diameter ≥2.5 mm) 150 patients suffering from acute myocardial infarction were randomized to either conservative treatment or stent. The primary endpoint of this trial was the composite clinical endpoint of death, reinfarction, or symptom-driven repeat target vessel revascularization. The secondary endpoint was angiographic evidence of restenosis at 6 months follow-up. The incidence of clinical events at 6 months was 9% in the stent group and 28% in the PTCA group (p = 0.003). Significant restenosis (≥50% diameter stenosis) or reocclusion occurred in 17% of the stent group and 43% of the PTCA group (p = 0.001).

Ongoing trials

The rationale for the design of the PAMI-Stent trial was based on the premise that since the heparin-coated stent reduces platelet deposition and reocclusion, it may be ideally suited to implantation in the thrombotic milieu of an acute myocardial infarction. The feasibility and safety of such an approach was shown in the PAMI-Stent Pilot study, in which 101 patients with an acute myocardial infarction received the Palmaz–Schatz heparin-coated stent as the primary reperfusion strategy.[49,50] Recruitment into the multicentre PAMI-Stent (Primary Angioplasty in Myocardial Infarction) trial was completed in November 1997. During the acute phase of a myocardial infarction, 901 patients at 64 international centres were randomized to either conventional primary PTCA or to heparin-coated Palmaz–Schatz stent implantation. The primary endpoint of the study is the six-months composite incidence of death, non-fatal reinfarction, disabling stroke, or ischaemia-driven target vessel revascularization. Six-months angiographic follow-up is being done to determine the incidence of reocclusion, restenosis, and left ventricular functional recovery in the primary PTCA and primary stent groups.

In the CADILLAC Trial (Controlled Abciximab and Device Investigation to Lower Late Angioplasty Complications) a total of 2000 consecutive patients with acute myocardial infarction will be prospectively randomized at 90 international centres to one of four treatment strategies:

- primary PTCA only;
- PTCA plus the glycoprotein IIb/IIIa inhibitor abciximab;
- primary stenting only;
- primary stenting plus abciximab.[51]

The low ionic strength contrast agent Ioxaglate is being used in all patients to minimize the risk of thromboembolic complications. The primary endpoint in CADILLAC is the cumulative composite incidence of death, reinfarction, ischaemia-driven target vessel revascularization (urgent or elective), and stroke at 6 months. Additional clinical follow-up data will be collected up to 12 months. Protocol angiography and left ventriculography will be done in a subset of 700 patients to assess angiographic restenosis rates and myocardial salvage. The stent being used in the CADILLAC trial is the MULTI-LINK stent. Two additional substudies in conjunction with the CADILLAC trial are being undertaken, one comparing the utility of the transluminal extraction catheter (TEC) with abciximab in patients in whom the vessel responsible for the acute myocardial infarction is a diseased saphenous vein graft, and a second substudy that will examine the potential role of intravascular ultrasound (IVUS) above and beyond that of angiography alone for the prediction of adverse events.

The PRISAM (PRImary Stenting for Acute Myocardial infarction) study has been designed to determine whether stenting with the Wiktor stent for acute myocardial infarction reduces the restenosis rate compared with balloon angioplasty. A total of 300 patients will be randomized into this nine-centre Japanese trial. Early results favour a benefit of Wiktor stent implantation over PTCA.[52,53]

The BESSAMI (BErlin Stent Study in Acute Myocardial Infarction) will randomize 250 patients with an acute myocardial infarction to either intravascular ultrasound (IVUS) guided balloon angioplasty alone, or IVUS guided stent implantation with the Wiktor GX Hepamed (heparin coated) stent.[54] The patients included in this trial will be divided into three groups. If after initial balloon dilatation there is no evidence of a residual dissection (as determined by angiography or IVUS) and normal blood flow is restored (TIMI 3), then no further treatment is performed. In angiography or IVUS reveals a dissection, or if TIMI 3 flow is not achieved, then the patients will be randomized to one of two groups. In one group the intervention will be considered concluded (balloon group) and IVUS guided stent implantation will be performed in the other group. Randomization into this trial is complete and results will soon be available.

STENTIM 2 (Stent In Myocardial infarction 2) is a French prospective randomized multicentre study that is comparing elective Wiktor stent implantation with conventional PTCA in acute myocardial infarction.[55] Randomization is performed prior to wire recanalization in suitable angiographic target vessels (>3 mm, absence of bifurcation lesion, left main disease or excessive calcification). The primary endpoint for this trial is a combined angiographic rate of restenosis and reocclusion at 6 months. A total of 211 patients have been included in 17 centres. Angiographic success (TIMI 2 & 3 flow with residual stenosis <50%) was achieved in 97% in both groups. Unilateral cross-over with rescue stenting (for dissection or a residual stenosis greater than 50%) was observed in 35.5% of patients in the PTCA group. Six months follow-up results will soon be available.

Stenting compared with directional atherectomy

Completed trials

The START (STent versus directional coronary Atherectomy Randomized Trial) trial is a single-centre Japanese study designed to compare angiographic outcome and chronic vessel response as assessed by serial IVUS between primary stenting and primary atherectomy.[56,57] A total of 122 lesions were randomly assigned to treatment with a Palmaz–Schatz stent or with directional coronary atherectomy (DCA). Single or multiple Palmaz–Schatz stents were implanted with high pressure in the stent group, and aggressive debulking using IVUS was done in the DCA group. Serial QCA and intravascular ultrasound were done preprocedure, immediately postprocedure, and at 3 and 6 months of follow-up. Results obtained at 3 months follow-up are striking.[58] Despite a similar acute gain in MLD (1.87 ± 0.45 mm DCA *vs* 1.79 ± 0.49 mm stent, p = not significant), vessels treated with DCA exhibited a significantly larger MLD than those treated with stents (2.33 ± 0.63 mm DCA *vs* 1.95 ± 0.65 mm stent, p = 0.0015). The restenosis rate was also lower for the DCA-treated group (8.5% *vs* 23%), due to a decrease in the neointimal proliferative response (loss index DCA *vs* stent; 0.31 ± 0.34 *vs* 0.49 ± 0.39, p = 0.009). These favourable results persisted to 6 months follow-up.[59]

Evaluation of adjunctive therapy

Adjunctive pharmacotherapy — acute and subacute thrombosis

Completed trials

The EPISTENT (Evaluation of Platelet IIb/IIIa Inhibitor for STENTing) trial[61] was a multicentre North American trial in which 2399 patients with ischaemic heart disease and suitable coronary lesions were randomly assigned to stenting plus placebo (n = 809), stenting plus abciximab (n = 794), or balloon angioplasty plus abciximab. Abciximab is a monoclonal Fab fragment directed against the glycoprotein IIb/IIIa[61] (GPIIb/IIIa) receptor on the external surface of platelets. The GPIIb/IIIa receptors on adjacent platelets bind fibrinogen and von-Willibrand factor, thereby mediating platelet aggregation. The antithrombotic effect of abciximab is a result of direct inhibition of the binding of these proteins to the platelet receptors, which leads to a dose-dependent inhibition of platelet aggregation. The activity of abciximab is not limited to the GPIIb/IIIa receptor, and it may interact with vitronectin receptors on the vessel wall. This may account for the reduction in the clinical restenosis rate that was observed with its use in conjunction with coronary angioplasty.[62] All patients in the EPISTENT trial received aspirin, heparin, and standard pharmacological therapy. The angiographic inclusion criteria were quite broad in this trial, and included all elective or urgent percutaneous revascularization cases if the target lesion exhibited stenosis of at least 60% amenable to balloon angioplasty or stenting and if the target lesion was not an unprotected left-mainstem stenosis. The primary endpoint of the trial was a composite of death from any cause, myocardial infarction or re-infarction, or need for urgent revascularization within the first 30 days of intervention. Secondary endpoints were death or myocardial infarction, and death and/or large myocardial infarction, defined as new pathological Q waves, or a creatinine kinase (or its MB isoenzyme fraction) of at least five times the upper laboratory limit in the participating hospital. The primary endpoint occurred in 87 (10.8%) of 809 patients in the stent plus placebo group, 42 (5.3%) of 794 in the stent plus abciximab group (p < 0.001 *vs* placebo), and 55 (6.9%) of 796 in the balloon plus abciximab group (p = 0.007 *vs* control) (figure 3.2). Major bleeding complications occurred in 2.2% of patients assigned to stent plus placebo, 1.5% assigned to stent plus abciximab, and 1.4% assigned to balloon angioplasty plus abciximab (p = 0.38). The results of this study clearly show that platelet IIb/IIIa blockade with abciximab improves the safety of coronary stenting procedures, and that balloon angioplasty with abciximab results in a better 30-day outcome than stenting without abciximab.

The prospective, randomized ISAR (Intracoronary Stenting and Antithrombotic Regimen) trial[63] was designed to test the premise, suggested by earlier observational trials, that inhibition of platelet function may be superior to

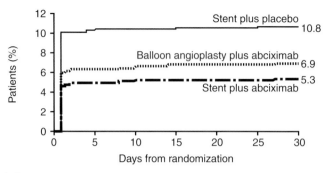

Figure 3.2: *Cumulative event rate (death, myocardial infarction, or urgent revascularization) for the three patient groups in the EPISTENT trial. (From The EPISTENT Investigators. Randomised placebo-controlled and balloon angioplasty controlled trial to assess safety of coronary stenting with use of platelet glycoprotein-IIb/IIIa blockade.* Lancet *1998; 352: 87–92.)*

anticoagulant therapy for the prevention of stent occlusion. In this trial, 517 patients were randomized after successful Palmaz–Schatz stent implantation to either antiplatelet therapy with aspirin and ticlopidine or to anticoagulant therapy with heparin, the vitamin K antagonist phenprocoumon, and aspirin. The population of patients crossed the spectrum of symptomatic coronary artery disease, including patients with stable angina and acute ischaemic syndromes, and those patients with complex coronary-artery lesions. Intravascular ultrasound assessment after stent placement was not required by the protocol, and was rarely done in this trial. High-pressure balloon inflation was done within the stented segment. The clinical endpoints of this study were the incidence of cardiac, vascular, and bleeding events at 30 days after stent placement. A primary cardiac endpoint was reached by 6.2% of patients in the anticoagulant therapy group, compared with 1.6% in the antiplatelet therapy group (p = 0.01). Haemorrhagic events resulting in organ dysfunction, or requiring blood transfusion or surgical correction, occurred in 6.5% of patients treated with anticoagulant therapy, but patients receiving combined antiplatelet therapy were free of haemorrhagic complications (p < 0.001). Peripheral vascular events were also less common in the antiplatelet therapy group than in the group that received anticoagulants (0.8% antiplatelet *vs* 6.2% anticoagulant, p = 0.001, figure 3.3). These data clearly show that the risk–benefit ratio for stenting is improved with the use of combined antiplatelet therapy.

The high incidence of acute and subacute stent thrombosis seen in the early clinical stent trials, and the publication of the results of the ISAR trial that confirmed that intense anticoagulation for the prevention of thrombosis may not

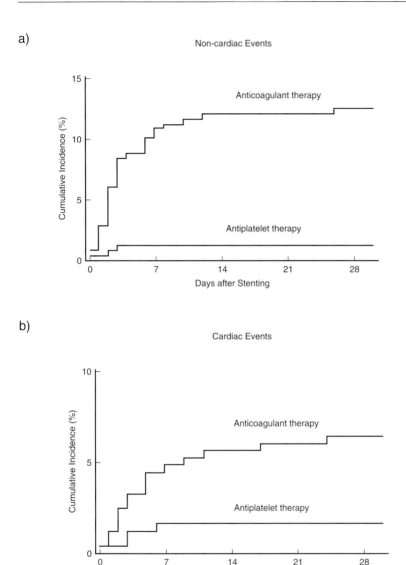

Figure 3.3: *Cumulative incidence of cardiac and non-cardiac events in the ISAR (Intracoronary Stenting and Antithrombotic Regimen) trial. A: Cardiac events (cardiac event = death due to cardiac causes or the occurrence of myocardial infarction, bypass surgery, or repeated balloon angioplasty, whichever occurred first). B: Non-cardiac events (non-cardiac event = death due to non-cardiac causes or the occurrence of a cerebrovascular accident, severe hemorrhagic or peripheral vascular complications, whichever occurred first). (From Schömig A, Neumann FJ, Kastrati A, et al. A randomized comparison of antiplatelet and anticoagulant therapy after the placement of coronary-artery stents. N Engl J Med 1996; **334:** 1084–89.)*

105

be necessary,[63] prompted the initiation of several randomized trials focused on the optimization of adjunctive pharmacotherapy. The STARS (Stent Anticoagulation Regimen Study) trial was a three-group multicentre randomized trial, with 550 patients per group. The trial compared the FDA-approved anticoagulation regimen of ASA 350 mg/day plus coumadin (INR 2.0–2.5) with two antiplatelet regimens (ASA 350 mg/day plus ticlopidine 250 mg twice daily for 4 weeks, ASA 350 mg/day alone) after optimum stent deployment (final angiographic stenosis <10%; no major dissections or abrupt in-lab closure) of one or two Palmaz–Schatz stents in native coronary lesions using high pressure (≥16 atmospheres) balloon deployment.[64,65] The primary endpoint was a composite surrogate for "stent thrombosis" comprised of death, Q-wave myocardial infarction, CABG, or repeat PTCA at 30 days. Both de-novo and restenotic lesions were included. Results showed a significant benefit of combination aspirin-ticlopidine therapy over aspirin alone and an aspirin-coumadin combination when both the primary endpoint and subacute closure with target vessel revascularization were considered (figure 3.4). No differences in mortality or the need for emergency bypass surgery were shown between the

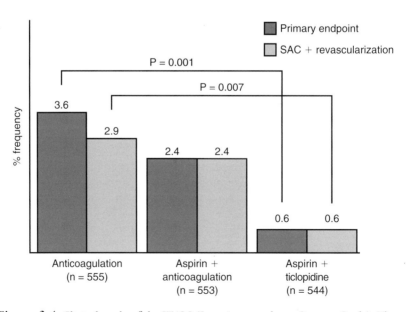

STARS Clinical Results

Figure 3.4: Clinical results of the STARS (Stent Anticoagulation Regimen Study). The primary endpoint was a composite surrogate for "stent thrombosis" comprised of death, Q-wave myocardial infarction, CABG, or repeat PTCA at 30 days. (SAC = subacute closure.)

groups; the benefit derived mainly from a reduction in the incidence of acute
Q-wave myocardial infarction (1.3% in the aspirin-only group, 0.4% in the
aspirin plus coumadin group, 0% in the aspirin plus ticlopidine group).
Haematologic dyscrasias with the use of ticlopidine were rare in this trial (0.4%)
and reversible with short-term therapy.

The MATTIS (Multi-centre Aspirin and Ticlopidine after Intracoronary
Stenting) trial[66] was designed to compare two different regimes (aspirin
250 mg/day plus ticlopidine 500 mg/day, and aspirin 250 mg/day plus
antivitamin K [INR 2.5–3]) in the treatment of high risk stent patients. A total
of 350 patients from 31 centres were randomized. Patients were considered
eligible (high risk) if any of the following were present:

- stent(s) implanted to treat abrupt closure after PTCA;
- suboptimum result on angiography after stenting;
- three or more stents used or the length of the stented segment 45 mm or
  more;
- nominal diameter of the largest balloon inflated in the stent 2.5 mm or less.

The primary composite endpoint in this trial was the occurrence of death, acute
myocardial infarction, CABG, or repeat intervention at 30 days. The secondary
endpoint was the occurrence of major vascular or bleeding complications.
Although not significant, there appeared to be a trend towards fewer clinical
events at 30 days with aspirin plus ticlopidine treatment compared with aspirin
plus antivitamin K (2.5% *vs* 11% respectively, p = 0.07). There was a significant
reduction in bleeding complications, however, in the aspirin plus ticlopidine
group compared with those treated with aspirin plus antivitamin K (1.7% *vs*
6.9% respectively, p = 0.02), indicating an advantage of combined antiplatelet
therapy for the treatment of high-risk stented patients.

The question of whether ticlopidine therapy added any additional benefit when
added to aspirin alone as antiplatelet therapy after optimum stent deployment
was addressed in a single-centre randomized trial reported by Hall and
colleagues.[67] In this study, 226 patients were randomly assigned to either aspirin
therapy alone or a combination of aspirin and ticlopidine therapy after successful
ultrasound-guided stent implantation. Six different tubular and coil stent types
were used: the Palmaz–Schatz stent, the Gianturco–Roubin stent, the Wiktor
stent, the Micro Stent, the Wallstent and the CrossFlex stent. Primary
angiographic and clinical endpoints were stent thrombosis, death, myocardial
infarction, the need for coronary artery bypass surgery or repeat angioplasty, and
significant side-effects of medical therapy requiring termination of the medication
within the first month after a successful procedure. At 1 month, the rate of stent
thrombosis was 2.9% in the aspirin-only group and 0.8% in the aspirin plus
ticlopidine group (p = 0.2). Cumulative major clinical events occurred in 3.9%
of the patients in the aspirin-treated group and in 0.8% of the aspirin plus

ticlopidine group (p = 0.1). There were no side-effects of medication reported in the aspirin-only group, while medication side-effects occurred in three patients in the aspirin plus ticlopidine group. The relatively small size of this study and the low incidence of events may have resulted in a failure to detect any differences in endpoints between the two groups.

Whether a postinterventional medical regimen of combined therapy with aspirin plus ticlopidine has advantages over ticlopidine monotherapy was assessed in a single-centre German trial.[68] A total of 243 patients were randomized after coronary stenting to either ticlopidine 2 × 200 mg/day or ticlopidine 2 × 200 mg/day plus aspirin 100 mg/day. The primary endpoint was defined as absence of the following events during hospitalization: death, subacute stent thrombosis, myocardial infarction, CABG, repeat PTCA, groin complications, or major bleeding. There were only 10 events in the entire cohort, five in each group. The conclusion that combined therapy with ticlopidine and aspirin has no advantages over monotherapy with ticlopidine must be made with caution, considering the low event-rate and small number of patients in this study.

The synergistic effects of aspirin and ticlopidine on platelet activation and aggregation was shown by a randomized trial in Germany.[69] In this study, 61 patients were randomized after implantation of a single Palmaz–Schatz stent to one of three groups: aspirin 300 mg/day plus ticlopidine 2 × 250 mg/day; ticlopidine 2 × 250 mg/day; or aspirin 300 mg/day. Platelet activation was measured at various times up to 14 days by flow cytometry, measurement of expression of CD62p (p-selectin), and the binding of fibrinogen to the platelet surface glycoprotein IIb/IIIa receptor. Platelet aggregation was induced by the addition of ADP or collagen. The results of this trial clearly showed the superiority of an aspirin plus ticlopidine combination over monotherapy with either drug on platelet aggregation and platelet activation markers.

Ongoing trials
The ENTICES (ENoxaprin, TIclopidine and aspirin versus the conventional Coumadin regimen after Elective Stenting) trial[70] has been designed to determine the effect of a reduced anticoagulation regimen on clinical outcomes after stent deployment. A total of 120 patients will be randomized 2:1 to enoxaprin 30–50 mg subcutaneously twice daily for 10 days plus aspirin plus ticlopidine versus aspirin, dipyridamole, dextran, and heparin plus coumadin. Surrogate haematological markers of platelet activation and thrombin activity are being measured 3 days after stent implantation, and will be correlated with clinical outcome at the completion of the trial. Interim analysis of the results of the first 40 patients show that thrombin and fibrin activity are suppressed to a greater extent in those treated with enoxaprin, ticlopidine, and aspirin.[70]

The CADILLAC Trial (Controlled Abciximab and Device Investigation to Lower Late Angioplasty Complications) was designed to investigate the potential and benefits of stenting and IIb/IIIa receptor inhibition in the setting of an acute MI. A total of 2000 consecutive patients with acute MI will be prospectively randomized at 90 international centres to one of four treatment strategies: (1) primary PTCA only, (2) PTCA plus the glycoprotein IIb/IIIa inhibitor abciximab, (3) primary stenting only or, (4) primary stenting plus abciximab. The primary endpoint in CADILLAC is the cumulative composite incidence of death, reinfarction, ischemia driven target vessel revascularization (urgent or elective), and stroke at 6 months.

Recognition of the inherent risk of neutropenia with ticlopidine therapy prompted the SALTS (Strategic ALternatives with Ticlopidine in Stenting) trial,[71] designed to compare the safety and efficacy of 10 days of ticlopidine therapy with 30 days of therapy. Electively stented patients were randomized to 10 or to 30 days of ticlopidine 250 mg twice daily plus ASA. Preliminary results show that 10 days of ticlopidine after stenting is a safe and effective treatment.[72]

Machraoui and colleagues[73] aim to assess the efficacy or safety of a postintervention medical regimen of coumadin plus aspirin compared with aspirin alone in their single-centre study. In this trial, 140 patients will be randomized after stent implantation to either coumadin plus aspirin or aspirin alone. The primary endpoint is the absence of cardiac events, major bleeding, and groin complications. Secondary endpoints include the rate of restenosis, cardiac events, and side-effects of the study medications during 3 months follow-up. Results of this trial will soon be available.

The primary objective of the CLASSICS (CLopidigrel ASpirin Stent International Co-operative Study) study is to test the relative safety of clopidogrel combined with aspirin *versus* ticlopidine combined with aspirin in patients treated for 28 days after coronary stenting. Clopidogrel is a thieno-pyridine inhibitor of platelet aggregation which is structurally related to ticlopidine. Unlike ticlopidine, clopidogrel therapy does not lead to neutropenia or thrombocytopenia. A total of 1005 patients are to be randomized into three parallel groups, 250 mg per day of ticlopidine plus aspirin, 75 mg per day of clopidogrel plus aspirin and 75 mg per day of clopidogrel with a loading dose of 300 mg of clopidogrel on the first day plus aspirin. Treatment will continue for 28 days, and the patients will be followed for 45 days. The secondary objective of this trial is an assessment of the incidence of death and major cardiac events to obtain data on the efficacy of clopidogrel in preventing subacute thrombosis.

The beneficial effect of trapidil, an inhibitor of PDGF-activated protein kinase, was evaluated in the 21 centre double blind, placebo controlled TRAPIST (TRAPidil In STent) trial. The primary endpoint of this trial was the in-stent neointimal volume measured by IVUS at 6 months follow-up. Secondary endpoints were: mean and minimal lumen diameter, diameter stenosis, mean and minimum lumen diameter, and late loss as determined by angiography, the incidence of adverse clinical events, bleeding complications and anginal status at 6 months follow-up. A total of 353 patients were randomized to receive trapidil

(200 mg three times a day) or placebo starting the day of the stent implantation procedure. Final results showed no difference in neointimal volume as measured by IVUS between the two treatment groups (228 mm^3 trapidil *vs* 226 mm^3 placebo). No difference was seen in any of the angiographic parameters or in the incidence of major adverse cardiac events (death, myocardial infarction, need for bypass surgery or target lesion revascularization). A significant difference was seen, however, in the incidence of unstable angina (6.1% *vs* 0.6%, p = 0.009) and silent ischemia (6.1% *vs* 1.2%, p = 0.03) between the two groups, with the placebo treated group showing a better outcome.

Restenosis

Completed trials
The efficacy of cilostazol, a 3'5'-cyclic nucleotide phosphodiesterase III inhibitor for the prevention of restenosis, was shown by a randomized Japanese trial.[74] Cilostazol is a potent platelet inhibitor, a vasodilator, and an inhibitor of smooth muscle proliferation. In this trial, 70 patients with a total of 82 lesions were randomized to either aspirin 81 mg/day (40 patients) or cilostazol 200 mg/day (30 patients) given 3 days before and an unspecified time after Palmaz–Schatz stenting. Follow-up angiography was done after a mean of 5 months. The MLD of the aspirin group was 1.89 ± 1.08 mm compared with 2.34 ± 0.74 mm in the cilostazol-treated group (p < 0.05). Restenosis (≥50% diameter stenosis) occurred in 11 patients (26.85) in the aspirin group, compared with three patients (8.6%) in the cilostazol group (p = 0.05).

The preventative effect of combined treatment with probucol, an antioxidant, and cilostazol against post-stenting restenosis was assessed in a single centre trial performed in Japan.[75] A total of 136 patients were randomized to four groups 1 week before stent implantation, control, probucol (500 mg/day), cilostazol (200 mg/day), and probucol (500 mg/day) plus cilostazol (200 mg/day). All patients received aspirin (81 mg/day). The study was conducted in a prospective, randomized manner, but was not blinded. Treatment began 5 days before stent implantation and continued until the 6 months follow-up evaluation. A total of 126 patients with 165 coronary artery lesions were randomized. The restenosis rate at 6 months follow-up was 31.7% for controls, 16.7% for the probucol group, 12.5% for the cilostazol group (p<0.05 *vs* control), and 9.5% for the combined treatment group (p<0.05 *vs* control). Further studies are necessary to confirm the efficacy of probucol and cilostazol for the prevention of restenosis.

A single-centre trial in The Netherlands examined the potential for locally delivered antisense oligonucleotides to prevent restenosis. The ITALICS (Investigation by the Thoraxcenter on Antisense DNA given by Local delivery and assessed by IVUS after Coronary Stenting) trial examined the effects on restenosis of a synthetic 15-mer antisense phosphorothioate oligodeoxynucleotide (LR-3280,

Lynx Therapeutics) directed against the translation-initiation region of the *c-myc* nuclear proto-oncogene.[76] Antisense to *c-myc* has been shown to inhibit smooth muscle cell migration, proliferation, and matrix protein synthesis in vitro, and to inhibit the restenosis process effectively in several animal models of vascular injury.[77] In this trial, 84 patients were randomized after successful placement of a Wallstent, to receive either placebo or the antisense compound using a local drug delivery catheter (Transport™, SciMed Life Systems) inside the stented segment. The primary endpoint for this trial was the in-stent neointimal volume at 6-months follow-up as assessed by intravascular ultrasound. Secondary endpoints included angiographic assessment of the target lesion at 6-months follow-up, and the occurrence of adverse cardiac events. Results of this trial showed that 10 mg LR-3280, given by the Transport catheter immediately after Wallstent implantation, did not reduce the clinical event rate or decrease the neointimal proliferative response as determined by IVUS and QCA (table 3.4).

The HIPS (Heparin Infusion Prior to Stenting) trial was a multicentre trial designed to test the hypothesis that local delivery of heparin prior to stent placement reduces subsequent restenosis.[79] A total of 179 patients were randomized to either a bolus of intracoronary heparin or heparin delivered intramurally with a local-delivery catheter. In this trial, 5000 units of heparin was given at the stented site using a LocalMed InfusaSleeve™ (LocalMed, Paolo Alto CA, USA) local-delivery device. No significant differences were seen in the primary endpoint of IVUS measured neointimal volume at 6 months. The secondary endpoints of angiographically determined restenosis at 6 months, and the need for lesion revascularization were also similar between the two treatment modalities.

Ongoing trials

The ERASER (Evaluation of ReoPro and Stenting to Eliminate Restenosis) study is a multicentre trial designed to ascertain whether the combined use of stents and abciximab (a glycoprotein IIb/IIIa blocker) yields additive or synergistic benefit against neointimal proliferation.[78] In this trial, 225 patients with optimum stent implantation in vessels of 2.5 mm diameter or more, as determined by IVUS criteria, will be randomized in a double-blind fashion to:

- bolus plus 12 hours abciximab 0.25 mg/kg (0.125 mg/kg/min);
- bolus plus 24 hours abciximab 0.25 mg/kg (0.125 mg/kg/min);
- placebo.

The primary objective of this trial is to determine if there is an absolute or dose-related difference in neointimal volume, as determined by IVUS, at 6 months after stent implantation, between patients treated systemically with abciximab or placebo. The secondary endpoints of this trial include an assessment of the occurrence of major adverse cardiac events and angiographic outcome at 6 months. Enrollment in this study is complete and results will soon be available.

Table 3.4 Angiographic results of the ITALICS trial

Treatment	Minimum luminal diameter (mm)			Treated length (mm)	Loss index	Volume obs (%)	Restenosis rate (%)
	pre-	post-	6 months				
Placebo	0.84 ± 0.4	2.70 ± 0.4	1.50 ± 0.6	27 ± 14	0.66 ± 0.3	44 ± 16	38
LR-3280	0.90 ± 0.5	2.80 ± 0.4	1.50 ± 0.5	28 ± 13	0.71 ± 0.3	46 ± 14	34
P	0.6	0.3	0.98	0.8	0.5	0.6	0.8

Loss index = Late loss in minimum luminal diameter divided by the procedural gain in minimum luminal diameter (MLD at f/u minus MLD post)/(MLD post minus MLD pre); obs = obstructon.

The effect on restenosis of locally administered heparin delivered using the Dispatch™ (SciMED Life Systems, Maple Grove MN, USA) is being assessed in a trial with a similar design. The DISTRESS (DISpatch STent REStenosis Study) is a single-centre randomized pilot study at the Washington Cardiology Centre. In total, 100 patients will be randomized to one of two groups. Patients in one group of this trial will receive 6000 units of locally delivered heparin, and patients randomized to the other group will undergo conventional stent implantation. The primary endpoint of this trial is the difference in neointimal volume between the two groups at 6 months as assessed by intravascular ultrasound. Secondary endpoints include acute and late clinical events, and the angiographically determined rate of restenosis.

Locally delivered enoxaprin is being compared with systemic heparin in patients treated with NIR stent implantation in a Polish trial.[80–82] A total of 100 patients have been randomized to either systemic heparin plus 10 mg enoxaprin given via a Transport™ (SciMED Life Systems, Minneapolis MN, USA) local drug-delivery catheter before stent implantation, or to systemic heparin only. Acute results show no major adverse events in either group. Six-months follow-up results will be available soon.

Another single-centre trial examining local drug delivery after coronary stenting for the prevention of restenosis is underway in Milan, Italy. In this trial, 200 patients will be randomized to stent only or to the local delivery of long-acting steroid into the vessel wall using the Infiltrator™ (Interventional Technologies, San Diego CA, USA) local drug-delivery balloon prior to stent implantation. Primary endpoints for this trial are angiographic restenosis and target lesion revascularization at 6 months follow-up. Secondary endpoints include acute procedural complications, subacute stent thrombosis, major adverse cardiac events, and the degree of intimal hyperplasia at follow-up as determined by IVUS.

Bleeding and vascular complications

Ongoing trials
The FANTASTIC (Full ANticoagulation versus Ticlopidine plus Aspirin after STent Implantation) trial is a multicentre European trial designed to determine whether two-pronged antiplatelet therapy can significantly reduce bleeding complications seen with anticoagulation therapy.[83] All patients undergoing Wiktor stent implantation were eligible for enrollment in this trial. After successful stent implantation, patients were randomized to receive either aspirin plus ticlopidine or aspirin plus coumadin (target INR 2.5–3.0). A secondary endpoint of this trial was to establish if the antiplatelet regimen would compromise the patency of the stented segment. A total of 485 patients have been randomized, and enrollment has ended. Six-months angiographic follow-up

results on the angiography subset show a significantly better outcome for those patients treated with antiplatelet agents (restenosis rate of 15%) than for the group treated with full anticoagulation (restenosis rate 39%, p < 0.05).[84]

Adjunctive rotational atherectomy

Ongoing trials
The RotaStent trial is a randomized trial to assess the safety and efficacy of stent placement with adjunctive atherectomy in patients with calcified lesions or diffuse lesions in native coronary arteries. In this trial, 400 patients will be randomized in 15 centres in the USA and Europe to either stent alone or stent plus pretreatment with rotational atherectomy. Primary and secondary endpoints include the incidence of major adverse cardiac events at 30 days, angiographic restenosis, and the need for target vessel revascularization at 6 months' follow-up. Enrollment of patients in this trial is currently underway.

The Edres trial is a small single-centre trial that has randomized 150 patients to either stand-alone stenting (Micro Stent II) or rotational atherectomy followed by stenting.[85] Inclusion criteria for patients in this trial were broad, and all elective cases with lesions amenable to stent implantation were considered. Enrollment has been completed and results will soon be available.

Adjunctive Doppler flow measurement

Ongoing trials
The aim of the multi-centre FROST (French Randomized Optimal STenting) trial is to compare the outcome of systematic stenting with coronary velocity reserve (CVR) guided stenting.[86,87] A total of 250 patients with short (<15 mm) stenoses of large (≥3 mm) vessels suitable for PTCA will be randomly assigned to systematic stenting using Palmaz–Schatz stents or to CVR-guided PTCA using a Doppler guidewire. In the latter group, after PTCA, CVR is measured and QCA is done. Stents are implanted only in patients with a CVR of less than 2.2 and/or residual stenosis of more than 35%. Endpoints of this trial include in-hospital and 6-months clinical outcome (death, myocardial infarction, re-PTCA, bypass surgery, functional status) and 6-months quantitative angiographic follow-up.

Adjunctive radiotherapy

Completed trials
The SCRIPPS trial (Scripps Coronary Radiation to Prevent Restenosis), undertaken by the group at the Scripps Foundation in California, has recently been completed.[88,89] A total of 55 patients were enrolled in this study and

randomized to conventional therapy or to treatment with intracoronary gamma irradiation using [192]Iridium radiation (^{192}Ir). The criteria for enrollment included a target segment in a restenotic lesion that either already contained a stent or was a candidate for Palmaz–Schatz stent placement, and previous treatment of the lesion more than 4 weeks before enrollment. The reference vessel had to be between 3 mm and 5 mm in diameter, with a target lesion that was 30 mm or less in length. A non-centred ^{192}Ir source delivered 800 cGy (centiGray) to the target (media) furthest from the source provided that 3000 cGy or less was delivered to the near field. At 6-months follow-up angiography the mean MLD was larger in the ^{192}Ir group than in the placebo group (2.43 ± 0.78 mm *vs* 1.85 ± 0.89 mm; p = 0.02). Late loss index was significantly lower in the ^{192}Ir-treated lesions (0.12 ± 0.63 mm *vs* 0.60 ± 0.43 mm; p < 0.01), indicating a significant reduction in the hyperplastic response. The angiographically determined restenosis rate (≥50% diameter stenosis) was significantly lower in the radiation treated than in the placebo treated group (17% *vs* 54%; p = 0.01). Clinical follow-up data at 12 months showed that fewer patients in the ^{192}Ir group reached the composite clinical endpoint (death, myocardial infarction, stent thrombosis, target lesion revascularization) than in the placebo group (15% *vs* 48%, p = 0.01). These data indicate that brachytherapy using gamma radiation is a promising new treatment for patients with restenosis. Subgroup analysis of the SCRIPPS trial suggests that intracoronary gamma radiation is more effective in smaller diameter vessels, native vessels, and diabetics.[90] Although of some interest, this analysis must be interpreted with caution due to the small sample size.

Ongoing trials
Currently underway is the SCRIPPS II trial. The original SCRIPPS trial included patients with lesions up to 30 mm in length, while SCRIPPS II will examine the effect of four different doses of gamma irradiation from an ^{192}Ir source in diffusely diseased vessels with diseased segments up to 65 mm in length.[91]

The IRIS (IsoStent for Restenosis Intervention Study) trial is designed to examine the safety and efficacy of low dose β-irradiation emitted from the surface of the radioactive IsoStent for the prevention of clinical and angiographic restenosis. In total, 1200 patients will be randomized to non-radioactive (control) stent implantation and to one of three activity ranges of [32]P. Endpoints in this trial are clinical events including target lesion revascularization and angiographic results determined at 6 months' follow-up.

The WRIST trial (Washington Radiation for In-Stent restenosis Trial) was designed to test the benefit of gamma radiation using ^{192}Ir as an adjunct therapy in the treatment of in-stent restenosis, for the reduction of 6-months clinical events and angiographic restenosis.[92,93] A total of 130 patients with in-stent restenosis have been randomized (100 native vessel; 30 saphenous vein graft lesions).

Patients underwent PTCA, atheroablative therapy (laser or rotational atherectomy) and/or additional stents until a residual in-stent stenosis of 20% or less was obtained. Patients were randomly assigned to either a ribbon with ^{192}Ir seeds or a placebo ribbon with non-radioactive seeds. The prescribed dose was 15 Gy to a 2 mm radial distance from the centre of the source in arteries between 3.0–5.0 mm in diameter. Results of the WRIST trial will soon be available.

Stenting compared with surgery

Ongoing trials

The SIMA (Stenting *vs* Internal Mammary Artery) trial is a multicentre prospective trial comparing clinical results of stent implantation and coronary bypass surgery (CABG) (left internal mammary artery grafting) for proximal left anterior descending (LAD) coronary artery stenosis in patients with left ventricular function >0.45.[94] Between 1994 and 1998, 123 patients with de novo, isolated, proximal LAD lesions were randomized. There were five cross-overs from surgery to stent implantation at the request of the patients after randomization. Palmaz–Schatz, Micro Stent II, NIR, MULTILINK, beStent and JoStent stents were implanted in this trial. In hospital minor complications (bleeding and arrythmias) were significantly more frequent after CABG than after stent implantation (28% *vs* 3%, p<0.0001). The incidence of in-hospital major adverse events (death, myocardial infarction, cerebrovascular accident or re-PTCA) was not different between the two groups.

A randomized trial comparing coronary bypass surgery with coronary stent implantation employing the Cordis/Johnson and Johnson Crown Stent for multiple vessel coronary disease is underway. This multicentre trial, given the acronym ARTS (Arterial Revascularization Therapies Study), will randomize a total of 1200 patients to either CABG or stent implantation. The primary objective of ARTS is an assessment of the effectiveness of each treatment as measured by freedom from major adverse cardiac and cerebrovascular events over a period of 1 year. Secondary objectives are to compare both strategies with respect to adverse events at 30 days, 3 years and 5 years, and cost-effectiveness and quality of life over 1, 3, and 5 years follow-up.

The SOS (Stent Or Surgery) trial is a large multicentre international trial which is currently underway. The trial plans to randomize 1800 patients with multivessel stenoses to either stent implantation or CABG to determine whether the benefits of stenting will translate to the management of multivessel coronary artery disease. Primary endpoints of this trial are myocardial-infarction-free survival at 1–4 years after stent implantation. Secondary endpoints include death, need for repeat revascularization, anginal symptoms, medication requirements, quality-of-life analysis, cognitive function, psychological assessment, and cost analysis. Randomization is underway in Europe and in the USA.

Comparison of stents

Completed trials
The direct comparison of clinical and angiographic outcomes of two stent designs in a randomized fashion eliminates the confounding influences of differences in patient selection criteria, indications for use, and lesion characteristics. The results of a small, single-centre, randomized trial comparing the Wiktor and the Palmaz–Schatz stents in patients with de-novo stenoses of the right coronary artery have been reported by Goy and colleagues.[95] In this study, a subgroup of 133 patients of the BENESTENT cohort (PTCA, 73 patients; Palmaz–Schatz stent, 60 patients) was compared with a group of 84 patients randomized to PTCA or stent with the Wiktor stent (PTCA, 42 patients; stent, 42 patients). Both clinical and angiographic endpoints at 6 months were considered. No differences were seen between any group in the incidence of death, myocardial infarction, or need for CABG. The group treated with a Palmaz–Schatz stent showed a significant reduction in need for repeat PTCA compared with the PTCA-alone or Wiktor-stent-treated groups. Angiographic results showed no significant differences between any of the groups with respect to acute gain or late loss at 6 months follow-up, although the restenosis rate of the Palmaz–Schatz-treated patients was significantly lower than the other groups (23% in the Palmaz–Schatz group *vs* 47% in the Wiktor-stent-treated group; $p < 0.05$). Based on these findings the investigators have questioned the ability of the Wiktor stent to prevent restenosis when implanted in the right coronary artery.[95]

Another small trial from the same centre compared the Palmaz–Schatz stent with the Wiktor stent in the setting of abrupt vessel closure following PTCA.[96] In this study, 65 patients were randomly assigned to either Wiktor or Palmaz–Schatz stent implantation. Stenting was technically feasible in all but one patient, and was immediately successful in reversing ischaemia and vessel closure in 60 patients. Endpoints for this trial were evaluated at hospital discharge and at 6 months follow-up, and included the clinical endpoints of death, myocardial infarction, and the need for CABG, and the angiographic endpoints of acute and subacute thrombosis. Clinical complication rates were similar at hospital discharge (any clinical endpoint 18% [Wiktor] *vs* 22% [Palmaz–Schatz], $p = 0.53$) and at 6-months follow-up. The endpoints of acute and subacute thrombosis were likewise similar between the two groups, as was the angiographically determined restenosis rate (38% Wiktor *vs* 27% Palmaz–Schatz, $p = 0.42$), in contrast to the results of the elective stent placement trial. Baseline, postprocedural, and follow-up quantitative angiographic measurements were similar for the two groups, except for the postprocedural percent residual stenosis which was slightly greater in the patients receiving the Wiktor stent (28% Wiktor *vs* 21% Palmaz–Schatz). These results showed that there is no difference between the use of Wiktor and Palmaz–Schatz stents for bailout management. The major limitation of this trial was its small size, and therefore the results should be interpreted with caution.

The Magic Wallstent was compared with the NIR stent in patients with native coronary lesions (greater than 3 mm diameter) longer than 20 mm on quantitive coronary angiography in the single centre randomized RENEWAL trial.[97] High pressure stent deployment techniques were used and adequate stent deployment was confirmed with intravascular ultrasound. A total of 82 patients with de novo coronary lesions were randomized to either Wallstent or NIR stent implantation. Three patients in the NIR stent group required crossover to Wallstent implantation. Mean stent length was 35.4 ± 2.5 mm in the NIR stent group and 41.6 ± 2.9 mm in the Wallstent group. At 6 months follow-up, the target vessel revascularization rate was similar for both groups (7.9% NIR stent *vs* 7.3% Wallstent). Restenosis rates for the two groups were also not significantly different, although there was a trend for a better outcome with the NIR stent (24% NIR *vs* 44% Wallstent, p=0.1). A larger trial is necessary in order to determine whether stent design influences the rate of restenosis in long lesions.

To resolve the issue of whether stent configuration can affect long-term outcome, large randomized trials have been designed to compare various stents "head to head". There are currently at least 10 of these equivalency trials completed or in progress. The equivalency design of these trials in simple "BENESTENT-like" lesions is predicated on showing similarity in safety and efficacy between the test stent and the Palmaz–Schatz stent, which serves as the standard to which all others are compared. These trials were not designed to test for subtle, and perhaps clinically unimportant, differences between stent designs, since an unreasonably large sample size would be required. Three trials have been completed. In all of these, stents were implanted in non-complex lesions with a length of less than 25 mm in native coronary vessels. Routine high-pressure post-dilatation and ASA/Ticlid regimens were used. In addition to clinical endpoints, angiography was obtained in a subset of the patients.

The ASCENT trial included 1040 patients from 16 US and four Canadian centres randomized to either Palmaz–Schatz or MULTILINK stent implantation.[98–100] Statistical equivalence in both the late clinical (figure 3.5) and angiographic (table 3.5) outcomes were shown for the MULTILINK and the Palmaz–Schatz stents. There was a trend towards a lower restenosis rate in the group treated with the MULTILINK stent, but similarity in the loss index (indicative of the late proliferative response) shows that the small restenosis benefit is a result of the larger acute lumen diameter. Likewise, equivalence

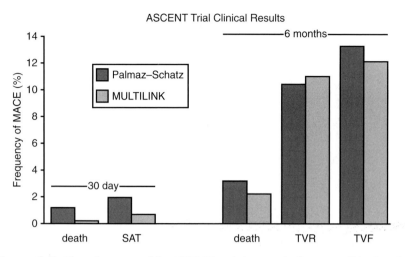

Figure 3.5: *Clinical outcome of the ASCENT trial showing the frequency of death and subacute thrombosis (SAT) at 30 days and the frequency of death, target vessel revascularization (TVR), and target vessel failure (TVF) (death, target vessel revascularization, myocardial infarction) at 9 months. No differences can be seen in the clinical outcome with implantation of either the Palmaz–Schatz stent or the MULTILINK stent. MACE = Major Adverse Coronary Events.*

between the Palmaz–Schatz stent and the Micro Stent II was shown in the SMART trial (Study of Microstent's Ability to limit Restenosis Trial), in which 613 patients with focal de-novo or restenotic native coronary lesions were randomized (figure 3.6, table 3.5).[101,102] Equivalence between Gianturco-Roubin II (GR II) and the Palmaz–Schatz stents was not shown in the GRII trial.[103,104] Differences at 6-months follow-up were seen in the 6-months clinical outcomes of target vessel revascularization and target vessel failure – a composite of death, myocardial infarction, and target vessel revascularization (figure 3.7). Significant differences were also seen in the 6-month follow-up angiographic parameters of MLD, percent diameter stenosis, and binary restenosis rate (table 3.5). The reasons for these differences are not clear, but may be due in part to a higher acute residual stenosis after stent implantation, or a higher loss index in the GR II-treated vessels (0.76 *vs* 0.57; p = 0.007), or as a result of GR II stent undersizing or longer stent length in the GR II group.[105]

Ongoing trials
Other equivalency trials which are currently underway are the NIRVANA trial (NIR vs Palmaz–Schatz),[106,107] the SCORES (Stent COmparative REStenosis) trial

Table 3.5 Angiographic follow-up of STENT VERSUS STENT trials

	ASCENT		SMART		GR II	
	Palmaz–Schatz	*MULTILINK*	*Palmaz–Schatz*	*Micro Stent II*	*Palmaz–Schatz*	*GR II*
Acute results						
Number of patients	520	520	331	330	364	364
ACC B2/C (%)	60§	63§	63§	62§	48#	45#
LAD (%)	43	43	42	47	40	43
Reference diameter (mm)	2.97	2.95	2.93	2.93	3.08	3.07
Post-stent stenosis (%)	10	8	8	5**	10	16**
Follow-up results						
MLD (mm)	1.91	1.97	2.00	1.86	1.92	1.51*
Diameter stenosis (%)	35	32	34	37	35	50*
Binary restenosis rate	21	17	23	25	19	45

ACC B2/C=Lesion morphology; ACC/AHA Task Force Report, *J Am Coll Cardiol* 1993; 22: 2033–54; LAD = Left anterior descending artery; MLD = Minimum luminal diameter; Binary restenosis rate = Diameter stenosis > 50% at follow-up; § Graded by angiographic core lab; # Graded on site; * p > 0.001 versus Palmaz–Schatz; ** p < 0.05 versus Palmaz–Schatz.

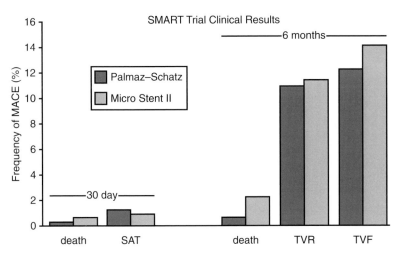

Figure 3.6: *Clinical outcome of the SMART trial showing the frequency of death and subacute thrombosis (SAT) at 30 days, and the frequency of death, target vessel revascularization (TVR), and target vessel failure (TVF) (death, target vessel revascularization, myocardial infarction) at 9 months. No differences can be seen in the clinical outcome with implantation of either the Palmaz–Schatz stent or the Micro Stent II. MACE = Major Adverse Coronary Events.*

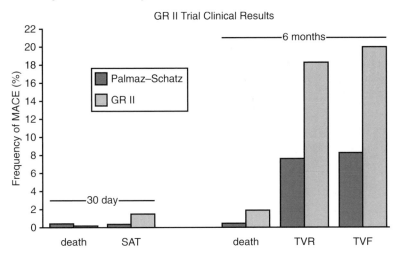

Figure 3.7: *Clinical outcome of the GR II trial showing the frequency of death and subacute thrombosis (SAT) at 30 days and the frequency of death, target vessel revascularization (TVR), and target vessel failure (TVF) (death, target vessel revascularization, myocardial infarction) at 9 months. Significant differences can be seen in the frequency of both target vessel failure (p <0.01) and target vessel revascularization (p <0.001) between the Palmaz–Schatz stent and the GR II stent. MACE = Major Adverse Coronary Events.*

(Radius vs Palmaz–Schatz),[108,109] Wiktor vs GR II, the Wallstent vs Palmaz–Schatz and the EXTRA (Evaluation of the XT stent for Restenosis in native Arteries) trials.

The EXTRA equivalency trial compared clinical and angiographic outcome in patients randomized to the Palmaz–Schatz coronary stent or the operator-mounted Bard XT stent.[110] A total of 650 patients with coronary ischemia and lesions (greater than 70% diameter stenosis and less than 25 mm in length) in native coronary arteries were randomized to the Palmaz–Schatz or XT stents. All XT stents were mounted and crimped by the operator, and all Palmaz–Schatz stents were premounted on a sheathed delivery system. The primary endpoint was target vessel failure at 9 months. Procedural success was similar for the implantation of both stents (96.7% XT vs 95.0% Palmaz–Schatz), and there were no episodes of stent embolization in either group. At 6 months follow-up, there was no difference in the need for target vessel revascularization (8.5% XT vs 8.7% Palmaz–Schatz). No differences were seen between the two stents with respect to the clinical endpoints of death, myocardial infarction, bypass surgery, or stent thrombosis. The restenosis rate at 6 months follow-up was not different between the two groups (36% XT vs 26% Palmaz–Schatz). Nine months follow-up results will soon be available.

A large German trial, in which the primary objective was to assess whether differences in stent design translated into differences in clinical outcome, has recently been completed.[111] In this trial, 1147 patients were randomly assigned to receive one of five types of stainless steel stents: Inflow (n = 231), MULTI-LINK (n = 227), NIR (n = 229), Palmaz–Schatz (n = 233), and PURA-A (n = 233). The primary endpoint of this trial was event-free survival at 1 year. Secondary endpoints of the study were the incidence of stent thrombosis at 30 days, and quantitative indices of restenosis (diameter stenosis, late lumen index, restenosis rate) at 6-months follow-up angiography. Results at 30-days follow-up showed no difference in overall success rate without major adverse cardiac events between any of the devices. Six-months and 1-year follow-up results are pending.

Assessment of the role of intravascular ultrasound (IVUS)

Completed trials
The aim of the single centre randomized SIPS (Strategy of Intracoronary ultrasound guided PTCA and Stenting) trial was to determine if the everyday use of intracoronary ultrasound (ICUS) improves the acute and chronic outcome after stent placement at an acceptable cost.[112,113] In this single center study conducted between 2/1996 and 5/1996, 296 patients were randomized to ICUS – guided or standard angiographically guided interventions. A special

combination catheter model (ICUS + PTCA-balloon in one single device, Oracle Focus™, Endosonics®) was used for the ICUS guided interventions and standard PTCA equipment was used for the angiography guided procedures. The goal of therapy in the ICUS group was a >65% minimal lumen area in comparison to the lumen area in the artery's unaffected reference segment. If this goal could not be achieved by PTCA alone a stent was deployed. Stents were deployed in 48% of the ICUS-guided group and in 49% of the angiography guided group. The primary angiographic endpoints of this trial were the acute MLD and the MLD at follow-up; the clinical endpoints were the occurrence of major cardiac events (death, myocardial infarction, and repeat revascularization) at 6 months follow-up. Stent use was not regulated and occurred in 52% of each group. Results show that procedural ICUS guidance leads to an improved net gain in MLD (1.25 ± 0.95 mm for ICUS guidance vs 0.78 ± 0.89 mm for angiographic guidance), and a trend towards lower target lesion revascularization procedures and restenosis rates[114–116] at 6 months follow-up.

A French group has reported similar results of a trial of IVUS-guided stent implantation.[117,118] In this study, 155 patients were randomized into one of two groups, with and without IVUS guidance. Optimum stent deployment was defined as cross-sectional area within the stent of more than 80% of the average cross-sectional area of the proximal and distal reference segments. In the group randomized to IVUS (n = 71), overdilatations were done when IVUS criteria were not reached. In the group randomized to no IVUS guidance (n = 73), blinded IVUS was done. Of the patients, 39% (37/79) in the IVUS guidance group had IVUS-guided overdilatation. At 6 months follow-up there was no difference in restenosis rate (≥50% diameter stenosis) between the IVUS-guided group and the group without IVUS guidance (22.5% vs 28.8% respectively, p = 0.39).

A single-centre German study has assessed the potential benefit of IVUS-guided coronary stent deployment with IVUS analysis after every interventional step, compared with angiographic coronary stent deployment with final IVUS assessment only.[119] Acute procedural success and 6-months angiographic follow-up were compared in both groups. A total of 84 patients were prospectively randomized to IVUS guidance (n = 42) or angiography plus final IVUS only (n = 43). Criteria for optimum stent deployment (complete stent opposition, complete coverage of dissection, >90% in-stent lumen area compared with reference) were achieved in 54% of the IVUS-guidance group and 57% of the final IVUS-only group (p = not significant). There was no significant difference in restenosis rate (33% IVUS guided vs 35% final IVUS, p = not significant) between the groups (applying ≥50% diameter stenosis criteria). There was also no difference in minimum in-stent luminal area at baseline, or at follow-up. When restenosis rates were compared considering the achievement of IVUS criteria, there were also no significant differences. The conclusion of this trial was that with regard to immediate procedural lumen gain and rate of restenosis, multiple IVUS examinations during the procedure show no benefit compared to final IVUS assessment only.

Ongoing trials

The need for IVUS guidance of stent placement is being assessed in two studies, in which patients are randomized to either IVUS or angiography guided stent implantation and expansion. In the AVID (Angiography Versus Intravascular ultrasound Directed coronary stent placement) trial,[120,121] patients are randomized to further angiographic guidance or IVUS guidance after an optimum angiographic result (<10% diameter stenosis on visual estimate and full stent apposition). In the angiography group, blinded IVUS is done and the patients are discharged on aspirin and ticlopidine. In the IVUS-directed group, patients who fail the IVUS criteria (<10% stenosis, absence of dissection, and full stent apposition) are treated with larger balloons. Patients who fulfil the IVUS criteria are discharged on aspirin and ticlopidine. Patients who fail angiographic or IVUS criteria receive enoxaprin for 2 weeks in addition to aspirin and ticlopidine. Enrollment is near completion, with a total of 800 patients planned for randomization. Preliminary results from the first 218 patients have been reported.[121] In the angiography group, the IVUS results were unblinded in 2.6% of the patients and an additional stent placed for dissection. Results at 30 days show no difference in clinical outcome between the two groups. Stent thrombosis was observed in 1.8% of the angiography-guided group and in 1.9% of the IVUS-guided cohort. One patient in the angiography group and two patients in the IVUS group required CABG. These results were seen despite the observation that 33% of patients with optimum stenting by angiographic criteria failed to satisfy IVUS criteria. No complications from IVUS therapy were seen in this trial. These data suggest that IVUS-directed stent implantation can indeed improve acute stent dimensions (32% increase in cross-sectional area in those who underwent larger balloon inflation for an underdilated stent in the IVUS group) but that it does not influence the 30-day clinical event rate.

The OPTICUS (OPTimization with IntraCoronary UltraSound to reduce stent restenosis) trial is a multicentre randomized study designed to test the hypothesis that IVUS guidance during stent implantation reduces the restenosis rates.[122] The study will enroll 550 patients with stable or unstable angina (Braunwald Class 1-2, A-C) and a single lesion suitable for Palmaz–Schatz stent implantation. The primary endpoints of the OPTICUS trial are diameter stenosis and angiographic MLD at 6 months follow-up, and the secondary endpoints are 12-months clinical follow-up and an economic assessment. Recruitment into this study is currently underway.

Assessment of the role of high-pressure stent deployment

Ongoing trials
Although high-pressure stent expansion has been widely recommended for the prevention of subacute stent thrombosis, there has been only one randomized trial designed to test this contention.[123,124] In this study, slotted-tube stents of five different types were used. Early results show that at 30-days follow-up of 900 patients, high-pressure implantation is associated with more favourable acute angiographic results, although the rate of complications is not significantly different between groups.

Comparison of access site

Completed trials
The BRAFE (Brachial RAdial FEmoral) trial is a multicentre trial that included 150 male patients at six different Belgian sites.[125] Since women often have a small radial artery, the study was limited to men in order to avoid access failure and postprocedural thrombosis with the radial approach. Patients were randomized to three different approaches (femoral puncture (n = 56), branchial cutdown (n = 56), radial puncture (n = 38)), using 6F guiding catheters for the elective implantation of Palmaz–Schatz stents. The primary endpoints of this trial were the entry-site complication rate (bleeding, haematoma, need for blood transfusion, thrombotic occlusion, need for vascular surgery, nerve damage) and average duration of post-stent hospitalization. Secondary endpoints included the success, failure, and subacute thrombosis rates, and the clinical endpoints of death, myocardial infarction, cerebrovascular accident, and the requirement for repeat revascularization. The vitamin K antagonist acenocoumarol was given to all patients on the day before stenting (7 mg) and was continued for 30 days with the International Normalized Ratio (INR) maintained at 2.5–3.5 for 30 days. All patients had clinical follow-up 30 days after the stenting procedure. Results showed no statistically significant differences between the three groups for procedural characteristics, in-hospital outcome, average hospitalization time after stenting or during the month after the stenting, or local complications at 1-month follow-up, although there was a clear trend towards more technical difficulties and more problems with the radial approach (eg, failure at entry site, failure of the guiding catheter, failure of angioplasty, failure of stent delivery, readmission to hospital, etc.). The only statistically significant difference was the arterial time of the procedure (from puncture of the vessel until removal of the last guiding catheter), with a mean time of 31.0 ± 10.2 minutes in the brachial group, 42.2 ± 21.8 minutes in the femoral group, and 55.8 ± 31.3 minutes in the radial group. One of the limitations of this study is the small sample size. It is likely that with a larger population, many of the "trends" that did not reach

statistical significance, such as unsuccessful stenting in the transradial group, may have become significant. In addition, this study was done with a full anticoagulation regimen, and therefore the major determinant of hospital stay was the anticoagulation target level. It might be expected that with antiplatelet therapy alone, the hospital stay may be shorter with the brachial and radial approaches.

Treatment of in-stent restenosis

Completed trials

The ROSTER (ROtablater *vs* balloon for STEnt Restenosis) trial was designed to evaluate the benefit of atheroablation using rotational atherectomy prior to adjunctive PTCA compared with PTCA alone, for the treatment of in-stent restenosis.[126,127] A total of 84 patients with in-stent restenosis (≥50% diameter stenosis, >8 weeks post-stent implantation) were randomized (42 rotational atherectomy, 42 PTCA). Patients randomized to the atherectomy group were treated with the Rotablator, which was followed by balloon dilatation up to 6 atmospheres. Balloon-only treated patients were treated with high pressure PTCA (12–16 atmospheres). There were no procedural complications in either group, and the CK-MB release was not different between treatments (16% in the atherectomy group *vs* 12% in the PTCA group). At 6 (±3) months follow-up the incidence of "clinical" restenosis (composite of angiographic restenosis, target lesion revascularization, recurrent angina Canadian Cardiovascular Society (CCS) class III-IV) was significantly higher in the PTCA treated group (36%) than in the group treated with rotational atherectomy (19%; p = 0.08).

Ongoing trials

Pullback atherectomy (PA) with or without adjunctive balloon angioplasty is also being compared with balloon angioplasty for the treatment of focal (less than 20 mm long) in-stent restenosis in the multicentre randomized PAIR (Pullback Atherectomy for In-stent Restenosis) trial. The primary objective of this trial is to compare the minimum lumen diameter as assessed by quantitative coronary angiography at 6 months follow-up. Secondary efficacy endpoints are also being monitored and include the incidence of adverse clinical events at 9 months follow-up, as well as objective assessments of the recurrence of ischemic symptoms.

Stenting in small vessels

Completed trials
The clinical efficacy of Wiktor stent compared to cutting balloon angioplasty for small vessel disease was assessed in the WCUS trial.[128] 127 patients with lesions in vessels less than 3.0 mm in diameter were randomized to cutting balloon angioplasty or Wiktor stent implantation. The initial success rate, the clinical complication rates, the restenosis rate, changes in per cent stenosis and minimal luminal diameter at 6 months post-treatment were the trial endpoints. The initial success rates were favourable in both groups with 98% for the cutting balloon group and 99% for the Wiktor stent group. Acute occlusion was observed in 6% of the Wiktor stent group and coronary dissection was observed in 5% of the cutting balloon group. Pre-procedure stenosis was 68.4% in the cutting balloon group, which decreased to 33.4% immediately post-procedure and increased to 46.4% at late follow-up. Corresponding values for the Wiktor stent treated group were 69.8% pre-procedure, 22.3% immediately post-procedure and 33.4% at follow-up. Late loss was 0.3 mm for the cutting balloon group and 0.8 mm for the Wiktor stent group. The restenosis rates at follow-up were similar for the two groups (34% for the cutting balloon group and 32% for the Wiktor stent group).

References

1. Serruys PW, de Jaegere P, Kiemeneij F et al, for the Benestent Study Group. A comparison of balloon-expandable-stent implantation with balloon angioplasty in patients with coronary artery disease. *N Engl J Med* 1994; **331**: 489–95.

2. Fischman DL, Leon MB, Baim DS et al, for the Stent Restenosis Study investigators. A randomised comparison of coronary-stent placement and balloon angioplasty in the treatment of coronary artery disease. *N Engl J Med* 1994; **331**: 496–501.

3. George CJ, Baim DS, Brinker JA et al. One-year follow-up of the Stent Restenosis (STRESS I) Study. *Am J Cardiol* 1998; **81**: 860–65.

4. Macaya C, Serruys PW, Ruygrok P et al. Continued benefit of coronary stenting versus balloon angioplasty: one year clinical follow-up of Benestent trial. *J Am Coll Cardiol* 1996; **27**: 255–61.

5. Masotti M, Serra A, Fernandez-Avilés F et al. Stent versus angioplasty restenosis trial (START): angiographic results at six month follow-up [abstract]. *Eur Heart J* 1996; 17 (suppl): 120.

6. Serruys PW, van Hout B, Bonnier H et al. Effectiveness, costs and cost-effectiveness of a strategy of elective heparin-coated stenting compared with

balloon angioplasty in selected patients with coronary artery disease: The Benestent II Study. *Lancet* 1998 (in press).

7. Legrand V, Serruys PW, Emanuelsson H et al. BENESTENT-II Trial – final results of visit I: a 15-day follow-up [abstract]. *J Am Coll Cardiol* 1997; 29 (suppl A): 170A.

8. Garcia E, Serruys PW, Dawkins K et al. BENESTENT-II trial: final results of visit II & III: a 7 month follow-up [abstract]. *Eur Heart J* 1997; 18 (suppl): 350.

9. van Hout B, van der Woude T, de Jaegere PT et al. Cost effectiveness of stent implantation versus PTCA: the BENESTENT experience. *Semin Intervent Cardiol* 1996; **1:** 263–68.

10. Penn IM, Ricci DR, Almond DG et al. Coronary artery stenting reduces restenosis: final results from the Trial of Angioplasty and Stents in Canada (TASC) I [abstract]. *Circulation* 1995; 92 (suppl I): I-279.

11. Heuser RR, Wong SC, Chuang YC et al. The LAD subgroup in the Stent Restenosis Study (STRESS): the most pronounced antirestenosis effect of stenting [abstract]. *Eur Heart J* 1995; 16 (suppl): 291.

12. Versaci F, Gaspardone A, Tomai F, Crea F, Chiariello L, Gioffrè PA. A comparison of coronary-artery stenting with angioplasty for isolated stenosis of the proximal left anterior descending coronary artery. *N Engl J Med* 1997; **336:** 817–22.

13. Rodriguez AE, Bernardi VH, Ayala FP et al. Optimal Coronary Balloon Angioplasty vs Stent (OCBAS): angiographic long term follow-up results of a randomized trial [abstract]. *Circulation* 1997; 96 (suppl): I-593.

14. Foley D, Serruys PW. Provisional stenting – stent-like balloon angioplasty evidence to define the continuing role of balloon angioplasty for percutaneous coronary revascularization. *Semin Intervent Cardiol* 1996; **1:** 269–73.

15. Knight CJ, Curzen N, Groves PH et al. Stenting suboptimal results following balloon angioplasty significantly reduces restenosis: results of a single centre randomised trial [abstract]. *Circulation* 1997; 96 (suppl): I-709.

16. Bilodeau L, Schreiber T, Hilton JD et al. The Wallstent In Native coronary arteries (WIN) multicenter randomized trial: in-hospital acute results [abstract]. *J Am Coll Cardiol* 1998; 31 (suppl): 80A.

17. Bilodeau L, Schreiber T, Hilton JD et al. The Wallstent in native coronary arteries (WIN) multicenter randomized trial: in-hospital acute results [abstract]. *Eur Heart J* 1998; 19 (suppl): 48.

18. Ambrose JA, Sharma SK, Marmur JD et al. Balloon Angioplasty vs Stent Study (BOSS): a prospective randomized trial. *Circulation* 1997; 96 (suppl): I-592.

19. Douglas JS, Savage MP, Bailey SR et al, for the SAVED Trial Investigators. Randomized trial of coronary stent and balloon angioplasty in the treatment of saphenous vein graft stenosis [abstract]. *J Am Coll Cardiol* 1996; 27 (suppl A): 178A.

20. Savage MP, Douglas JS, Fischman DL et al, for the Saphenous Vein De Novo Trial Investigators. Stent placement compared with balloon angioplasty for obstructed coronary bypass grafts. *N Engl J Med* 1997; **337:** 740–47.

21. Erbel R, Haude M, Höpp HW et al, on behalf of the REST Study Group. REstenosis ST (REST)-Study: randomized trial comparing stenting and balloon angioplasty for treatment of restenosis after balloon angioplasty. *J Am Coll Cardiol* 1996; 27 (suppl A): 139A.

22. Shah V, Haude M, Erbel R et al, for the REST Investigators. Long-term follow-up of "stent-like" post-PTCA results ($\leq$30% residual diameter stenosis) in the restenotic lesions: results of the REST trial [abstract]. *J Am Coll Cardiol* 1997; 29 (suppl A): 77A.

23. Hamburger JN, de Feyter PJ, Serruys PW. The laser guidewire experience: "crossing the Rubicon". *Semin Interven Cardiol* 1996; **1:** 163–71.

24. Sirnes PA, Golf S, Myreng Y et al, for the SICCO Study Group. Stenting in chronic coronary occlusion (SICCO): a multicenter, randomized, controlled study [abstract]. *J Am Coll Cardiol* 1996; **27** (suppl): 139A.

25. Sirnes PA, Golf S, Myreng Y et al. Stenting in chronic coronary occlusion (SICCO): a randomized controlled trial of adding stent implantation after successful angioplasty. *J Am Coll Cardiol* 1996; **28:** 1444–51.

26. Sirnes PA, Golf S, Myreng Y et al. Sustained benefit of stenting in chronic occlusions: long-term follow-up of the SICCO Study [abstract]. *J Am Coll Cardiol* 1998; **31** (suppl): 237A.

27. Höher M, Grebe O, Wöhrle J et al. Stenting *vs* PTCA after recanalization of chronic total occlusions: results of the SPACTO trial with the Wiktor® stent [abstract] *Eur Heart J* 1998; 19 (suppl): 47.

28. Sato Y, Nosaka H, Kimura T, Nobuyoshi M. Randomized comparison of balloon angioplasty versus coronary stent implantation for total occlusion [abstract]. *J Am Coll Cardiol* 1996; 27 (suppl): 152A.

29. Rubartelli P, Niccoli L, Verna E et al, for the Gruppo Italiano Sullo Stent Nelle Occlusioni Coronariche (GISSOC). Stent implantation versus balloon angioplasty in chronic total coronary occlusions: results from the GISSOC trial. *J Am Coll Cardiol* 1998; **32:** 90–96.

30. Thomas M, Hancock J, Holmberg S, Wainwright R, Jewitt D. Coronary stenting following successful angioplasty for total occlusions: preliminary results of a randomised trial [abstract]. *J Am Coll Cardiol* 1996; 27 (suppl): 153A.

31. Lotan C, Krakover R, Turgeman Y et al. The STOP study: a randomized multicentre Israeli study for stents in total occlusion and restenosis prevention [abstract]. *Eur Heart J* 1998; 19 (suppl): 471.

32. Guérin Y, Chevalier B, Tron C et al, on behalf of the CORSICA investigators. Preliminary results of a randomized study between balloon versus stent in chronic coronary occlusion [abstract]. *Eur Heart J* 1997; 18 (suppl): 382.

33. Ray SG, Penn IM, Ricci DR et al. The CORSICA trial: short and mid-term outcome [abstract] *Eur Heart J* 1998; **19** (suppl): 471

34. Penn IM, Ricci DR, Brown RI et al. Randomized study of prolonged balloon dilatation in failed angioplasty (PTCA): preliminary data from the trial of angioplasty and stents in Canada (TASC II) [abstract]. *Circulation* 1993; **88**: I-601.

35. Keane D, Roubin G, Marco J, Fearnot N, Serruys PW. GRACE – Gianturco Roubin stent Acute Closure Evaluation: substrate, challenges and design of a randomized trial of bailout management. *J Interven Cardiol* 1994; **7**: 333–39.

36. Haude M, Erbel R, Hoepp HW, Heublein B, Sigmund M, Meyer J, and the STENT-BY Study group. STENT-BY Study: a prospective randomized trial comparing immediate stenting versus conservative treatment strategies in abrupt vessel closure or symptomatic dissections during coronary balloon angioplasty [abstract]. *Eur Heart J* 1996; 17 (suppl): 172.

37. Rodríguez A, Bernardi V, Fernández M et al, on behalf of the GRAMI Investigators. In-hospital and late results of coronary stents versus conventional balloon angioplasty in acute myocardial infarction (GRAMI Trial). *Am J Cardiol* 1998; **81**: 1286–91.

38. Rodríguez AE, Bernardi VH, Santaera OA et al. Coronary stents improve outcome in acute myocardial infarction: immediate and long term results of the GRAMI Trial [abstract]. *J Am Coll Cardiol* 1998; 31 (suppl): 64A.

39. Rodriguez A, Fernandez M, Bernardi V et al, on behalf of the GRAMI investigators. Coronary stents improved hospital results during coronary angioplasty in acute myocardial infarction: preliminary results of a randomized controlled study (GRAMI Trial) [abstract]. *J Am Coll Cardiol* 1997; 29 (suppl A): 221A.

40. Rodriguez A, Bernardi V, Santaera O, Mauvecin C, Roubin G, Ambrose J, on behalf of the GRAMI investigators. Coronary stents improved hospital outcome in patients undergoing PTCA in acute myocardial infarction: results of a randomized multicenter study (GRAMI trial) [abstract]. *Am J Cardiol* 1997; 80 (suppl 7A): 21S.

41. Saito S, Hosokawa G. Primary Palmaz–Schatz stent implantation for acute myocardial infarction: the final results of Japanese PASTA (Primary Angioplasty *vs* Stent Implantation in AMI in Japan) trial [abstract]. *Circulation* 1997; 96 (suppl): I-595.

42. Saito S, Hosokawa G, Suzuki S, Nakamura S, for the Japanese PASTA trial study group. Primary stent implantation is superior to balloon angioplasty in acute myocardial infarction – the result of the Japanese PASTA (Primary Angioplasty Versus Stent Implantation in Acute Myocardial Infarction) trial [abstract]. *J Am Coll Cardiol* 1997; 29 (suppl A): 390A.

43. Hoorntje JC, Suryapranata H, de Boer M-J, Zijlstra F, van't Hof AW, van den Brink L. ESCOBAR: primary stenting for acute myocardial infarction: preliminary results of a randomized trial [abstract]. *Circulation* 1996; 94 (suppl): I-570.

44. Suryapranata H, van't Hof AW, Hoorntje JC, de Boer MJ, Zijlstra F. Randomized comparison of coronary stenting with balloon angioplasty in selected patients with acute myocardial infarction. *Circulation* 1998; **97:** 1502–05.

45. Suryapranata H, Hoorntje JCA, Boer MJ de, Zijlstra F. Randomized comparison of primary stenting with primary balloon angioplasty in acute myocardial infarction [abstract]. *Circulation* 1997; 96 (suppl): I-327.

46. Antoniucci D, Santoro GM, Bolognese L et al. Stenting in acute myocardial infarction: preliminary results of the FRESCO study (Florence Randomized Elective Stenting in Acute Coronary Occlusions) [abstract]. *Eur Heart J* 1997; 18 (suppl): 586.

47. Antoniucci D, Santoro GM, Bolognese L et al. Elective stenting in acute myocardial infarction: preliminary results of the Florence randomized elective stenting in acute coronary occlusions (FRESCO) study [abstract]. *J Am Coll Cardiol* 1997; 29 (suppl A): 456A.

48. Antoniucci D, Santoro GM, Bolognese L, Valenti R, Trapani M, Fazzini PF. Clinical trial comparing primary stenting of the infarct-related artery with optimal primary angioplasty for acute myocardial infarction: results from the Florence Randomized Elective Stenting in Acute Coronary Occlusions (FRESCO) Trial. *J Am Coll Cardiol* 1998; **31:** 1234–39.

49. Stone GW, Brodie B, Griffin J et al. A prospective, multicenter trial of primary stenting in acute myocardial infarction – the PAMI Stent Pilot Study [abstract]. *Circulation* 1996; 94 (suppl): I-570.

50. Serruys PW, Garcia-Fernandez E, Kiemeney F et al. Heparin-coated stent in acute myocardial infarction: a pilot study as a preamble to a large randomized trial comparing balloon angioplasty and stenting [abstract]. *Eur Heart J* 1997; 18 (suppl): 272.

51. Stone GW. Stenting and IIb/IIIa receptor blockade in acute myocardial infarction: an introduction to the CADILLAC Trial. *J Invas Cardiol* 1998; 10 (suppl B): 36B–47B.

52. Nishida Y, Nonaka H, Ueda K et al. In-hospital outcome of primary stenting for acute myocardial infarction using Wiktor Coil Stent: results from a multicenter randomized PRISAM study [abstract]. *Circulation* 1997; 96 (suppl): I-397.

53. Ueda K, Nishida Y, Iwase T et al. Quantitative angiographic restenosis of primary stenting using Wiktor Coil Stent for acute myocardial infarction: results from a multicenter randomized PRISAM study [abstract]. *Circulation* 1997; 96 (suppl): I-531.

54. Monassier JP, Elias J, Meyer P, Morice MC, Royer T, Cribier A. STENTIM I: the

French registry of stenting at acute myocardial infarction [abstract]. *J Am Coll Cardiol* 1996; 27 (suppl): 68A.

54. Horstkotte D, Piper C, Andresen D et al. Stent implantation for acute myocardial infarction: results of a pilot study with 80 consecutive patients [abstract]. *Eur Heart J* 1996; 17 (suppl): 297.

55. Maillard L, Hamon M, Monassier JP, Raynaud P, for the Stentim 2 Investigators. STENTIM 2-hospital outcome: elective Wiktor stent implantation in acute myocardial infarction versus balloon angioplasty [abstract]. *Eur Heart J* 1998; 19 (suppl): 59.

56. Tsuchikane E, Sumitsuji S, Funamoto M et al. Acute results of stent versus directional atherectomy randomized trial (START) [abstract]. *Eur Heart J* 1997; 18 (suppl): 349.

57. Tsuchikane E, Sumitsuji S, Nakamura T et al. Impact of superficial calcification of coronary plaque on lumen dilation: comparison of stenting and atherectomy from acute results of stent *vs* directional coronary atherectomy randomized trial (START) [abstract]. *Circulation* 1997; 96 (suppl): I-81.

58. Tsuchikane E, Sumitsuji S, Nakamura T, Awata N, Kobayashi K. Angiographic follow-up results of STent versus Atherectomy Randomized Trial (START) [abstract]. *J Am Coll Cardiol* 1998; 31 (suppl): 379A.

59. Kobayashi T, Sumitsuji S, Tsuchikane E, Awata N, Kobayashi T. The influence of stent implantation on the increase of plaque area (Stent vs Atherectomy Randomized Trial; START) [abstract]. *J Am Coll Cardiol* 1998; 31 (suppl): 315A.

60. Kobayashi T, Tsuchikane E, Sumitsuji S et al. Comparison of intimal proliferation between primary stenting and optimal directional coronary atherectomy: a serial intracoronary ultrasound study from START (Stent versus directional coronary Atherectomy Randomized Trial) [abstract]. *Eur Heart J* 1998; 19 (suppl): 47.

61. The EPISTENT Investigators. Randomised placebo-controlled and balloon angioplasty controlled trial to assess safety of coronary stenting with use of platelet glycoprotein-IIb/IIIa blockade. *Lancet* 1998; **352:** 87–92.

62. The EPIC Investigators. Use of a monoclonal antibody against the platelet glycoprotein IIb/IIIa receptor in high-risk coronary angioplasty. *N Engl J Med* 1994; **330:** 956–61.

63. Schömig A, Neumann FJ, Kastrati A et al. A randomized comparison of antiplatelet and anticoagulant therapy after the placement of coronary-artery stents. *N Engl J Med* 1996; **334:** 1084–89.

64. Mehran R, Popma JJ, Baim DS et al. Routine high pressure post-stent dilatation did not influence clinical restenosis in STARS [abstract]. *J Am Coll Cardiol* 1998; 31 (suppl): 80A.

65. Kuntz RE, Baim DS, Popma JJ et al. Late clinical results of the stent anticoagulation regimen study (STARS) [abstract]. *Circulation* 1997; 96 (suppl): I-594.

66. Urban P, Macaya C, Rupprecht H-J et al, for the MATTIS investigators. Multicenter Aspirin and Ticlopidine Trial after Intracoronary Stenting in high risk patients [abstract]. *J Am Coll Cardiol* 1998; 31 (suppl): 397A.

67. Hall P, Nakamura S, Maiello L et al. A randomized comparison of combined ticlopidine and aspirin therapy versus aspirin therapy alone after successful intravascular ultrasound-guided stent implantation. *Circulation* 1996; **93:** 215–22.

68. Machraoui A, Germing A, von Dryander S et al. Efficacy and safety of ticlopidine alone *vs* ticlopidine and aspirin in post-stenting medical treatment: results of a randomized clinical trial [abstract]. *Circulation* 1997; 96 (suppl): I-593.

69. Rupprecht HJ, Darius H, Borkowski U et al. Comparison of antiplatelet effects of aspirin, ticlopidine, or their combination after stent implantation. *Circulation* 1998; **97:** 1046–52.

70. Kruse KR, Greenberg CS, Tanguay J-F et al. Thrombin and fibrin activity in patients treated with enoxaprin, ticlopidine and aspirin versus the conventional coumadin regimen after elective stenting: the ENTICES trial [abstract]. *J Am Coll Cardiol* 1996; 27 (suppl A): 334A.

71. Szto GYF, Linnemeier TJ, Lewis SJ et al. A randomized trial of 10 or 30 days of ticlopidine after coronary stenting: Strategic ALternatives with Ticlopidine in Stenting Pilot Study (SALTS) [abstract]. *Am J Cardiol* 1997; 80 (suppl 7A): 64S.

72. Szto GYF, Linnemeier TJ, Lewis SJ et al. Safety of 10 days of ticlopidine after coronary stenting – a randomized comparison with 30 days: Strategic ALternatives with Ticlopidine in Stenting Study (SALTS) [abstract]. *J Am Coll Cardiol* 1998; 31 (suppl): 352A.

73. Machraoui A, Germing A, von Dryander S et al. High pressure coronary stenting: efficacy and safety of aspirin versus coumadin plus aspirin. *J Invas Cardiol* 1997; **9:** 171–76.

74. Kunishima T, Musha H, Eto F et al. A randomized trial of aspirin versus cilostazol after successful coronary stent implantation. *Clin Ther* 1997; **19:** 1058–66.

75. Sekiya M, Funada J, Watanabe K, Miyagawa M, Akutsu H. Effects of probucol and cilostazol alone and in combination on frequency of poststenting restenosis. *Am J Cardiol* 1998; **82:** 144–7.

76. Kutryk MJB, Serruys PW, Bruining N et al. Randomized trial of antisense oligonucleotide against *c-myc* for the prevention of restenosis after stenting: results of the Thoraxcenter "ITALICS" trial [abstract]. *Eur Heart J* 1998; 19 (suppl): 569.

77. Bennet MR, Schwartz SM. Antisense therapy for angioplasty restenosis: some critical considerations. *Circulation* 1995; **92:** 1981–93.

78. Ellis SG, Serruys PW, Popma JJ et al. Can abciximab prevent neointimal proliferation in Palmaz–Schatz stents? The final ERASER results [abstract]. *Circulation* 1997; 96 (suppl): I-87.

79. Wilensky RL, Tanguay J-F, Ito S et al. The Heparin Infusion Prior to Stenting (HIPS) trial: procedural, in-hospital, 30 day, and 6 month clinical, angiographic and IVUS results [abstract]. *J Am Coll Cardiol* 1998; 31 (suppl): 457A.

80. Kiesz RS, Deutsch E, Buszman P et al. Prospective randomized study of local enoxaparin delivery versus systemic heparin for NIR stent placement [abstract]. *Am J Cardiol* 1997; 80 (suppl 7A): 19S.

81. Kiesz RS, Deutsch E, Buszman P et al. Results of prospective randomized study of local enoxaparin delivery versus systemic heparinization for NIR stent placement [abstract]. *J Am Coll Cardiol* 1998; 31 (suppl): 495A.

82. Kiesz RS, Deutsch E, Buszman P et al. Prospective randomized study of local enoxaparin delivery vs systemic heparinization for NIR stent placement [abstract]. *Circulation* 1997; 96 (suppl): I-654.

83. Bertrand M, Legrand V, Boland J et al. Full anticoagulation versus ticlopidine plus aspirin after stent implantation: a randomized multicenter European study: the FANTASTIC trial [abstract]. *Circulation* 1996; 94 (suppl): I-685.

84. Anzuini A, Legrand V, Fleck E et al. Full anticoagulation versus ticlopidine plus aspirin after Wiktor implantation (Fantastic trial): angiographic results at 6 months follow-up [abstract]. *Eur Heart J* 1997; 18 (suppl): 622.

85. Niazi KA, Patel AA, Nozha F et al. A prospective randomized study of the effects of debulking on restenosis (Edres trial) [abstract]. *Circulation* 1997; 96 (suppl): I-709.

86. Steg PG, the FROST Study Group. Should we stent all the patients? Preliminary answer from the multicenter randomized FROST study [abstract]. *J Am Coll Cardiol* 1998; 31 (suppl): 317A.

87. Lafont AM, Dubois-Rande JL, Steg PGG. The French Optimal Stenting Trial (FROST): a multicenter, prospective randomized study comparing systematic stenting to angiography/coronary flow reserve guided stenting [abstract]. *Circulation* 1998; 96 (suppl): I-222.

88. Teirstein PS, Massullo V, Jani S et al. Radiation therapy following coronary stenting – 6 month follow-up of a randomized clinical trial [abstract]. *Circulation* 1996; 94 (suppl): I-210.

89. Teirstein PS, Massullo V, Jani S et al. Catheter-based radiotherapy to inhibit restenosis after coronary stenting. *N Engl J Med* 1997; **336:** 1697–703.

90. Teirstein PS, Massullo V, Jani S et al. Radiotherapy to reduce restenosis: subgroup analysis of the SCRIPPS randomized trial [abstract]. *Circulation* 1997; 96 (suppl): I-218.

91. Teirstein PS, Massullo V, Jani S et al. Initial report of gamma radiotherapy for diffuse coronary restenosis: the SCRIPPS II Trial [abstract]. *J Am Coll Cardiol* 1998; 31 (suppl): 238A.

92. Waksman R, White RL, Chan RC et al. Intracoronary radiation therapy for patients with in-stent restenosis: interim report from a randomized clinical study [abstract]. *J Am Coll Cardiol* 1998; 31 (suppl): 222A.

93. Waksman R, White RL, Chan RS et al. Localized intracoronary radiation therapy for patients with in-stent restenosis: preliminary results from a randomized clinical study [abstract]. *Circulation* 1997; 96 (suppl): I-219.

94. Kaufmann U, Gaspardone A, Bertel O et al, on behalf of the SIMA investigators. Design and acute results of the SIMA trial [abstract]. *Eur Heart J* 1998; 19 (suppl): 136.

95. Goy JJ, Eeckhout E, Debbas N, Stauffer JC, Vogt P. Stenting of the right coronary artery for de novo stenosis: a comparison of the Wiktor and the Palmaz–Schatz stents [abstract]. *Circulation* 1995; 92 (suppl I): I-596.

96. Goy JJ, Eeckhout E, Stauffer J-C, Vogt P, Kappenberger L. Emergency endoluminal stenting for abrupt vessel closure following coronary angioplasty: a randomized comparison of the Wiktor and the Palmaz–Schatz stents [abstract]. *Cathet Cardiovasc Diagn* 1995; **34:** 128–32.

97. de Belder A, Thomas MR, Nageh T, Williams I, Wainwright RJ. The RENEWAL study; a randomised trial of endoluminal reconstruction using the NIR stent or Wallstent in angioplasty of long segment native coronary disease [abstract]. *Eur Heart J* 1998; 19 (suppl): 48.

98. Baim DS. ASCENT Trial – evaluation of the ACS Multi-Link stent. *J Invas Cardiol* 1998; 10 (suppl B): 53B–54B.

99. Baim DS, Cutlip DE, Midei M et al. Acute 30-day and late clinical events in the randomized parallel-group comparison of the ACS Multi-Link coronary stent system and the Palmaz–Schatz stent [abstract]. *Circulation* 1997; 96 (suppl): I-593.

100. Popma JJ, Curran MJ, Abizaid AS et al. Early quantitative angiographic outcomes in the randomized ACS multilink stent *vs* Palmaz–Schatz coronary stent trial for the treatment of de novo coronary lesions [abstract]. *Circulation* 1997; 96 (suppl): I-593.

101. Heuser RR, Kuntz RE, Lansky AJ et al. The SMART trial: acute outcome indicates superior efficacy with the AVE stent [abstract]. *Circulation* 1997; 96 (suppl): I-593.

102. Heuser R, Kuntz R, Lansky A et al. Six-month clinical and angiographic results of the SMART trial [abstract]. *J Am Coll Cardiol* 1998; 31 (suppl): 64A.

103. Dean LS, Roubin GS, O'Shaughnessy CD et al, for the GR II Clinical Investigators. Equivalent late clinical outcomes in "STRESS-like" lesions: results of a randomized trial comparing GR II and Palmaz–Schatz stents [abstract]. *Am J Cardiol* 1997; 80 (suppl 7A): 21S.

104. Dean LS, Roubin GS, O'Shaughnessy CD et al, on behalf of the GRII Clinical

Investigators. Elective stenting of de novo lesions: randomized, multicentre trial comparing two stent designs [abstract]. *Eur Heart J* 1997; 18 (suppl): 349.

105. Dean LS, Holmes DR, Roubin GS et al, on behalf of the GRII Clinical Investigators. Does stent type determine clinical outcome? Final results of the Gianturco Roubin II randomized trial. *Eur Heart J* 1998; **19** (suppl): 47.

106. Baim DS. Acute and 30-day clinical results of the NIRVANA Trial [abstract]. *Circulation* 1997; 96 (suppl): I-594.

106. Lansky AJ, Popma JJ, Mehran R et al. Late quantitative angiographic results after NIR stent use: results from the NIRVANA randomized trial and registries [abstract]. *J Am Coll Cardiol* 1998; 31 (suppl): 80A.

108. Goldberg S, Schwartz RS, Mann JT III et al. Comparison of a novel self-expanding Nitinol stent (RADIUS™) with a balloon expandable (Palmaz–Schatz™) stent: initial results of a randomized trial (SCORES) [abstract]. *Circulation* 1997; 96 (suppl): I-654.

109. Han RO, Schwartz RS, Mann JT et al. Comparative efficacy of self expanding and balloon expandable stents for the reduction of restenosis [abstract]. *J Am Coll Cardiol* 1998; 31 (suppl): 314A.

110. Carrozza J, Kereiakes D, Caputo R et al. Acute, 30-day and 6-month clinical outcome from the randomized US EXTRA trial comparing the operator-mounted Bard XT stent and the Palmaz–Schatz coronary stent [abstract]. *Eur Heart J* 1998; 19 (suppl): 136.

111. Hausleiter J, Dirschinger J, Schühlen H et al. A multicenter randomized trial comparing five different types of slotted-tube stents [abstract]. *J Am Coll Cardiol* 1998; 31 (suppl): 80A.

112. Hodgson JMcB, Frey AW, Roskamm H. Net gain after six month angiographic follow-up is greater when IVUS is used to guide initial interventions: chronic SIPS trial results [abstract]. *Am J Cardiol* 1997; 80 (suppl 7A): 17S.

113. Hodgson JMcB, Frey AW, Müller C, Roskamm H. Comparison of acute procedure cost and equipment utilization with strategies of ICUS guided *vs* angiographic guided PTCA and stenting: preliminary results of the Strategy of ICUS-guided PTCA and Stenting (SIPS) study [abstract]. *Circulation* 1996; 94 (suppl): I-235.

114. Frey AW, Roskamm H, Hodgson JMcB. IVUS-guided stenting: does acute angiography predict long term outcome? Insights from the strategy of IVUS-guided PTCA and stenting (SIPS) trial [abstract]. *Circulation* 1997; 96 (suppl): I-222.

115. Frey AW, Grove A, Suciu A et al. Reduction of restenosis rates after ICUS guided interventions: QCA results of the SIPS study [abstract]. *Eur Heart J* 1998; 19 (suppl): 136.

116. Frey AW, Hodgson JMcB, Roskamn H. Reductions of revascularization procedures

after ICUS-guided interventions: results from the 6-month follow-up of the SIPS study [abstract]. *Eur Heart J* 1998; 19 (suppl): 126.

117. Schiele F, Meneveau N, Vuillemont A et al. Restenosis after intracoronary ultrasound-guided stent deployment; a randomized multicentric study: results on the 6 month angiographic restenosis rate [abstract]. *J Am Coll Cardiol* 1998; 31 (suppl): 103A.

118. Schiele FJ, Meneveau NF, Vuillemont AR et al on behalf of the RESIST study group: Impact of intravascular ultrasound guidance in stent deployment on 6-month restenosis rate: a multicenter randomized study comparing two strategies – with and without intravascular ultrasound guidance. *J Am Coll Cardiol* 1998; **32:** 320–8.

119. Jeremias A, Ge J, Konorza T, Simon HU, Welge D, Gorge G. Six months' angiographic outcome after stepwise versus "final look" IVUS guided coronary stent deployment [abstract]. *Circulation* 1998; 96 (suppl): I-223.

120. Russo RJ, Teirstein PS, for the AVID Investigators. Angiography versus intravascular ultrasound-directed stent placement [abstract]. *J Am Coll Cardiol* 1996; 27 (suppl A): 306A.

121. Russo RJ, Teirstein PS, for the AVID Investigators. Angiography versus intravascular ultrasound-directed stent placement [abstract]. *Circulation* 1996; 94 (suppl): I-263.

122. Mudra H, Henneke K-H, Zeiher AM, de Jaegere P, di Mario C. Acute and preliminary follow-up results of the "OPTimization with ICUS to reduce stent restenosis" (OPTICUS) Trial [abstract]. *J Am Coll Cardiol* 1998; 31 (suppl): 494A.

123. Dirschinger J, Schuehlen H, Hausleiter J et al. A randomized trial of low versus high balloon pressure for coronary stent placement: analysis of early outcome [abstract]. *Circulation* 1997; 96 (suppl): I-653.

124. Dirschinger J, Hausleiter J, Schühlen H et al. High versus normal balloon pressure dilatation for coronary stent placement: 6-month clinical and angiographic results from a randomized multicenter trial [abstract]. *J Am Coll Cardiol* 1998; 31 (suppl): 17A.

125. Benit E, Missault L, Eeman T et al. Brachial, radial or femoral approach for elective Palmaz–Schatz stent implantation: a randomized comparison. *Cathet Cardiovasc Diagn* 1997; **41:** 124–30.

126. Sharma SK, Kini A, Duvvuri S et al. Randomized trial of rotational atherectomy *vs* balloon angioplasty for in-stent restenosis (ROSTER) [abstract]. *J Am Coll Cardiol* 1998; 31 (suppl): 142A.

127. Sharma SK, Kini A, Garapati A et al. Randomized trial of rotational atherectomy *vs* balloon angioplasty for in-stent restenosis (ROSTER) [abstract]. *Eur Heart J* 1998; 19 (suppl): 115.

128. Muramatsu T, Tsukahara R, Ho M, Ito S, Inoue T. A prospective randomized study of Wiktor stent and cutting balloon angioplasty for small vessel disease – WCUS study [abstract]. *Eur Heart J* 1998; 19 (suppl): 48.

4. Current Indications for Stenting

The use of coronary stent implantation as a primary treatment in interventional cardiology is increasing at a staggering rate. The rapid increase in the use of stents is primarily a result of their use in treatment categories not included in the completed controlled randomized trials. In most interventional centres, stents are used in 50% or more of all coronary angioplasty procedures. There is an enormous mismatch between clinical practice and trial-based evidence. This "stentomania" is driven by both the gratifying acute results seen by the interventionist when using these devices and the results extrapolated from observational and randomized trials. The initial zeal for coronary-stent implantation was based on the encouraging reduction in restenosis reported by the BENESTENT and STRESS trials.[1,2] The lesion types in the very highly selected cohorts of patients in these studies are found in only a fraction of the patients considered for percutaneous revascularization procedures. As an example, in a series of 700 consecutive patients with 745 lesions treated with coronary stents, Sawada and colleagues[3] found that only 20% of lesions would have been eligible for inclusion in the BENESTENT and STRESS studies. Although the restenosis rate for the BENESTENT/STRESS equivalent lesions was 11%, restenosis occurred in more than 30% of lesions that would have been excluded from these randomized trials. Several other observational series have likewise shown a reduction in the relative advantages of stent implantation when applied to a less select group of patients than those studied in the two landmark randomized trials.[4-6] The "bigger is better" attitude first proposed by Kuntz and colleagues[7] has also been adopted by many operators, who feel that the greater the acute gain in lumen diameter, the smaller the chances of short-term and long-term failure.[8] Inherent in this attitude is the concept that the stent is merely a means to an end, and therefore, irrespective of the particular stent or other dilating or debulking device employed, success of the procedure is determined solely by the acute results. Whether differences between various stent designs and materials are sufficient to affect their clinical effects remains to be shown in controlled "stent versus stent" trials.

The positive results of the completed randomized trials have been enthusiastically applied to almost every other sub-category of patients and lesions. Although randomized trials remain the reference standard for comparing therapies, they are designed to include relatively homogenous populations and have many clinical and angiographic exclusions. Registries also have the same limitation, although they tend to have a broader scope. Comparison of the results of registries and randomized trials of different time-frames can also prevent any definite conclusions from being drawn. Continual improvements in operator experience and periprocedural management of patients can result in apparently conflicting results. Data from the observational and randomized studies must be carefully scrutinized, since many of these studies are multicentre studies with a relatively small number of procedures done by a large number of operators, or are reports from low-volume centres. In view of these limitations, several indications for stenting have been supported by observational and randomized studies, although these are limited to very few stent types. The definitive evidence for the use of stents for several specific clinical indications is still lacking. As the results of the many ongoing randomized stent trials become available, the indications for stenting will need to be adapted accordingly.

Currently, there is solid evidence from observational studies and randomized trials to support the use of coronary stents for five indications:

1. Treatment of abrupt or threatened vessel closure during angioplasty;
2. primary reduction in restenosis in de-novo focal lesions in vessels greater than 3.0 mm in diameter;
3. focal lesions in saphenous vein grafts;
4. treatment of chronic total coronary occlusions;
5. as the primary treatment of myocardial infarctions.

Treatment of abrupt or threatened vessel closure during angioplasty

Despite increased operator experience and improved catheter technology, abrupt vessel closure continues to limit the safety and efficacy of coronary angioplasty. Acute closure is usually defined as TIMI grade 0 or 1 flow after percutaneous transluminal coronary angioplasty (PTCA). A consensus has not been reached for the definition of threatened closure, which may include one or more of the following; 50% or more residual stenosis, dissection 15 mm or more in length, extraluminal contrast, angina, or electrocardiographic changes of ischaemia. Overall, an incidence of acute or threatened closure of 4–10% has been reported, although the determination of the exact incidence is hampered by the use of different criteria to define acute occlusion and by differences in the characteristics of patients in the various trials.[9,10] The aetiology of abrupt closure is multifactorial and includes arterial dissection, elastic recoil, formation of thrombus, vascular spasm, and intramural haemorrhage.[11,12] The clinical consequences of abrupt vessel closure are significant. The National Heart, Lung, and Blood Institute 1985–86 PTCA Registry reported that 20% of all deaths, 40% of all myocardial infarctions, and 25% of coronary bypass operations recorded at 1-year follow-up occurred in the 6.8% of patients who had periprocedural coronary occlusion.[10,13] Successful redilatation can be achieved in around 44% of these patients, however, 4% of them still die, 20% sustain an acute myocardial infarction, and 7% require urgent bypass surgery, which after failed PTCA is associated with a myocardial infarction rate of 25–50% and a mortality ranging from 2% to 25%.[9,14–17] In some cases of acute or threatened closure, conventional balloon redilatation may be effective, but in most instances prolonged inflation times with an autoperfusion balloon is necessary in order to avoid ischaemic complications. Perfusion balloon rescue PTCA with prolonged dilatation has a reported success rate of 41–95%, but in high-grade complex dissections, deterioration after perfusion PTCA is frequent.

The rationale for using intracoronary stents as a bailout technique in acute or threatened closure is based on their ability to scaffold intimal/medial flaps away from the lumen. They therefore repair the dissected and re-occluded artery, and maintain radial support to offset elastic recoil. Clinical experience with bailout stent implantation was first reported by Sigwart and colleagues.[18] The Wallstent was implanted in a limited number of patients, which resulted in an immediate restoration of flow, normalization of the electrocardiogram (ECG) and relief of symptoms with no evidence of acute myocardial infarction. Further experience, restricted to bailout stenting, was subsequently reported by this group in 1988.[19] At that time, many centres began implanting stents in bailout circumstances as a bridge to cardiac surgery, and not as a definitive procedure, in order to avoid the risks of subacute thrombosis. Since these early reports, several observational and retrospective trials have used different stent types for the treatment of abrupt closure[19–44] (table 4.1). The technical success rate of these observational trials was quite high, although significant differences in the incidence of adverse events was apparent. These differences may be attributed to ambiguity in the definition of subacute closure, to differences in the populations of patients studied, and to variability in the techniques for stent deployment and periprocedural pharmacotherapy. A French multicentre study,[39] which examined stent implantation without the use of postprocedural oral anticoagulant therapy in 529 consecutive patients treated since November 1993, showed that in the subgroup of 112 patients stented for bailout indications, coronary events that were related, or possibly related, to stent thrombosis and that were recorded up to 30 days post-procedure, occurred in 5.4% of patients. The overall cardiac complication rate, including the need for emergency CABG in these patients, was 18.8%, which compares very favourably to the complication rate seen after autoperfusion balloon therapy. Since this initial report, several other studies have also shown the safety and efficacy of bailout stenting with antiplatelet therapy only.[40–43]

Results of a case-control analysis, which compared clinical outcome after stenting with that after conventional therapy for abrupt or threatened closure, have been reported by Lincoff and colleagues.[44] For this analysis, 61 patients treated by stenting for acute closure were matched according to angiographic

Table 4.1 Events following stent implantation for threatened or acute closure after percutaneous transluminal coronary angioplasty

Study	Study period	Patients (n)	Implantation success (%)	Complications (%) Death	Complications (%) AMI	Complications (%) Urgent CABG	Occlusion (%) Incidence	Occlusion (%) Time interval	Restenosis (%)
Wallstent									
Sigwart et al[19]	1986–88	11	100	9	9	0	9	NR	–
de Feyter et al[21]	1989–90	15	100	7	13	60	20	day 0–7	–
Goy et al[22]	1986–89	17	100	0	6	0	6	day 0	25
Eeckhout et al[23]	1986–91	33	100	3	30	9	24	NR	9
Gianturco-Roubin									
George et al[24]	1988–91	518	95	2	6	7	9	day 0–29	–
Hearn et al[25]	1987–90	116	89	4	35.5	11	9	NR	53
Roubin et al[20]	1989–91	115	96	2	7	4	8	NR	–
Sutton et al[26]	1989–91	415	NR	3	5	12	NR	NR	–
Lincoff et al[44]	1989–91	61	97	3	4	5	NR	NR	46
Chan et al[27]	1991–94	42	95	0	5	7	24	NR	–
Palmaz–Schatz									
Haude et al[28]	NR	15	100	0	0	7	7	day 0	21
Herrmann et al[29]	1988–91	50	98	4	20	13	16	day 1–10	–

Table 4.1 continued

Maiello et al[30]	1990–92	32	100	6	6	6	6	NR	54
Kiemeneij et al[31]	1990–91	52	89	7	NR	15	23	NR	29
Colombo et al[32]	1989–92	56	100	4	4	5	2	NR	36
Foley et al[33]	1990–92	60	100	0	22	7	17	NR	50
Schömig et al[34]	1989–93	327	97	4	4	1	7	day 2–22	30
Alfonso et al[35]	1990–93	42	93	0	5	3	5	NR	–
Chauhan et al[41]	1993–95	82	100	0	7	0	5	day 0–30	–
Chauhan et al[43]	1994–95*	65	100	0	5	0	0	day 0–30	–
Wiktor									
Vrolix and Piessens[36]	1991	119	95	3	NR	3	17	NR	–
Strecker									
Reifart et al[37]	1990–91	48	97	10	2	6	21	day 0–19	–
Several									
Witkowski et al[40]	1994–96*	32	97	3	13	3	3	day 0–30	46
Metz et al[38]	1988–93	88	94	3	26	8	9	NR	–
Antoniucci et al[42]	1995–96*	120	100	6	7	1	3	NR	28

* Study used antiplatelet therapy only. NR = not reported.

143

features of closure and estimated left ventricular mass at risk for ischaemia, with patients treated conventionally before stent availability. Despite better immediate angiographic results, there was no difference in the likelihood or severity of myocardial infarction in patients with established vessel closure. In this subset of patients, the need for urgent bypass surgery was significantly lower in those treated with stenting (4.9% *vs* 18% in the conventionally treated group, p = 0.02). Patients with threatened vessel closure could not be shown to benefit from stent treatment.

By contrast to the case-control study of Lincoff and colleagues,[44] registry results from the New York Hospital-Cornell Medical Centre suggested a benefit of stenting for the treatment of acute vessel closure.[45] Using registry data, angioplasty complication rates in 2242 consecutive patients at this tertiary-care referral centre were compared before and after coronary stents became available. Major complications (composite of in-hospital death, Q-wave myocardial infarction, and need for emergency bypass surgery) occurred in 4.1% of patients treated before stents were available and in 2.0% of patients afterwards (p < 0.01), which suggests a benefit of coronary stenting.

Although the results of the TASC II trial and preliminary results from the STENT-BY trial suggest a benefit for stenting over other treatments for acute or threatened closure, the GRACE trial will provide clear information on the direct comparison between the two preferred treatments – stent implantation and autoperfusion balloon treatment. Despite the lack of conclusive results from completed randomized trials, because of the additional catheterization time required with prolonged balloon inflation, and because of the significant crossover to stenting with this strategy, early stenting for the treatment of acute and threatened closure may indeed be the best approach. The timing of stent implantation for abrupt closure also appears to be important. The risk of myocardial infarction is nearly three times higher when stents are used for established acute closure than when they are used for threatened closure.[46]

Stent design may make a profound difference in clinical and angiographic medium-term outcome. This was recently suggested by the results of a trial in which the Gianturco–Roubin and the Palmaz–Schatz stents were compared.[47] Twenty-five patients were included in each group and matched according to vessel size, location of the target lesion, and dissection type. These results showed a greater late loss in those lesions treated with the coil Gianturco–Roubin stent than with the Palmaz–Schatz stent (0.96 ± 0.75 mm *vs* 0.62 ± 0.55 mm respectively, p = 0.05). Angiographic restenosis (>50% diameter stenosis) occurred in four (16%) lesions treated with the tubular stent and in 10 (40%) lesions treated with the coil stent (p < 0.05). This result suggests that stent design may have a significant influence on 6-months outcome. Clearly, further randomized trials are necessary to confirm this interesting finding. In addition, information on the long-term outcome after stent implantation for acute or threatened closure is still lacking.

Primary reduction in restenosis in de-novo focal lesions in vessels greater than 3.0 mm in diameter

Histological studies have shown that irrespective of the type of vessel wall injury, neointimal hyperplasia as a non-specific tissue reaction will occur, and may lead to restenosis when excessive. Intracoronary stent implantation may reduce the restenosis rate by optimizing the acute angiographic results, which allows greater accommodation of the neointimal tissue.[48] One factor that may account for the improved immediate results is the prevention of elastic recoil. Elastic recoil has been reported to account for a 32%–47% loss of the maximum achievable vessel diameter or cross-sectional area immediately after balloon angioplasty.[49,50] In contrast, the recoil is 4%–18% with Palmaz–Schatz stent implantation and 20%–22% with Gianturco–Roubin or Wiktor stent implantation.[51,52] In addition to prevention of acute recoil, stent implantation may have favourable effects on vessel wall remodeling.[53,54]

There are eight completed trials comparing stenting with PTCA in de-novo lesions in the native circulation.[1,2,55–67] All of these trials show a significant benefit in the rate of restenosis seen at follow-up for Palmaz–Schatz stent implantation compared with balloon angioplasty alone. The favourable results of these trials have been used to justify the enormous increase in the use of stents as the first choice of treatment strategy in patients referred for balloon angioplasty. Caution must be exercised, however, in the interpretation of the results of these trials. The observed benefits of stent implantation may only apply to a select group of patients, as dictated by the inclusion and exclusion criteria of the studies. The conclusions of these trials may not apply to patients with different lesion characteristics (long, multiple, mainstem) or to patients in whom the technical approach differs (stent type, multiple stents, periprocedural management). In these subgroups, additional data are needed. Care must also be exercised when assessing the patients included in these studies. For instance, meta-analysis of the BENESTENT and STRESS I and II trials suggests that stent placement in vessels less than 2.6 mm in diameter and in those greater than 3.4 mm in diameter gives no advantage in either restenosis rates or in clinical events when compared with angioplasty alone.[68] Similarly, working on the premise that "bigger is better", stratification of the patients in the BENESTENT trial, based on acute angiographic results, suggested that in those patients treated with balloon angioplasty in whom a 30% or less diameter stenosis was obtained at the time of the intervention, 1-year outcome was similar to stented patients with comparable acute angiographic results.[39] The expression "stent-like" was coined in reference to such an agreeable angioplasty result. The strategy of striving for and accepting a stent-like result with balloon angioplasty has been termed "provisional stenting".[69,70] In the BENESTENT trial, stent-like results were achieved in 35% of patients treated with angioplasty alone. Thus, not all patients similar to those included in the BENESTENT study may benefit from primary stent implantation. A strategy of balloon angioplasty in vessels with a diameter of less than 2.6 mm, and acceptance of postprocedural stent-like results in those vessels above 2.6 mm diameter, may result in long-term outcomes comparable with non-selective stenting. The results of several recently reported randomized trials support the application of the principles of provisional stenting.[65-67] However, a clinically relevant consensus on the definition of what constitutes optimum balloon angioplasty is required before clinical guidelines can be instituted.

Saphenous vein graft disease

The growing numbers of patients with previous cardiac surgery and aged bypass grafts have made the management of patients with recurrent angina after coronary bypass surgery an increasing clinical challenge. Attrition rates of saphenous vein grafts of 15%–20% in the first year after bypass surgery, of 1%–2% per year from 1 to 6 years after surgery, and of 4% per year between years 6 and 10, have been reported.[71] By 10 years, about 50% of the grafts are occluded. As a result of attrition and progression of coronary artery disease, 10%–15% of bypass patients will require repeat surgery within 10 years of the initial operation. Re-operation is technically more difficult and is associated with a higher mortality (3%–7%) and a higher perioperative myocardial infarction rate (3%–12%).[71] For these reasons, percutaneous treatments of patients with bypass graft disease have been developed.

In selected cases, balloon angioplasty is associated with a high initial success rate of between 75% and 94%, with a combined overall success rate of 88%.[71] Although the consequences of balloon dilatation of saphenous bypass grafts are less predictable than angioplasty in the native coronary circulation, the complication rate is relatively low, with a procedure-related death rate of less than 1%, a myocardial infarction rate of around 4%, and a need for urgent surgery of less than 2%. These comparatively good immediate results are offset by a high restenosis rate and poor long-term clinical outcome. The reported restenosis rate is 28% for lesions in the distal end of the graft, but 58% for ostial or very proximal lesions, and 52% for lesions in the body of the graft. The reported 5-year survival and event-free survival (freedom from myocardial infarction, repeat bypass surgery, and angioplasty) are 74% and 26%, respectively.[72]

Results of several observational studies have shown a high procedural success rate for stenting of vein grafts, and an improved long-term graft patency and in-hospital clinical outcome[73-95] (table 4.2). The incidence of restenosis in the early observational trials was as high as 47%,[80] but in the later studies restenosis rates below 20% were reported.[83,84] The restenosis rate after stenting of non-ostial lesions (29%) is significantly lower than stenting of ostial lesions (60%–62%, $p=0.008$)[95,96] – this is similar to findings with balloon angioplasty. The results of the SAVED (SAphenous VEin graft De novo) trial are in agreement with those of the observational studies, showing an improved clinical outcome at 6-months follow-up in patients with vein graft disease treated with stent implantation.[97,98] Based on the results of the observational series and the SAVED study, stenting with the Palmaz–Schatz stent in short, non-restenotic, non-ostial vein graft lesions is associated with better acute and intermediate-term outcomes compared with PTCA.

There are very few data available on the long-term results of stenting in saphenous vein graft disease. A single-centre observational trial recently reported 5-years follow-up results of 62 post-bypass patients treated with stent implantation.[99] Overall survival at 5 years was 83%, and event-free survival was 30%. Analysis of pooled data from the medical literature shows similar results, with 5-years event-free survival of 26% after balloon angioplasty, 30% after stent implantation, and 63%–76% after repeat surgery.[99] Results of medium-term and predicted long-term clinical outcomes of a single-centre American observational series have also been reported.[86] In that study, patients judged to be at high risk for repeat surgical repair or repeat angioplasty were followed-up (high surgical risk: severe or multiple comorbid conditions, poor left ventricular function, more than one previous CABG; high procedural risk: unstable angina, recent myocardial infarction, age >70 years, type C lesions). Mean follow-up was 19.1 ± 13.5 months. Kaplan-Meier estimated survival at 4 years was predicted to be reasonably high at 0.79 ± 0.06. Recurrent events, however, were quite frequent, with an estimated event-free survival of only 0.29 ± 0.07.

Chronic total occlusions

Balloon angioplasty of chronically occluded arteries is associated with a high incidence of luminal renarrowing, reocclusion and restenosis.[100,101] The failure of PTCA to produce a favourable long-term outcome has prompted the search for alternative treatments for this subset of lesions. Available observational data suggest that coronary stent implantation is feasible and may show benefit with respect to reocclusion and restenosis when compared with historical data of standard angioplasty after resolution of flow in an occluded vessel[102–118] (table 4.3). Despite the relative paucity of observational results, three randomized trials have reported compelling data that show a significant benefit of stenting a successfully opened chronic total occlusion over balloon angioplasty alone. Unfortunately, both the SICCO[119,120] and GISSOC[121] trials used the outdated stenting techniques of relatively low-pressure stent deployment and postprocedural anticoagulation, and most (63%) of the patients in the SPACTO trial were also treated with these outmoded methods.[122,123] Only two observational studies that used high inflation pressures for final stent expansion, and postprocedural antiplatelet therapy without anticoagulation, have been reported.[111,114] Both of these studies showed very encouraging results, with rates of restenosis of under 30%. Multivariate analysis of stent implantation in chronic

Table 4.2 Events following stent implantation in saphenous vein bypass grafts

| Study | Report year | Patients (lesions) | Implantation success (%) | In-hospital complications (%) | | | Subacute occlusion (%) | Restenosis (%) |
				Death	AMI	Urgent CABG		
Wallstent								
Keane et al[75]	1994	29 (30)	97	0	0	0	3.4	32
Strauss et al[73]	1992	101 (135)	NR	4	NR	NR	8	39
Urban et al[76]	1989	13 (14)	100	0	0	0	0	20
Stewart et al[74]	1992	58 (68)	99	1.7	1.7	NR	3.4	NR
Joseph et al[77]	1997	53 (59)	NR	5.6	NR	NR	0	27
Nordrehaug et al[78]	1994	19 (19)	100	0	5.3	0	10.5	17
de Jaegere et al[79]	1996	62 (62)	98	3.2	3.2	4.8	NR	53
de Scheerder et al[80]	1992	69 (95)	100	1.4	7.2	5.8	10	47
Gianturco–Roubin								
Dorros et al[94]	1994	96 (101)	99	3.1	8.3	0	1.1	–
Bilodeau et al[93]	1992	37 (37)	NR	0	13.5	0	NR	35

Table 4.2 continued

Palmaz–Schatz								
Wong et al[91]	1995	589 (624)	99	1.7	5.1	0.9	1.4	30
Fenton et al[90]	1994	198 (209)	99	0.4	0	0	0.5	34
Leon et al[82]	1993	589 (NR)	97	1.7	0.3	0.9	1.4	30
Strumpf et al[83]	1992	26 (30)	100	0	7.7	0	3.8	13
Maiello et al[85]	1994	43 (50)	94	2	4	2	NR	11
Frimerman et al[86]	1997	186 (244)	97	1.1	1.1	0.5	1.6	NR
Pomerantz et al[85]	1992	69 (84)	99	0	0	0	0	25
Palmaz–Schatz/Biliary								
Rechavia et al[216]	1995	29 (29)	100	0	0	0	0	NR
Wong et al[88]	1995	234 (309)	99	1.3	0.9	0.4	1.7	NR
Piana et al[84]	1994	111 (145)	99	0.6	7.3	0	0.6	17
Wiktor								
Fortuna et al[92]	1993	101 (NR)	95	1	3	1	2	NR
Mixed								
Eeckhout et al[81]	1994	40 (58)	100	2	0	2	NR	25

NR = not reported.

Table 4.3 Events following stent implantation in chronic total occlusions

Study	Study period	Lesions (n)	Implantation success (%)	In-hospital complications (%) Death	AMI	Urgent CABG	Acute/subacute thrombosis (%)	Restenosis %
Wallstent								
Ozaki et al[103]	NR	20	100	0	0	0	3.3	29
Palmaz–Schatz								
Almagor et al[105]	NR	65	97	1.5	1.5	0	3.1	24
Nienaber et al[110]	NR	100	NR	NR	NR	NR	0	19
Medina et al[102]	NR	30	100	0	0	0	6.7	22
Goldberg et al[104]	1989–93	60	98	0	1.7	0	5.1	20
Mori et al[115]	1992–95	43	100	0	0	NR	2.3	27.9
Wiktor								
Anzuini et al[113]	1993–96	91	98	0	1.1	1.1	6	32
Anzuini et al[116]	1993–97	93	98	0	4	NR	4	27

Table 4.3 continued

Various

Rau et al[114]	1994–95	121	NR	NR	NR	NR	NR	22
Gambhir et al[112]	1995–97	42	100	0	0	0	0	25
Moussa et al[111]	1993–95	94	95	0	5.3	3.2	3	27
Suttorp et al[109]	1995	39	97	0	0	0	0	40
Etuso et al[108]	NR	126	100	NR	NR	NR	NR	76

NR = not reported.

total coronary occlusions, using high-pressure deployment techniques and postprocedural antiplatelet therapy, has shown four variables to have an independent, statistically significant influence on the likelihood of a restenosis or a reocclusion: 1) the presence of a dissection after balloon angioplasty; 2) a minimum luminal diameter (MLD) post-stenting of 2.54 mm or less; 3) a stented vessel segment length of more than 16 mm; and 4) a balloon/vessel diameter ratio for final stent expansion of 1.00 or less.[111] These data suggest that the MLD after stenting should be at least 2.5 mm and that the balloon diameter for stent expansion should exceed the vessel reference diameter by 25%.[111] However, over-expansion of a vessel carries a risk of severe dissection, and to prevent this complication two precautions have been advanced. First, the length of the balloon used for stent expansion must not exceed the length of the stented vessel segment. Second, in the situation of a calcified lesion, debulking techniques should be considered.[111] Long-term follow-up of the SICCO patients to 33 months showed a continued benefit for stenting over angioplasty alone for total occlusions.[124–126] Thus, although existing data overwhelmingly support stent implantation after successful recanalization for the treatment of chronic total occlusions, future randomized trials are needed to confirm the superiority of stent placement over PTCA alone in the era of high-pressure stent deployment and postprocedural antiplatelet therapy, and prospective studies are needed to define further the clinical factors that will lead to a more favourable outcome.

Acute myocardial infarction

To overcome the limitations of thrombolytic therapy (TIMI 3 flow achieved around 55% of the time, rare but often serious haemorrhagic complications), balloon angioplasty has been introduced as an alternative for the treatment of patients with an acute myocardial infarction.[127–129] Results of a meta-analysis of 10 prospective randomized trials show that compared with thrombolytic therapy, primary PTCA (balloon angioplasty without antecedent thrombolytic therapy) results in a more frequent restoration of TIMI 3 flow, and reduces rates of mortality, reinfarction, and stroke.[130,131] Despite these promising results, balloon treatment is associated with reocclusion of the infarct artery in 5%–10% of the patients, and gives a reinfarction rate of 3%–5%.[132–134] At 6-months follow-up, 10%–15% of the patients show a total occlusion of the treated artery, and angiographic restenosis is present in 30%–50% of patients.[135] Reports that the implantation of a metallic endoprosthesis into a thrombogenic environment increases subacute thrombosis rates[136] resulted in an early reluctance for their use in acute myocardial infarction. With improved stent-implantation techniques and the introduction of ticlopidine, several reports of stent implantation in the setting of failed primary PTCA for acute myocardial infarction have shown that stenting is feasible, safe, and effective, and has low subacute occlusion rates comparable with those of bailout stenting after elective balloon angioplasty.[137–152] The advantage of antiplatelet therapy only after stent placement was suggested in a trial by Neumann and colleagues.[137] In that trial, 80 patients with complicated angioplasty for acute myocardial infarction were treated with stent implantation, the last 30 of whom were treated without postprocedural oral anticoagulants with very good outcomes.

The very low subacute occlusion rates observed with stent implantation in the setting of acute myocardial infarction for bailout purposes, or for suboptimal results after PTCA, prompted investigations to focus on the utility of stents as primary treatment for acute myocardial infarction. A small, single-centre Italian registry[153] treated 22 patients who had acute myocardial infarction, with primary stenting. Inclusion criteria into this trial were very selective (<6 hours after onset of chest pain, culprit vessel diameter >3 mm, single vessel disease, target lesion length <15 mm). The results of the trial were quite good, with all stents patent at 24 hours, and recurrence of symptoms in only one patient at intermediate-term follow-up. Postprocedure pharmacotherapy included intravenous heparin, aspirin, ticlopidine, and subcutaneous low-molecular-weight heparin. Angiographic follow-up was only done in 50% of the patients, and restenosis was observed in only one patient studied. Numerous subsequent reports from other observational trials with primary stent implantation in acute myocardial infarction have also been favourable.[154–175]

The results of the prospective pilot study STAMI (STenting in Acute Myocardial Infarction) were also encouraging.[176,177] The inclusion criteria in this trial were broader than those in the Italian trial (chest pain <12 hours, ST segment elevation, target vessel diameter ≥3.0 mm). A total of 55 patients were enrolled. In-hospital death occurred in 4.2% of patients. At 6-months follow-up there was one additional death. Chest pain recurred in 33% of patients, myocardial infarction in 4%, and 15% required target vessel revascularization. All patients in this trial were treated with aspirin, ticlopidine, and coumadin.

The results of the STENTIM I Study (French Registry of Stenting in Acute Myocardial Infarction),[178] the prelude to the larger randomized STENTIM II Study, are now available. STENTIM I was a prospective observational study in 20 centres, that included 648 consecutive patients who underwent PTCA with stent implantation for acute myocardial infarction. Of the 648 patients, 269 (41.5%) were dilated early (<24 hours) after the onset of symptoms, and 379 (58.5%) were dilated between 24 hours and 14 days after their myocardial infarction. Combined ticlopidine/aspirin antiplatelet therapy was used after the procedure. Successful stent implantation, as determined by angiographic criteria, was successful in both groups of patients (96% and 97% respectively). During the in-hospital follow-up period, there were 14 (5.2%) deaths in the group dilated early, and 11 (3.9%) deaths in the group dilated later. Stent thrombosis occurred in eight (3%) patients in the early group, compared with six (1.6%) patients in the later group. Multivariate analysis of this cohort identified bailout stenting as the sole predictor of stent thrombosis.

A prelude to the larger randomized PAMI-Stent trial, the PAMI-Stent pilot study was a prospective pilot study which examined the role of primary stenting as a reperfusion strategy for patients with acute myocardial infarction.[179] A total of 312 consecutive patients treated with primary PTCA for acute myocardial infarction at nine international centres were prospectively enrolled. After PTCA, stenting was attempted in all eligible lesions (vessel size ≥ 3 mm and ≤ 4 mm; lesion length <2 stents; absence of excessive thrombus burden after PTCA; major side branch jeopardy; or proximal tortuosity or calcification). Patients were treated with aspirin, ticlopidine, and a 60-hour tapering heparin regimen. Stenting (primarily with the Palmaz–Schatz stent) was found to be feasible in 240 (77%) of the 312 consecutive patients, with a 98% procedural success rate.[179] Patients with stents had a low rate of in-hospital death (0.8%), reinfarction (1.7%), recurrent ischaemia (3.8%), and predischarge target vessel revascularization for ischaemia (1.3%).[179,180] At 30-days follow-up, no additional deaths or reinfarctions occurred among patients with stents, and target vessel revascularization was required in only one additional patient (93.7% were event free). At 6-months follow-up, 83.3% were event-free (alive, without reinfarction or target vessel revascularization).[181] Nine-months angiographic follow-up is underway. Similarly favourable results were reported from the 18-centre PAMI Heparin Coated Stent Pilot Trial, in which the 30-days and 7-months event-free survival rates in 101 patients with acute myocardial infarction were 97.0% and 81.2% respectively, after implantation of heparin-coated Palmaz–Schatz stents.[182–185] Restenosis rates at 6 months were reported as 15.3%.[183,184] Despite these encouraging preliminary results, differences in outcome between the two groups could be due to differences in the population of patients and investigator bias. This underscores the importance of the results of randomized trials designed to compare PTCA alone with stent implantation.

The results of four small randomized trials of stenting in the setting of acute myocardial infarction have been reported (GRAMI,[187–190] PASTA,[191,192] Zwolle Myocardial Infarction,[193–195] and FRESCO[196–198]), and five other larger trials are nearing completion (PAMI-Stent,[199,200] CADILLAC,[201] PRISAM,[202] STENTIM II,[203] and BESSAMI[204]). The favourable reports of the randomized trials, although impressive must be judged with some caution. The published trials are all relatively small, the largest being the GRAMI trial that enrolled 227 patients. The entry criteria of these trials must be carefully scrutinized. For example, the exclusive entry criteria of the Zwolle trial resulted in 50% of the patients with acute myocardial infarction undergoing primary PTCA being judged clinically and anatomically ineligible for stenting.[194] Of the ineligible patients, 27% were excluded because of small vessel size or diffuse disease. A large-scale German registry failed to show any benefit of coronary stenting over balloon angioplasty in the setting of acute myocardial infarction.[175] That registry analysed data from 2331 direct interventional procedures, lending validity to the findings despite the observational design of the study. Unlike the reported randomized trials that treated selected patients in highly specialized centres, large-scale observational studies are more likely to represent "real world" patients in a more diverse range of hospitals.

Although the randomized trials show a benefit, it is still not clear which patient and lesion characteristics respond best to acute infarct stenting. A prospective German study, in which stenting was attempted in 560 patients with acute myocardial infarction admitted within 72 hours from onset of pain, has examined the risk factors for stenting[205]. The occurrence of death, non-fatal repeat acute myocardial infarction or stroke during the first month represented the combined endpoint of this study. Results showed that the strongest risk factors by Cox analysis were cardiogenic shock before the procedure, reduced left ventricular function, and post-stenting therapy without ticlopidine. The study endpoint was reached by 3.4% of 494 patients without shock, and by only 1.96% of 407 patients without shock and with ticlopidine therapy. Whether stents should be used empirically or only when the balloon-angioplasty results are suboptimal (the concept of provisional stenting) must also be considered. Results of an observational study, and of the FRESCO randomized trial suggest a potential benefit of coronary stenting over stent-like PTCA in acute myocardial infarction, with both short-term and long-term outcomes being better in the stented patients.[172,196–198] Large-scale randomized trials need to be done to answer this very important question.

The compelling results of the randomized trials reported to date clearly show a benefit of direct stent implantation over balloon angioplasty for the treatment of acute myocardial infarctions. The results of the large-scale registry studies are much less favourable, which suggests that further randomized trials are needed to define the subset of patients that will show the greatest benefit from stent implantation. The results of the ongoing trials should help establish the role of primary stent implantation in patients undergoing catheter-based intervention for the treatment of acute myocardial infarction.

Data from randomized trials, and from observational studies and case reports show that there may be a benefit for the use of stents in:

1. the treatment of restenotic lesions;
2. ostial and left main disease;
3. bifurcation lesions.

Restenotic lesions after previous balloon angioplasty

Irrespective of the definition of restenosis, it is estimated that approximately 25% of all percutaneous coronary interventions are done for the treatment of restenosis of a previously dilated lesion.[206] Previous studies evaluating treatment with balloon angioplasty for restenosis have found that the procedure can be done safely, without complications or a higher risk of subsequent restenosis.[207–211] The pathological substrate of the restenotic lesion is different from that of a primary stenosis, and therefore the favourable results of the primary restenosis prevention trials probably cannot be extrapolated to secondary restenosis prevention. There have been several published reports from observational studies which have addressed stent placement in restenotic lesions, although in many of these trials stent placement was not the main focus, and most were done in the early days of stenting.[212–220] Several of these trials showed higher restenosis rates for stenting for restenotic narrowings compared with de-novo lesions. Savage and colleagues[217] analysed 300 consecutive patients with elective stent implantation in native vessels. They reported a restenosis rate of 14% in de-novo lesions compared with 39% in restenotic lesions. Moscucci and colleagues[219] also reported a higher second restenosis rate for restenotic narrowings (37% *vs* 24%) treated with either stent placement or atherectomy, although they believed that the difference may have been due to a preselection of patients in the restenotic group for factors predisposing to restenosis. Mittal and colleagues[220] studied 114 consecutive patients. In their series, 37% of the stents were deployed in de-novo lesions and 63% in restenotic lesions. They observed a higher restenosis rate in the restenotic group than in those with de-novo lesions (15% *vs* 37%, $p = 0.05$), although the two groups of patients were similar with regard to factors associated with restenosis.

Results of one of these observational trials[218] showed that the number of balloon angioplasty procedures done before stent implantation did not influence the risk for subsequent restenosis after stenting. The odds for restenosis in the situation of stent implantation for a second, third, or fourth restenosis compared with stent implantation for a first restenosis was 0.8 (95% CI 0.4–1.8) according to the 0.72 mm criterion, and 1.5 (95% CI 0.6–3.7) based on the 50% diameter stenosis criterion. The only significant predictor of recurrence of restenosis was the relative gain when it exceeded 0.48 (odds ratio 2.7, 95% CI 1.1–6.4) based on the 0.72 mm criterion. This result confirms earlier data that showed that deep arterial injury is associated with more extensive neointimal proliferation.

In a recent prospective analysis, the long-term outcome of some of the first patients to be stented were reported.[221] A total of 113 stents (78 Wallstents, 29 Palmaz–Schatz, 6 Wiktor) were implanted in 106 patients to treat restenosis following angioplasty in both native coronaries (86 cases) and in vein grafts (20 cases). Follow-up at 6 months showed a combined angiographic and restenosis rate of 18%, and a clinical-event rate of 20%. Long-term follow-up at a mean of 65 months showed that an additional 9% of patients experienced a clinical event and 14% showed angiographic restenosis that occurred between 6 and 65 months.

The results of observational studies and the REST trial show that stent implantation may be superior to balloon angioplasty for a reduction in recurrent restenosis. Further trials are currently underway to verify the favourable results in patients with stent-like results after balloon angioplasty that were observed in the REST trial.

Ostial and left main disease

Aorto-ostial stenoses are not amenable to treatment with balloon angioplasty because of the elasticity of the aorta. There are only a few small, uncontrolled, observational studies that suggest that stent implantation is feasible and that it results in good angiographic results in aorto-ostial saphenous vein graft lesions[78,86,222–227] and ostial right coronary lesions.[222,224,228] In these situations, results of observational series suggest that stenting may be superior to both directional atherectomy[227] and balloon angioplasty.[228] Stent implantation in the aorto-ostial position is technically difficult, and this is a situation where IVUS (intravascular ultrasound) assessment may help to assess the degree of calcification before stenting, to guide proper stent sizing, and to ensure adequate stent expansion and apposition to the vessel wall.

Two trials that report on stent placement in the ostium of the LAD (left anterior descending artery)[222,228] show encouraging results. In a small trial analysing Palmaz–Schatz stent placement in 23 ostial LAD lesions, no acute adverse events occurred.[227] There was one case of subacute thrombosis, and at follow-up the restenosis rate was 22%. The anatomical characteristics differ between aorto-ostial vein graft lesions, aorto-ostial right coronary artery lesions, and ostial circumflex and LAD lesions, which probably contributes to differences in behaviour post-stenting, with restenosis rates as high as 62% in ostial vein-graft stents. Although the results to date look promising, large registry series or randomized trials are necessary to support conclusively the use of stents for ostial stenoses.

Left main stenosis is the most serious manifestation of coronary artery disease. The prognosis of medically treated patients with left main disease is poor, with a 3-year mortality rate of around 50%.[230] Left main stenosis has long been regarded as an absolute indication for coronary artery bypass surgery. Although bypass surgery significantly improves survival, patients with left main coronary artery disease are in the highest risk group. Results of the CASS study show an overall operative mortality of 3.5%, with risk increased with more severe stenoses and when a larger myocardial territory is in jeopardy.[231,232] Patients with left main coronary artery disease can be divided into two groups; protected (those with at least one patent bypass graft to the left anterior descending or circumflex coronary arteries), and unprotected. Experience with balloon angioplasty of left main coronary stenoses reported varying degrees of procedural success, but uniformly poor long-term results.[233–235] The use of adjuvant therapies such as percutaneous cardiopulmonary bypass,[236] autoperfusion catheter,[237] and intra-aortic balloon counterpulsation[238] have all failed to improve the poor long-term prognosis of percutaneously treated left main coronary artery disease.[239] These unfavourable findings led most interventionists to agree with a 1988 report by an American College of Cardiology/American Heart Association Task Force[240] that judged unprotected left main coronary artery disease an absolute contraindication to percutaneous treatment.[240] However, for critically ill patients in whom operative risk is prohibitive, stenting of unprotected left main coronary stenoses has been attempted.[241–249] There have also been a few reports of unprotected left main stenting in bailout situations.[250–252] Elective stenting in patients with unprotected lesions of the left main coronary artery has generally been judged to be contraindicated, primarily due to the potential for catastrophic consequences of abrupt closure and the poor clinical tolerance to restenosis. However, with recent improvement in stent-implantation techniques, post-stent antithrombotic regimens, and operator experience, this contraindication to stenting is being re-evaluated. Park and colleagues[253] have reported the results of elective stent placement in 42 patients with unprotected left main coronary stenoses and normal left ventricular function treated from 1995 to 1997. All but one were considered good surgical candidates but had refused bypass surgery, and all were treated with both aspirin and ticlopidine after stent implantation. The procedural success rate was 100%. There were no episodes of subacute stent thrombosis and angiographic restenosis occurred in seven patients (22%) at 6-months follow-up. The only death occurred 2 days after elective coronary bypass surgery for in-stent restenosis. Similarly favourable results have been reported by Laruelle and colleagues,[254] who reported their experience with left main stent implantation in 18 patients. Elective stent implantation was done in 10 patients, of whom seven were considered good surgical candidates. Of the patients in whom stents were electively implanted, the procedural success rate was 100%. There were no procedural complications and only one patient experienced an in-hospital myocardial infarction and required additional PTCA of the proximal circumflex artery. In the emergency group, however, a high rate of major events during the hospital stay was noted. Two patients died, one experienced a non-Q wave myocardial infarction, and one required urgent surgical revascularization. During clinical follow-up (average of 10 months) no major cardiac events were seen in either group. Romero and colleagues[255] treated 42 patients who had left main coronary disease with elective stent implantation. All patients received an antithrombotic regimen of low-molecular-weight heparin, ticlopidine, and aspirin. In 11 patients, the lesion involved the bifurcation, and nine patients needed additional balloon dilatation of ostium of the circumflex through the metallic structure of the stent. Primary success was obtained in 40 (95%) patients. Major in-hospital complications were a non-Q wave myocardial infarction (one patient) and a peri-interventional death (one patient). There were no episodes of subacute stent thrombosis. At 9-months angiographic follow-up, four (15%) patients showed restenosis at the treated segment. Similar small retrospective analyses by Barragan and colleagues,[256] Tamara and colleagues,[257,258] and Silvestri and colleagues[259] have also shown encouraging results in selected patients. The results of studies of elective stent implantation in an unprotected left main coronary artery of patients judged to be good surgical candidates are summarized in table 4.4. The 16-centre ULTIMA (Unprotected Left main Trunk Intervention Multicentre Assessment) registry is also currently underway. This study will collect data on consecutive unprotected left main transcatheter treatments from 1994 to the present.[260] Results from this registry will provide further information on the feasibility and success of all modes of transcatheter treatment for left main disease, which may affect the design of future trials.

In summary, results from the few available observational analyses show that elective stenting of unprotected left main coronary artery stenoses can be done with a high success rate and a low complication rate, and suggest that stenting is a reasonable revascularization option in elective cases. The data must be interpreted with caution, however, because selection bias and the small numbers of patients may have contributed to the favourable results. At present, however, CABG surgery remains the treatment of choice for all patients with significant left main disease other than for those who are clearly not surgical candidates. The available data strongly support the initiation of randomized trials to compare left main coronary artery stenting with surgical management for those patients who are good surgical candidates.

Bifurcation lesions

A bifurcation lesion is defined as the presence of a greater than 50% stenosis involving both a parent vessel and the ostium of its side branch. Balloon angioplasty of such stenoses is associated with a significant risk of side branch occlusion[261] through plaque shift, dissection, or elastic recoil of the treated ostium, and several techniques have been developed in an attempt to reduce the treatment failure rate.[262–267] If a stent is to be deployed in the parent vessel, compression and extrusion of plaque may compromise flow in the side-branch where it originates from the treated segment. Fischman and colleagues[268] reported a 5% incidence of occlusion of side-branches as a result of Palmaz–Schatz stenting in the main artery. However, 14% of side-branches were occluded if the ostium of the side-branch had a stenosis of 50% or more. For relatively small side-branches (≤ 20 mm in diameter), worsening of ostial stenoses after stenting does not usually lead to major clinical events, although if there is concern, these stenoses can be dilated before stent implantation in the main vessel.[269] In the event that symptomatic closure does occur in small side-branch vessels, dilatation through the struts of certain stents with low profile balloons is possible, and may be required.[268,269] Experimental studies have tested

Table 4.4 Events following elective stent implantation in unprotected left main stenoses in patients considered to be good surgical candidates

| Study | Patients (n) | Implantation success (%) | In-hospital complications (%) | | | Acute/subacute thrombosis (%) | Restenosis (%) |
			Death	AMI	Urgent CABG		
Park et al[255]	42	100	0	0	0	0	22
Laruelle et al[254]	7	100	0	14	0	0	NR
Romero et al[255]	42	95	2	2	0	0	NR
Tamura et al[258]	11	100	0	0	0	0	18
Barragan et al[256]	21	100	0	0	0	0	NR
Silvestri et al[259]	29	100	0	0	0	0	NR

NR = not reported.

several balloons that will pass through a deployed Palmaz–Schatz stent and return intact without damaging the stent.[270] Some stent designs allow passage of a second balloon and stent through the struts of the first.[271] Stent implantation in bifurcation lesions in which both branches are 2.0 mm or more in diameter requires an approach that will ensure easy access to both the main and side-branch vessels, and that will give optimum final results.

Borrowing from the experience with angioplasty, new stenting techniques are being investigated for the treatment of bifurcation stenoses. A "kissing stent" procedure has been described,[272,273] which is analogous to the "kissing balloon" technique introduced by Gruentzig in 1981 and presented by Meier[267] in 1984 (figure 4.1). This procedure involves simultaneous inflation of two separate balloons, one in the parent vessel and one in the side-branch, followed by simultaneous stent deployment. The stents are positioned so that they lie side by side in the main vessel proximal to the crotch, and each of their distal ends extends into the one leg of the bifurcation. The stents are expanded alternately in a step-wise fashion to maintain correct stent position. Final expansion is done with the simultaneous inflation of two balloons at the same pressure to minimize obstruction to flow.

Other approaches that have been recently described include the "Y" technique, a "T" technique, and the "Culotte" technique. The "Y" technique, a modification of the "kissing stent" procedure, involves the simultaneous deployment of stents at the ostia of the side-branch and the parent vessel distal to the take-off of the side-branch, followed by placement of a third stent proximal to the crotch[274,275] (figure 4.2). The (proximal) third stent can either be crimped on two balloons and advanced to the carina, or it can be mounted on a single balloon with final kissing-balloon expansion. None of the stents in the resultant "Y" configuration are overlapping. A variant of the "Y" stenting approach has been described by Khoja and colleagues.[276] They took advantage of the design of the tantalum Tensum stent, which is fashioned with subunits connected with short bridges. A single stent was bent at the articulation site and mounted on two balloons. The folded stent on the two balloons was introduced as a unit and advanced such that one portion was positioned in the ostium of the side-branch and the other distal to the carina in the main vessel, to cover both legs of the bifurcation simultaneously. The connecting bridge of both parts of the stent enabled precise positioning of the stent exactly at the bifurcation site. A second stent was inserted to cover the main vessel proximal to the bifurcation over the same two balloons. Although a Tensum stent was used by these investigators, any tubular crimpable stent with a single articulation can be used (eg, Palmaz–Schatz). A technique in which all three stents are introduced in a single manoeuvre has also been described, in what has been called the "inverted Y" technique (figure 4.3).

In the "T" stenting technique, two coil or tubular stents can be used. The first

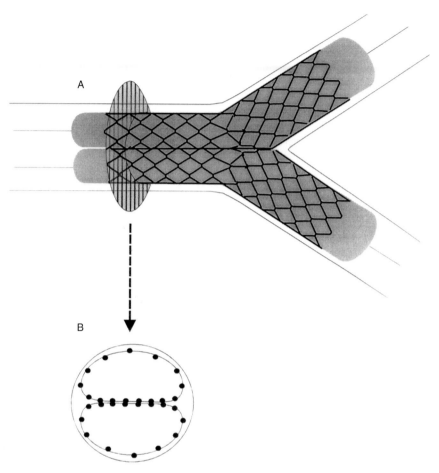

Figure 4.1: *The kissing stent technique for the treatment of bifurcation lesions. A. Two stents are implanted, which cover the main vessel proximal to the bifurcation and both branches. The two balloons are dilated alternately in a stepwise fashion to maintain correct position during deployment. The final expansion is done with the simultaneous inflation of the two balloons at the same pressure. B. Cross-section through the main vessel showing the metal flow-divider created by the abutting stents. (Modified from di Mario C, Colombo A. Trouser-Stents: how to choose the right size and shape? Cathet Cardiovasc Diagn 1997;* **41:** *197–99.)*

stent is normally implanted in the main vessel, and a second stent is inserted in the side branch through the struts of the previously deployed stent.[277,278] Alternatively, in situations where the angle of separation of the bifurcation is large, the side-branch can be stented first. This may be necessary since the second stent may not be able to negotiate the acute bend into the side-branch.[279]

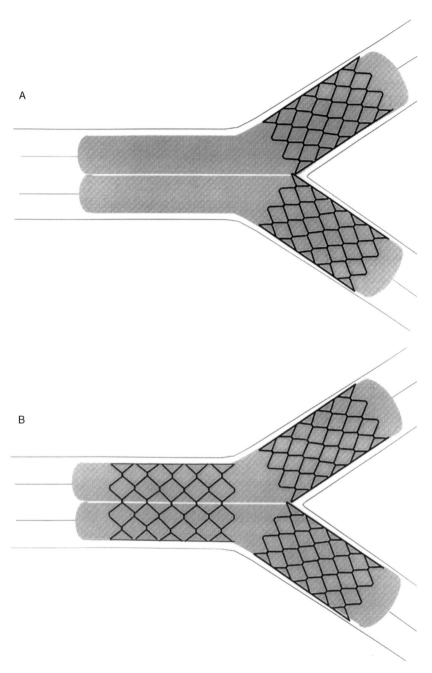

Figure 4.2: *The "Y" technique for the treatment of bifurcation lesions. A. Two stents are implanted from the ostium of both branches. B. A stent crimped on two balloons is advanced to both branches. Alternatively, the third stent can be mounted on one balloon with a final kissing balloon expansion.*

163

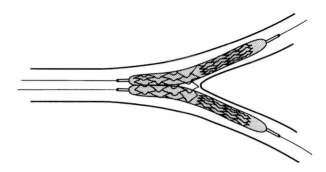

Figure 4.3: *The Colombo "Inverted Y" technique for the treatment of bifurcation lesions. Three stents are mounted on suitably long balloons, one stent being mounted on both balloons. The entire "bifurcation stent" is placed in one manoeuvre.*

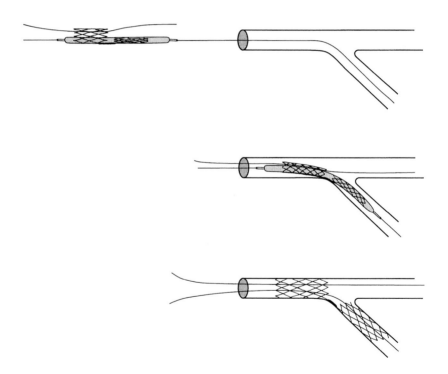

Figure 4.4: *A modification of the "T" stenting technique for the treatment of bifurcation lesions. This method takes advantage of the central bridge of articulated stents. The stent is positioned in both the main vessel and the most angulated leg of the bifurcation, ensuring that the central articulation is positioned at the most proximal portion of the ostium of the side branch. After deployment, a second stent is introduced through the proximal portion of the first.*

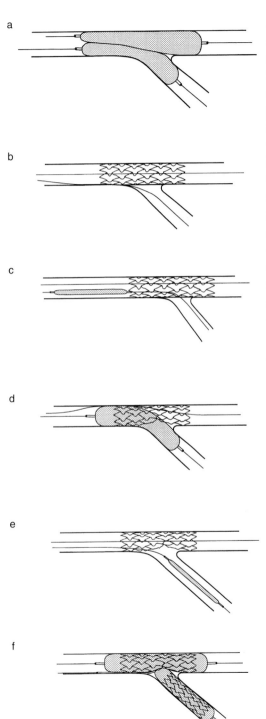

Figure 4.5: *The "Monoclonal Antibody" technique for the treatment of bifurcation lesions. Guidewires are placed in the two vessels and a "kissing balloon" pre-dilatation is performed (a). A stent is then placed in the main vessel with entrapment of the side branch wire (b). The side branch wire is withdrawn and reintroduced through the stent struts (c). The stent struts are separated with balloon inflation (d). A short balloon with a crimped stent is introduced through the stent struts (e), and a second balloon is introduced and inflated in the main vessel (f). The side branch balloon is then pulled against this balloon and inflated as appropriate to deploy the second stent.*

165

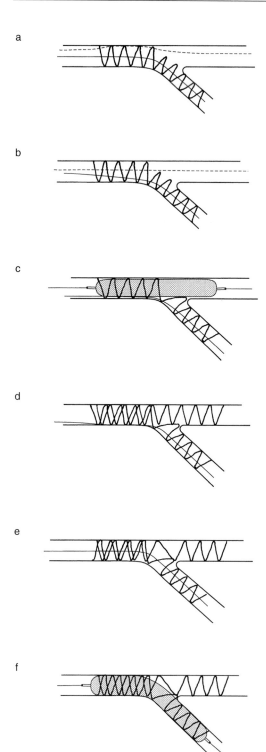

Figure 4.6: The "Culottes" technique for the treatment of bifurcation lesions. The first coil stent is placed in the main artery and the side-branch and post-dilated (a). This temporarily traps the main vessel guidewire (b) which is retracted and readvanced through the stent struts. The stent is further post-dilated to further open the struts (c). A second stent is placed in the main vessel across the bifurcation, with proximal overlap of the two stents (d), which traps the side-branch wire. The wire is removed and repositioned (e), and the bifurcation is then appropriately post-dilated.

Table 4.5 Advantages and disadvantages of the various stenting techniques for the treatment of bifurcation lesions

Advantages	Disadvantages
Culottes stenting	
• Technically less demanding than other techniques	• Possible plaque prolapse through stent struts
• Coil and linked ring designs facilitate crossing with wire and balloon and dilatation through the struts	• Coil stents without longitudinal support may be damaged during recrossing and balloon dilatation
• Second stent deployed only if necessary	• On repositioning, the guidewire may recross on the outside of the initially deployed stent
T-stenting	
• Suitable for the treatment of large side-branches	• Access to side-branch is lost while stenting the main vessel
• Optimal coverage in the main vessel	• Positioning of the second stent is cumbersome (gaps or protrusion of the side-branch stent into the main vessel is possible)
Kissing stent	
• Suitable for the treatment of two large arteries (left main stenting)	• Creates a metal "neo-carina" in the middle of the vessel that is not in contact with the vessel wall
• Access to both vessels always maintained	
• Complete lesion coverage	

Table 4.5 continued

Y-stenting

- Complete lesion coverage
- Suitable for the treatment of two large arteries (left main stenting)
- Access to both vessels always maintained

- Technically difficult
- Leaves an unstented "gap" in the main vessel opposite the ostium of the side-branch vessel

Modified from di Mario C, Colombo A, *Cathet Cardiovasc Diagn* 1997; **41**: 197–99.

Although this technique was routinely applied with the Palmaz–Schatz stent, several of the newer stent designs facilitate passage of a second balloon and stent through the struts of the first.[271] Several modifications of the "T" stenting technique have been described. One of these involves the positioning of the side-branch stent first, then the main vessel stent, followed by their sequential deployment.[280] Another modification takes advantage of the central bridge of articulated stents. The stent is positioned in the main vessel with the distal portion placed in the most angulated leg of the bifurcation, ensuring that the central articulation is positioned at the ostium of the side branch. After deployment, there is relatively unobstructed access to the other leg (figure 4.4). The "Monoclonal Antibody" approach involves stenting of the main vessel followed by a "T" stenting technique of the side-branch with a balloon inflated in the main vessel stent[274] (figure 4.5).

The "Culottes" technique employs two coil or ring stents that are successively placed in the bifurcation such that the proximal ends of the two stents are nested within each other (figure 4.6). The first stent is deployed in the most angulated branch, and the guidewire from the other branch is removed and repositioned through the struts of the deployed stent. The second stent is introduced through the dilated struts of the first. Culottes stenting has been described with Freedom, GR II, Crossflex, Micro Stent II, GFX, Bard XT, and Wiktor stents, all of which allow interlocking of the devices without an undue excess of metal.[281–284] In general, those stents with longitudinal supports (GR II), with weld points between the stent loops, or those designed with multiple short subunits linked together, are more sturdy than the coil stents without such support, and are therefore more suitable for bifurcation stenting using the Culottes technique. All suffer from the drawback that displacement of the struts with a balloon to allow for side-branch access creates a short segment without metal strut coverage that is at risk for plaque protrusion. Another pitfall in the use of this technique may occur with repositioning of the wire through the struts of the first deployed stent, particularly in rapidly tapering vessels. In this situation, the guidewire may recross on the outside of the stent. The guidewire can be "bound" between the balloon and the initial stent, and therefore passage of the wire through the stent is ensured.[283]

All of the methods for bifurcation stenting are technically demanding, and their success is dependant upon the skill of the operator. The advantages and disadvantages of the various techniques are outlined in table 4.5. The medical-device industries have responded to the challenges of bifurcation stenting with the introduction of a number of innovative stents, all designed to allow the treatment of bifurcation lesions. Although preliminary work shows that bifurcation stenting may be superior to balloon angioplasty,[285,286] controlled studies must be done to confirm the feasibility and long-term success of such treatments.

Two new applications of coronary stents are currently being investigated. These are:

1. The treatment of symptomatic myocardial bridging;
2. the management of cardiac allograft vasculopathy.

Myocardial bridging

Myocardial bridging occurs when a segment of an epicardial coronary artery runs within myocardial tissue. Myocardial bridging almost exclusively involves the LAD and its prevalence in pathologic series varies from 15 to 85%.[287] In one angiographic series an incidence of 12% has been reported, but only a small number of patients (1.7%) demonstrated systolic narrowing of more than 50%.[288] Intravascular ultrasound studies have confirmed systolic constriction of the coronary arteries at the point of bridging, and have demonstrated delayed release of compression which may reduce diastolic blood flow and result in the occasionally observed clinical findings.[289] Bridging is generally asymptomatic, but has been associated with ventricular arrythmias,[290] myocardial ischemia,[289,291–294] acute myocardial infarction[295–299] and sudden cardiac death.[300,301]

In general, the long-term prognosis of myocardial bridging is excellent. However many patients suffer from angina.[288,289,291] The treatment of symptomatic myocardial bridging is controversial. Cases refractory to medical management have been successfully treated by coronary bypass grafting,[302] myotomy,[303–306] and PTCA.[307–311] There has been reluctance to use stents to treat myocardial bridges because of concern over the long term effects of rhythmic high pressure compressions on the stent. Two case reports have shown that stent implantation can completely normalize the pathophysiology and alleviate symptoms for up to one year after treatment.[312,313] The results of a small observational series reported by Schwarz and colleagues were not as favourable.[314] In their series, 11 patients were followed for a mean of 8 months after coronary stent implantation. Although all patients were asymptomatic immediately after treatment, 5 had developed recurrent angina by follow-up and 4 required repeat intervention due to in stent restenosis (2 repeat PTCA, 2 coronary bypass surgery). Clearly more short- and long-term information is needed before elective stent implantation can be considered as the preferred treatment for symptomatic myocardial bridging.

Cardiac allograft vasculopathy

Cardiac allograft vascular disease (CAVD) is characterized by diffuse and multifocal heterogenous intimal hyperplasia. It is the chief impediment to long-term survival in heart transplant patients. The actuarial survival rate of patients with discrete lesions in the proximal and mid-epicardial coronary arteries has been shown to be only 22% at 3 years.[315] The options for the treatment of allograft vasculopathy are limited, and cardiac retransplantation is regarded as the final option in advanced CAVD.[316] Catheter based palliative procedures such as balloon angioplasty have been used, however peri-procedural complications and high restenosis rates (around 55%) represent major limitations to the widespread application of this technique.[317–319] The efficacy of coronary stent implantation for other lesion types compared with balloon angioplasty suggests that stenting may have a role in the treatment of allograft vasculopathy. Little is known about the use of endovascular stents in CAVD. There have been two case reports of favourable short and intermediate-term outcome after stent implantation in heart transplant recipients.[320,321] In addition to these, two observational series have been reported. In a study of 27 patients (48 lesions) treated with coronary stents, all patients were event free at 7 months follow-up.[322] Sixteen patients (24 stents) had angiographic follow-up, and of these 25% showed restenosis (greater than 50% diameter stenosis). In an interesting study reported by Wong and co-workers, 12 patients underwent intervention for CAVD.[323,324] In this unique cohort, wherein patients served as their own controls, 17 stented lesions were compared with 17 balloon angioplasty treated lesions. At a mean follow-up of 345 ± 252 days, 7 of 16 (44%) stented and 12 of 14 (85%) balloon treated lesions had restenosed (p=0.046). Thus, coronary stent implantation may prove to be the treatment of choice for CAVD.

References

1. Serruys PW, de Jaegere P, Kiemeneij F et al, for the Benestent Study Group. A comparison of balloon-expandable-stent implantation with balloon angioplasty in patients with coronary artery disease. *N Engl J Med* 1994; **331**: 489–95.

2. Fischmann DL, Leon MB, Baim DS et al, for the Stent Restenosis Study investigators. A randomized comparison of coronary-stent placement and balloon angioplasty in the treatment of coronary artery disease. *N Engl J Med* 1994; **331**: 496–501.

3. Sawada Y, Nokasa H, Kimura T, Nobuyoshi M. Initial and six months outcome of Palmaz–Schatz stent implantation: STRESS/BENESTENT equivalent vs non-equivalent lesions [abstract]. *J Am Coll Cardiol* 1996; 27 (suppl): 252A.

4. Schwartz L, Blew B. Outcome of stenting in the real world [abstract]. *J Am Coll Cardiol* 1997; 29 (suppl): 496A.

5. Tilli F, Aliabadi D, Kinn J, Kaplan B, Benzuly K, Safian R. Real-life stenting: a comparison of target lesion revascularization in BENESTENT-STRESS lesions to non BENESTENT-STRESS lesions [abstract]. *Circulation* 1996; 94 (suppl): I-332.

171

6. George C, Kennard E, Holubkov R, Detre K. Are STRESS results generalizable? The NACI-PSS experience [abstract]. *J Am Coll Cardiol* 1997; 29 (suppl): 495A.

7. Kuntz RE, Gibson CM, Nobuyoshi M, Baim DS. Generalized model of restenosis after conventional balloon angioplasty, stenting and directional atherectomy. *J Am Coll Cardiol* 1993; **21**: 15–25.

8. Macaya C, Serruys PW, Ruygrok P et al. Continued benefit of coronary stenting versus balloon angioplasty: one year clinical follow-up of Benestent trial. *J Am Coll Cardiol* 1996; **27**: 255–61.

9. de Feyter PJ, de Jaegere PPT, Serruys PW. Incidence, predictors and management of acute coronary occlusion after coronary angioplasty. *Am Heart J* 1994; **127**: 643–51.

10. Detre KM, Holmes DR, Holubkov R et al, coinvestigators of the NHLBI PTCA registry. Incidence and consequences of periprocedural occlusion: the 1985–1986 National Heart, Lung and Blood Institute Percutaneous Transluminal Coronary Angioplasty Registry. *Circulation* 1990; **82**: 739–50.

11. Lincoff AM, Popma JJ, Ellis SG, Hacker JA, Topol EJ. Abrupt vessel closure complicating coronary angioplasty: clinical, angiographic and therapeutic profile. *J Am Coll Cardiol* 1992; **19**: 926–35.

12. Ellis SG, Roubin GS, King SB III et al. Angiographic and clinical predictors of acute closure after native vessel coronary angioplasty. *Circulation* 1988; **77**: 372–79.

13. Detre KM, Holubkov R, Kelsy SF et al, coinvestigators of the NHLBI PTCA registry. One year follow-up results of the 1985–1986 National Heart, Lung, and Blood Institute's Percutaneous Transluminal Coronary Angioplasty Registry. *Circulation* 1989; **80**: 421–28.

14. Stark KS, Satler LF, Krucoff MW, Rackley CE, Kent KM. Myocardial salvage after failed coronary angioplasty. *J Am Coll Cardiol* 1990; **15**: 78–82.

15. Talley JD, Weintraub WS, Roubin GS et al. Failed elective percutaneous coronary angioplasty requiring coronary artery bypass surgery: In hospital and late clinical outcome at 5 years. *Circulation* 1990; **82**: 1203–13.

16. Buffet P, Danchin N, Villemot JP et al. Early and long-term outcome after emergency coronary artery bypass surgery after failed coronary angioplasty. *Circulation* 1991; 84 (suppl III): III 254–III 259.

17. Craver JM, Weintraub WS, Jones EL, Guyton RA, Hatcher CR Jr. Emergency coronary artery bypass surgery for failed percutaneous coronary angioplasty: a 10-year experience. *Ann Surg* 1992; **215**: 425–33.

18. Sigwart U, Puel J, Mirkovitch V, Joffre F, Kappenberger L. Intravascular stents to prevent occlusion and restenosis after transluminal angioplasty. *N Engl J Med* 1987; **316**: 701–06.

19. Sigwart U, Urban P, Golf S et al. Emergency stenting for acute occlusion after coronary balloon angioplasty. *Circulation* 1988; **78**: 1121–27.

20. Roubin GS, Cannon AD, Agrawal SK et al. Intracoronary stenting for acute and threatened closure complicating percutaneous transluminal coronary angioplasty. *Circulation* 1992; **85:** 916–27.

21. de Feyter PJ, de Scheerder IK, van den Brand M, Larrman GJ, Suryapranata H, Serruys PW. Emergency stenting for refractory acute coronary occlusion during coronary angioplasty. *Am J Cardiol* 1990; **66:** 1147–50.

22. Goy JJ, Sigwart U, Vogt P, Stauffer JC, Kappenberger L. Long-term clinical follow-up of patients treated with the self-expanding coronary stent for acute occlusion during balloon angioplasty of the right coronary artery. *J Am Coll Cardiol* 1992; **19:** 1593–96.

23. Eeckhout E, Goy JJ, Vogt P, Stauffer JC, Sigwart U, Kappenberger L. Complications and follow-up after intracoronary stenting: critical analysis of a 6-year single-center experience. *Am Heart J* 1994; **127:** 262–72.

24. George BS, Voorhees WD III, Roubin GS et al. Multicenter investigation of coronary stenting to treat acute or threatened closure after percutaneous transluminal coronary angioplasty: clinical and angiographic outcomes. *J Am Coll Cardiol* 1993; **22:** 135–43.

25. Hearn JA, King SB III, Douglas JS, Carlin SF, Lembo NJ, Ghazzal ZMB. Clinical and angiographic outcomes after coronary artery stenting for acute or threatened closure after percutaneous transluminal coronary angioplasty: initial results with a balloon-expandable, stainless steel design. *Circulation* 1993; **88:** 2086–96.

26. Sutton JM, Ellis SG, Roubin GS et al, for the Gianturco–Roubin Intracoronary Stent Investigator Group. Major clinical events after coronary stenting: the multicenter registry of acute and elective Gianturco–Roubin stent placement. *Circulation* 1994; **89:** 1126–37.

27. Chan CNS, Tan ATH, Koh TH et al. Intracoronary stenting in the treatment of acute or threatened closure in angiographically small coronary arteries (<3.0 mm) complicating percutaneous transluminal coronary angioplasty. *Am J Cardiol* 1995; **75:** 23–25.

28. Haude M, Erbel R, Straub U, Dietz U, Schatz R, Meyer J. Results of intracoronary stents for the management of coronary dissection after balloon angioplasty. *Am J Cardiol* 1981; **67:** 691–96.

29. Herrmann HC, Buchbinder M, Clemen MW et al. Emergent use of balloon-expandable coronary artery stenting for failed percutaneous transluminal angioplasty. *Circulation* 1992; **86:** 812–19.

30. Maiello L, Columbo A, Gianrossi R, McCanny R, Finci L. Coronary stenting for treatment of acute or threatened closure following dissection after balloon angioplasty. *Am Heart J* 1993; **125:** 1570–75.

31. Kiemeneij F, Laarman GJ, van der Wieken R, Surwarganda J. Emergency coronary stenting with the Palmaz–Schatz stent for failed transluminal coronary angioplasty: results of a learning phase. *Am Heart J* 1993; **126:** 23–31.

32. Colombo A, Goldberg SL, Almagor Y, Maiello L, Finci L. A novel strategy for stent deployment in the treatment of acute or threatened closure complicating balloon coronary angioplasty: use of short or standard (or both) single or multiple Palmaz–Schatz stents. *J Am Coll Cardiol* 1993; **22:** 1887–91.

33. Foley JB, Brown RIG, Penn IM. Thrombosis and restenosis after stenting in failed angioplasty: comparison with elective stenting. *Am Heart J* 1994; **128:** 12–20.

34. Schömig A, Kastrati A, Mudra H et al. Four-year experience with Palmaz–Schatz stenting in coronary angioplasty complicated by dissection with threatened or present vessel closure. *Circulation* 1994; **90:** 2716–24.

35. Alfonso F, Hernandez R, Goicolea J et al. Coronary stenting for acute coronary dissection after coronary angioplasty: implications of residual dissection. *J Am Coll Cardiol* 1994; **24:** 980–95.

36. Vrolix M, Piessens J. Usefulness of the Wiktor stent for treatment of threatened or acute closure complicating coronary angioplasty. *Am J Cardiol* 1994; **73:** 737–41.

37. Reifart N, Langer A, Storger H, Schwarz F, Preuzler W, Hoffman P. Strecker stent as a bailout device following percutaneous transluminal coronary angioplasty. *J Interven Cardiol* 1992; **5:** 79–83.

38. Metz D, Urban P, Camenzind E, Chatelain P, Hoang V, Meier B. Improving results of bailout coronary stenting after failed balloon angioplasty. *Cathet Cardiovasc Diagn* 1994; **32:** 117–24.

39. Lablanche J-M, McFadden EP, Bonnet J-L et al. Combined antiplatelet therapy with ticlopidine and aspirin: simplified approach to intracoronary stent management. *Eur Heart J* 1996; **17:** 1373–80.

40. Witkowski A, Chmielak Z, Dabrowski M et al. High-pressure bail-out coronary stenting without anticoagulation: early outcome and follow-up results. *J Invas Cardiol* 1998; **10:** 83–88.

41. Chauhan A, Zubaid M, Buller CE et al. Reduced anticoagulation with antiplatelet therapy alone is safe and effective after "bail-out" stenting for failed angioplasty. *J Invas Cardiol* 1997; **9:** 398–406.

42. Antoniucci D, Valenti R, Santoro GM et al. Bailout coronary stenting without anticoagulation or intravascular ultrasound guidance: acute and six month angiographic results in a series of 120 consecutive patients. *Cathet Cardiovasc Diagn* 1997; **41:** 14–19.

43. Chauhan A, Zubaid M, Buller CE et al. Comparison of bailout versus elective stenting: time to reassess our benchmarks of outcome. *Cathet Cardiovasc Diagn* 1997; **41:** 40–47.

44. Lincoff AM, Topol EJ, Chapekis AT et al. Intracoronary stenting compared with conventional therapy for abrupt vessel closure complicating coronary angioplasty: a matched case-control study. *J Am Coll Cardiol* 1993; **21:** 866–75.

45. Altmann DB, Racz M, Battleman DS et al. Reduction in angioplasty complications after the introduction of coronary stents: results from a consecutive series of 2242 patients. *Am Heart J* 1996; **132:** 503–07.

46. Agrawal S, Liu M, Hearn J et al. Can preemptive stenting improve the outcome of acute closure? [abstract]. *J Am Coll Cardiol* 1993; 21 (suppl): 291A.

47. Fernández-Ortiz A, Goicolea J, Pérez-Vizcayno MJ et al. Six-month follow-up of successful stenting for acute dissection after coronary angioplasty: comparison between slotted tube (Palmaz–Schatz) and flexible coil (Gianturco–Roubin) stent designs. *J Interven Cardiol* 1998; **11:** 41–47.

48. de Jaegere PPT, Hermans WR, Rensing BJ, Strauss BH, de Feyter PJ, Serruys PW. Matching based on quantitative coronary angiography. A surrogate for randomized studies? Comparison between stent implantation and balloon angioplasty of a native coronary lesion. *Am Heart J* 1993; **125:** 310–19.

49. Rensing BJ, Hermans WR, Strauss BJ, Serruys PW. Regional differences in elastic recoil after percutaneous transluminal coronary angioplasty: a quantitative angiographic study. *J Am Coll Cardiol* 1991; **17:** 34B–38B.

50. Hanet C, Wijns W, Michel X, Schroeder E. Influence of balloon size and stenosis morphology in immediate and delayed elastic recoil after percutaneous transluminal coronary angioplasty. *J Am Coll Cardiol* 1991; **18:** 506–11.

51. Haude M, Erbel R, Issa H, Meyer J. Quantitative analysis of elastic recoil after balloon angioplasty and after intracoronary implantation of balloon-expandable Palmaz–Schatz stents. *J Am Coll Cardiol* 1993; **21:** 26–34.

52. de Jaegere P, Serruys PW, van Es GA et al. Recoil following Wiktor stent implantation for restenotic lesions of coronary arteries. *Cathet Cardiovasc Diagn* 1994; **32:** 147–56.

53. Mintz GS, Kovach JA, Pichard AD et al. Geometric remodelling is the predominant mechanism of clinical restenosis after coronary angioplasty [abstract]. *J Am Coll Cardiol* 1994; 25 (suppl): 138A.

54. Brott BC, Labinaz M, Culp SC et al. Vessel remodelling after angioplasty: comparative anatomic studies [abstract]. *J Am Coll Cardiol* 1994; 25 (suppl): 138A.

55. George CJ, Baim DS, Brinker JA et al. One-year follow-up of the Stent Restenosis (STRESS I) Study. *Am J Cardiol* 1998; **81:** 860–65.

56. Macaya C, Serruys PW, Ruygrok P et al. Continued benefit of coronary stenting versus balloon angioplasty: one year clinical follow-up of Benestent trial. *J Am Coll Cardiol* 1996; **27:** 255–61.

57. Masotti M, Serra A, Fernández-Avilés F et al. Stent versus angioplasty restenosis trial (START). Angiographic results at six month follow-up [abstract]. *Eur Heart J* 1996; 17 (suppl): 120.

175

58. Serruys PW, van Hout B, Bonnier H et al. Effectiveness, costs, and cost-effectiveness of a strategy of elective heparin-coated stenting compared with balloon angioplasty in selected patients with coronary artery disease: the Benestent II study. *Lancet* 1998 (in press).

59. Legrand V, Serruys PW, Emanuelsson H et al. BENESTENT-II Trial – final results of visit I: a 15-day follow-up [abstract]. *J Am Coll Cardiol* 1997; 29 (suppl A): 170A.

60. Garcia E, Serruys PW, Dawkins K et al. BENESTENT-II trial: final results of visit II & III: a 7 month follow-up [abstract]. *Eur Heart J* 1997; 18 (suppl): 350.

61. van Hout B, van der Woude T, de Jaegere PT et al. Cost effectiveness of stent implantation versus PTCA: the BENESTENT experience. *Semin Intervent Cardiol* 1996; **1**: 263–68.

62. Penn IM, Ricci DR, Almond DG et al. Coronary artery stenting reduces restenosis: final results from the Trial of Angioplasty and Stents in Canada (TASC) I [abstract]. *Circulation* 1995; 92 (suppl I): I-279.

63. Heuser RR, Wong SC, Chuang YC et al. The LAD subgroup in the Stent Restenosis Study (STRESS): the most pronounced antirestenosis effect of stenting [abstract]. *Eur Heart J* 1995; 16 (suppl): 291.

64. Versaci F, Gaspardone A, Tomai F, Crea F, Chiariello L, Gioffrè PA. A comparison of coronary-artery stenting with angioplasty for isolated stenosis of the proximal left anterior descending coronary artery. *N Engl J Med* 1997; **336**: 817–22.

65. Rodriguez AE, Ayala FP, Pardinas CA et al. Optimal Coronary Balloon Angioplasty vs Stent (OCBAS): preliminary results of a randomized trial [abstract]. *J Am Coll Cardiol* 1997; 29 (suppl): 311A.

66. Rodriguez AE, Bernardi VH, Ayala FP et al. Optimal Coronary Balloon Angioplasty vs Stent (OCBAS): angiographic long term follow-up results of a randomized trial [abstract]. *Circulation* 1997; 96 (suppl): I-593.

67. Knight CJ, Curzen N, Groves PH et al. Stenting suboptimal results following balloon angioplasty significantly reduces restenosis: results of a single centre randomised trial [abstract]. *Circulation* 1997; 96 (suppl): I-709.

68. Azar AJ, Detre K, Goldberg S, Kiemeneij F, Leon MB, Serruys PW, on behalf of the Benestent and Stent Restenosis Study. A meta-analysis on the clinical and angiographic outcomes of Stents vs PTCA in the different coronary vessel sizes in the Benestent-1 and Stress-1/2 trials [abstract]. *Circulation* 1995; 92 (suppl): I-475.

69. Foley DP, Serruys PW. Provisional stenting – "stent-like" balloon angioplasty. Evidence to define the continuing role of balloon angioplasty for percutaneous coronary revascularization. Submitted for publication.

70. Narins CR, Holmes DR, Topel EJ. A call for provisional stenting. The balloon is back! *Circulation* 1998; **97**: 1298–305.

71. de Feyter PJ, van Suylen RJ, de Jaegere PPT, Topol EJ, Serruys PW. Balloon angioplasty for the treatment of lesions in saphenous venous bypass grafts. *J Am Coll Cardiol* 1993; **21:** 1539–49.

72. Plokker HWT, Meester BH, Serruys PW. The Dutch experience in percutaneous transluminal angioplasty of narrowed saphenous veins used for aortocoronary bypass. *Am J Cardiol* 1991; **67:** 361–66.

73. Strauss BH, Serruys PW, Bertrand ME et al. Qualitative angiographic follow-up of the coronary Wallstent in native vessel and bypass grafts (European experience: March 1986–March 1990). *Am J Cardiol* 1992; **69:** 475–81.

74. Stewart J, Williams M, Goy JJ et al. Stenotic disease of saphenous vein coronary artery bypass grafts treated by self expanding stents [abstract]. *J Am Coll Cardiol* 1992; 19 (suppl): 49A.

75. Keane D, Buis B, Reifart N, Plokker TH. Clinical and angiographic outcome following implantation of the new less shortening Wallstent in aortocoronary vein grafts: introduction of a second generation stent in the clinical arena. *J Intervent Cardiol* 1994; **7:** 557–64.

76. Urban P, Sigwart U, Golf S, Kaufman U, Sadeghi H, Kappenberger L. Intravascular stenting for stenosis of aortocoronary venous bypass grafts. *J Am Coll Cardiol* 1989; **13:** 1085–91.

77. Joseph T, Loubeyre Ch, Fajadet J et al. Reconstruction of diffusely degenerated stenosed or occluded saphenous vein grafts with less-shortening Wallstents after aggressive antiplatelet-anticoagulant pre-treatment [abstract]. *Eur Heart J* 1997; 18 (suppl): 383.

78. Nordrehaug JE, Priestly KA, Chronos NAF et al. Self expanding stents for the management of aorto-ostial stenoses in saphenous vein bypass grafts. *Br Heart J* 1994; **72:** 285–87.

79. de Jaegere PP, Domburg RT, de Feyter PJ et al. Long-term clinical outcome after stent implantation in saphenous vein grafts. *J Am Coll Cardiol* 1996; **28:** 89–96.

80. de Scheerder IK, Strauss BH, de Feyter PJ et al. Stenting of venous bypass grafts: a new treatment modality of patients who are poor candidates for reintervention. *Am Heart J* 1992; **123:** 1046–54.

81. Eeckhout E, Goy JJ, Stauffer JC, Vogt P, Kappenberger L. Endoluminal stenting of narrowed saphenous vein grafts: long-term clinical and angiographic follow-up. *Cathet Cardiovasc Diagn* 1994; **32:** 139–46.

82. Leon MB, Wong SC, Pichard AD. Balloon expandable stent implantation in saphenous vein grafts. In: Clinical use of the Palmaz–Schatz Intracoronary Stent. Herrmann HC, Hirshfeld JW, eds. Mount Kisco, NY; Futura, 1993: 111–21.

83. Strumpf RK, Mehta SS, Ponder R, Heuser RR. Palmaz–Schatz stent implantation in stenosed saphenous vein grafts: clinical and angiographic follow-up. *Am Heart J* 1992; **123:** 1329–36.

84. Piana RN, Moscucci M, Cohen DJ et al. Palmaz–Schatz stenting for treatment of focal vein graft stenosis: immediate results and long-term outcome. *J Am Coll Cardiol* 1994; **23:** 1296–304.

85. Pomerantz RM, Kuntz RE, Carrozza JP et al. Acute and long-term outcome of narrowed saphenous vein grafts treated by endoluminal stenting and directional atherectomy. *Am J Cardiol* 1992; **70:** 161–67.

86. Frimerman A, Rechavia E, Eigler N, Payton MR, Makker R, Litvack F. Long-term follow-up of a high risk cohort after stent implantation in saphenous vein grafts. *J Am Coll Cardiol* 1997; **30:** 1277–83.

87. Maiello L, Colombo A, Gianrossi R, Goldenberg S, Martini G, Finci L. Favourable results of treatment of narrowed saphenous vein grafts with Palmaz–Schatz stent implantation. *Eur Heart J* 1994; **15:** 1212–16.

88. Wong SC, Popma JJ, Pichard AD et al. Comparison of clinical and angiographic outcomes after saphenous vein graft angioplasty using coronary versus "biliary" tubular slotted stents. *Circulation* 1995; **91:** 339–50.

89. Carrozza JP, Kuntz RE, Levine MJ et al. Angiographic and clinical outcome of intracoronary stenting: immediate and long-term results from a large single center experience. *J Am Coll Cardiol* 1992; **20:** 328–37.

90. Fenton SH, Fischman DL, Savage MP et al. Long-term and clinical outcome after implantation of balloon expandable stents in aortocoronary saphenous vein grafts. *Am J Cardiol* 1994; **74:** 1187–91.

91. Wong SC, Baim DS, Schatz RA et al, for the Palmaz–Schatz Stent Study Group. Acute results and late outcomes after stent implantation in saphenous vein graft lesions: the multicenter U.S. Palmaz–Schatz stent experience. *J Am Coll Cardiol* 1995; **26:** 704–12.

92. Fortuna R, Heuser RR, Garratt KN, Schwartz R, Buchbinder M. Wiktor intracoronary stent: experience in the first 101 vein graft patients [abstract]. *Circulation* 1993; 88 (suppl I): 309.

93. Bilodeau L, Iyer S, Cannon AD et al. Flexible coil stent (Cook Inc.) in saphenous vein grafts: clinical and angiographic follow-up [abstract]. *J Am Coll Cardiol* 1992; 19 (suppl): 264A.

94. Dorros G, Bates MC, Iyer S et al. The use of Gianturco–Roubin flexible metallic coronary stents in old saphenous vein grafts: in hospital outcome and 7 day angiographic patency. *Eur Heart J* 1994; **15:** 1456–62.

95. Fenton S, Fischman D, Savage M et al. Does stent implantation in ostial saphenous vein graft lesions reduce restenosis [abstract]. *J Am Coll Cardiol* 1994; 25 (suppl): 118A.

96. Wong SC, Hong MK, Popma JJ et al. Stent placement for the treatment of aorto-ostial saphenous vein graft lesions [abstract]. *J Am Coll Cardiol* 1994; 25 (suppl): 118A.

97. Douglas JS, Savage MP, Bailey SR et al, for the Saved Trial Investigators. Randomized trial of coronary stent and balloon angioplasty in the treatment of saphenous vein graft stenosis [abstract]. *J Am Coll Cardiol* 1996; 27 (suppl A): 178A.

98. Savage MP, Douglas JS, Fischman DL et al, for the Saphenous Vein De Novo Trial Investigators. Stent placement compared with balloon angioplasty for obstructed coronary bypass grafts. *N Engl J Med* 1997; **337:** 740–47.

99. de Jaegere PP, van Domburg R, de Feyter PJ et al. Long-term clinical outcome after stent implantation in saphenous vein grafts. *J Am Coll Cardiol* 1996; **28:** 89–96.

100. Berger PB, Holmes DR, Ohman M et al, for the MARCATOR Investigators. Restenosis, reocclusion and adverse cardiovascular events after successful balloon angioplasty of occluded versus nonoccluded coronary arteries: results from the Multicenter American Research Trial with Cilazapril after angioplasty to prevent Transluminal Coronary Obstruction and Restenosis (MARCATOR). *J Am Coll Cardiol* 1996; **27:** 1–7.

101. Violaris AG, Melkert R, Serruys PW. Long-term luminal renarrowing after successful elective coronary angioplasty of total occlusions: a quantitative angiographic analysis. *Circulation* 1995; **91:** 2140–50.

102. Medina A, Melian F, Suarez de Lezo J et al. Effectiveness of coronary artery stents for the treatment of chronic total occlusion in angina pectoris. *Am J Cardiol* 1994; **73:** 1222–24.

103. Ozaki Y, Violaris AG, Hamburger J et al. Short- and long-term clinical and quantitative angiographic results with the new less shortening Wallstent for vessel reconstruction in chronic total occlusion: a quantitative angiographic study. *J Am Coll Cardiol* 1996; **28:** 354–60.

104. Goldberg SL, Colombo A, Maiello L, Borrione M, Finci L, Almagor Y. Intracoronary stent insertion after balloon angioplasty of chronic total occlusions. *J Am Coll Cardiol* 1995; **26:** 713–19.

105. Almagor Y, Borrione M, Maiello L, Khlat B, Finci L, Colombo A. Coronary stenting after recanalisation of chronic total coronary occlusions [abstract]. *Circulation* 1993; 88 (suppl): I-504.

106. Bilodeau L, Iyer SS, Cannon AD et al. Stenting as an adjunct to balloon angioplasty for recanalization of totally occluded coronary arteries: clinical and angiographic follow-up [abstract]. *J Am Coll Cardiol* 1993; 21 (suppl): 292A.

107. Etsuo T, Osamu K, Masanobu F, Satoru O, Hitone T, Tohru K. Impact of stenting on PTCA of chronic total occlusions [abstract]. *Circulation* 1996; 94 (suppl): I-249.

108. Suttorp MJ, Mast G, Plokker HWT, Kelder JC, Ernst SMPG, Bal E. Primary coronary stenting after successful balloon angioplasty of chronic total occlusions: a single-center experience [abstract]. *Circulation* 1996; 94 (suppl): I-687.

109. Suttorp MJ, Mast G, Plokker HWT, Kelder JC, Ernst SMPG, Bal E. Primary

coronary stenting after successful balloon angioplasty of chronic total occlusions: a single-center experience. *Am Heart J* 1998; **135**: 318–22.

110. Nienaber CA, Fratz S, Lund GK, Stiel GM. Primary stent placement or balloon angioplasty for chronic coronary occlusions: a matched pair analysis in 100 patients [abstract] *Circulation* 1996; 94 (suppl): I-686.

111. Moussa I, di Mario C, Moses J et al. Comparison of angiographic and clinical outcomes of coronary stenting of chronic total occlusions versus subtotal occlusions. *Am J Cardiol* 1998; **81**: 1–6.

112. Gambhir DS, Sudha R, Singh S et al. Elective coronary stenting after recanalization for chronic total occlusion: clinical and angiographic follow-up results. *Indian Heart J* 1997; **49**: 163–68.

113. Anzuini A, Rosanio S, Legrand V et al. Wiktor stent for treatment of chronic total coronary occlusions: short- and long-term clinical and angiographic results from a large multicenter experience. *J Am Coll Cardiol* 1998; **31**: 281–88.

114. Rau T, Schofer J, Schlüter M, Seidensticker A, Berger J, Mathey DG. Stenting of nonacute total coronary occlusions: predictors of late angiographic outcome. *J Am Coll Cardiol* 1998; **31**: 275–80.

115. Mori M, Kurogane H, Hayashi T et al. Comparison of results of intracoronary implantation of the Palmaz–Schatz stent with conventional balloon angioplasty in chronic total coronary arterial occlusion. *Am J Cardiol* 1996; **78**: 985–89.

116. Anzuini A, Legrand VM, Kulbertus H et al. Medtronic™ Wiktor stent implantation in chronic coronary total occlusions: in-hospital and long-term outcomes [abstract]. *Circulation* 1997; 96 (suppl): I-268.

117. Elezi S, Kastrati A, Schuhlen H et al. Stent placement in chronic vs acute total coronary occlusion: six-month angiographic follow-up [abstract]. *Circulation* 1997; 96 (suppl): I-269.

118. Mehran R, Hong MK, Calabuig JS, Esfandiari NH, Keers B, Kent KM. Long term clinical follow-up after successful recanalization of chronic total occlusions [abstract]. *Circulation* 1997; 96 (suppl): I-269.

119. Sirnes PA, Golf S, Myreng Y et al, for the SICCO Study Group. Stenting in chronic coronary occlusion (SICCO): a multicenter, randomized, controlled study [abstract]. *J Am Coll Cardiol* 1996; 27 (suppl): 139A.

120. Sirnes PA, Golf S, Myreng Y et al. Stenting in chronic coronary occlusion (SICCO): a randomized controlled trial of adding stent implantation after successful angioplasty. *J Am Coll Cardiol* 1996; **28**: 1444–51.

121. Rubartelli P, Niccoli L, Verna E et al, for the Gruppo Italiano Sullo Stent Nelle Occlusioni Coronariche (GISSOC). Stent implantation versus balloon angioplasty in chronic total coronary occlusions: results from the GISSOC trial. *J Am Coll Cardiol* 1998; **32**: 90–96.

122. Hoher M, Grebe O, Woehrle J, Kochs M, Homback V, Buchwald AB. Wiktor stent implantation in chronic total occlusions reduces restenosis rate – initial results of the SPACTO trial [abstract]. *Circulation* 1997; 96 (suppl): I-268.

123. Höher M, Grebe OC, Wöhrle J, Kochs M, Hombach V, Buchwald AB. Stenting versus PTCA after recanalization of chronic total occlusions: results from the SPACTO trial with the Wiktor® stent [abstract]. *Eur Heart J* 1998; 19 (suppl): 47.

124. Sirnes PA, Golf S, Myreng Y et al. Sustained benefit of stenting in chronic occlusions: long-term follow-up of the SICCO study [abstract]. *Eur J Cardiol* 1998; 19 (suppl): 472.

125. Sirnes PA, Golf S, Myreng Y et al. Sustained benefit of stenting in chronic occlusions: long-term follow-up of the SICCO Study [abstract]. *J Am Coll Cardiol* 1998; 31 (suppl): 237A.

126. Sirnes PA, Golf S, Myreng Y et al. Sustained benefit of stenting chronic coronary occlusion: long-term clinical follow-up of the Stenting in Chronic Coronary Occlusion (SICCO) study. *J Am Coll Cardiol* 1998; **32:** 305–10.

127. Grines CL, Browne KR, Marco J et al, for the Primary Angioplasty in Myocardial Infarction Study Group. A comparison of primary angioplasty with thrombolytic therapy for acute myocardial infarction. *N Engl J Med* 1993; **328:** 673–79.

128. Zijlstra F, de Boer MJ, Hoorntje JCA, Reiffers S, Reiber JHC, Suryapranata H. A comparison of immediate coronary angioplasty with intravenous streptokinase in acute myocardial infarction. *N Engl J Med* 1993; **328:** 680–84.

129. Gibbons RJ, Holmes DR, Reeder GS et al, for the Mayo Coronary Care Unit and Catheterization Laboratory Groups. Immediate angioplasty compared with the administration of a thrombolytic agent followed by conservative treatment for myocardial infarction. *N Engl J Med* 1993; **328:** 685–91.

130. Michels KB, Yusuf S. Does PTCA in acute myocardial infarction affect mortality and reinfarction rates? A quantitative overview of the randomized clinical trials. *Circulation* 1995; **91:** 476–85.

131. Weaver WD, Simes RJ, Ellis SG et al. Comparison of primary coronary angioplasty and intravenous thrombolytic therapy for acute myocardial infarction: a quantitative review. *JAMA* 1997; **278:** 2093–98.

132. O'Neill WW, Weintraub R, Grines CL et al. A prospective placebo controlled randomized trial of intravenous streptokinase and angioplasty versus lone angioplasty therapy of acute myocardial infarction. *Circulation* 1992; **86:** 1710–17.

133. O'Neill WW, Brodie RR, Ivanhoe R et al. Primary coronary angioplasty for acute myocardial infarction. *Am J Cardiol* 1994; **73:** 627–34.

134. Brodie RR, Grines CL, Ivanhoe R et al. Six-month clinical and angiographic follow-up after direct angioplasty for acute myocardial infarction: final results from the primary angioplasty registry. *Circulation* 1994; **90:** 156–62.

135. Stone GW, Grines CL, Topol EJ. Update on percutaneous transluminal coronary angioplasty for acute myocardial infarction. In: Topol E, Serruys P (eds). Current Review of Interventional Cardiology, 2nd edn. Philadelphia, PA, Current Medicine; 1995: 1–56.

136. Agrawal SK, Ho DSW, Lie MW et al. Predictors of thrombolytic complications after placement of the flexible coil stent. *Am J Cardiol* 1994; **73:** 1216–19.

137. Neumann F-J, Walter H, Richardt G, Schmitt C, Schömig A. Coronary Palmaz–Schatz stent implantation in acute myocardial infarction. *Heart* 1996; **75:** 121–26.

138. Eeckhout E, Stauffer J-C, Vogt P, Seydoux C, Kappenberger L, Goy J-J. Unplanned use of intracoronary stents during rescue or direct PTCA following acute myocardial infarction [abstract]. *Transcath Cardiovasc Therapeutics* 1996; **8:** 43.

139. Lefèvre T, Morice M-C, Karrillon G, Aubry P, Zemour G, Valeix B. Coronary stenting during acute myocardial infarction: results from the stent without coumadin French registry [abstract]. *J Am Coll Cardiol* 1996; 27 (suppl): 69A.

140. Savalle LH, Schalij MJ, Jukema W, Reiber JHC, Bruschke AVG. The Micro Stent in acute myocardial infarction: quantitative angiographic and procedural results [abstract]. *Transcath Cardiovasc Therapeutics* 1996; **8:** 57.

141. Steinhubl SR, Moliterno DJ, Teirstein PS et al. Stenting for acute myocardial infarction: the early United States multicenter experience [abstract]. *J Am Coll Cardiol* 1996; 27 (suppl): 279A.

142. Garcia-Cantu E, Spaulding C, Corcos T et al. Stent implantation in acute myocardial infarction. *Am J Cardiol* 1996; **77:** 451–54.

143. Rodriguez AE, Fernandez M, Santaera O et al. Coronary stenting in patients undergoing percutaneous transluminal coronary angioplasty during acute myocardial infarction. *Am J Cardiol* 1996; **77:** 685–89.

144. Walton AS, Oesterle SN, Yeung AC. Coronary artery stenting for acute closure complicating primary angioplasty for acute myocardial infarction. *Cathet Cardiovasc Diag* 1995; **34:** 142–46.

145. Ahmad T, Webb JG, Carere RR, Dodek A. Coronary stenting for acute myocardial infarction. *Am J Cardiol* 1995; **76:** 77–80.

146. Wong PH, Wong CM. Intracoronary stenting in acute myocardial infarction. *Cathet Cardiovasc Diagn* 1994; **33:** 39–45.

147. Benzuly KH, Goldstein JA, Almany SL et al. Feasibility of stenting in acute myocardial infarction [abstract]. *Circulation* 1995; 92 (suppl): I-616.

148. Iyer S, Bilodeau L, Cannon A et al. Stenting the infarct related artery within 15 days of the acute event: immediate and long term outcome using the flexible metallic coil stent [abstract]. *J Am Coll Cardiol* 1993; 21 (suppl): 291A.

149. Capers Q, Thomas C, Weintraub W, King S, Douglas J, Scott N. Emergent stent

placement: worse outcome in the patients with a recent myocardial infarction [abstract]. *J Am Coll Cardiol* 1994; 23 (suppl): 71A.

150. Levy G, De Boisgelin X, Volpiliere R, Gallay P, Bouvagnet P. Intracoronary stenting in direct infarct angioplasty: is it dangerous? [abstract]. *Circulation* 1995; 92 (suppl): I-139.

151. Katz S, Green SJ, Ong LY, Chepurko L. Intracoronary stenting in direct infarct angioplasty: experience with 117 consecutive cases [abstract]. *Circulation* 1996; 94 (suppl): I-576.

152. Hans-Jürgen R, Thomas V, Jürgen R, Christoph B, Dietz U, Christine E-K. Short and longterm results of stent implantation within 12 hours after failed PTCA in acute myocardial infarction [abstract]. *Circulation* 1996; 94 (suppl): I-577.

153. Sheiban I, Tonni S, Chizzoni A, Trevi P. Coronary stenting in primary angioplasty for acute myocardial infarction [abstract]. *Transcath Cardiovasc Therapeutics* 1996; **8:** 57.

154. Takayama M, Imaizumi T, Aoki S et al. Favorable progress on coronary stent implantation as an early treatment in patients with acute myocardial infarction [abstract]. *Circulation* 1996; 94 (suppl): I-576.

155. Medina A, Hernández E, Suárez de Lezo J et al. Primary stent treatment for acute evolving myocardial infarction [abstract]. *Circulation* 1996; 94 (suppl): I-576.

156. Katz S, Chepurko L, Ong LY, Green SJ, Rosenblad ME. Is stent deployment during acute myocardial infarction superior to balloon angioplasty? [abstract]. *Circulation* 1996; 94 (suppl): I-576.

157. Ong LY, Katz S, Green SJ, Padmanabhan V, Rosenblad ME, Chepurko L. Routine stenting for acute myocardial infarction results in 6 month outcomes comparable to patients with elective stenting [abstract]. *Circulation* 1996; 94 (suppl): I-577.

158. Glatt B, Diab N, Chevalier B, Royer T. Prospective primary stenting in acute myocardial infarction [abstract]. *Circulation* 1996; 94 (suppl): I-577.

159. Valeix BH, Labrunie PJ, Massiani PF. Systematic coronary stenting in the first eight hours of acute myocardial infarction [abstract]. *Circulation* 1996; 94 (suppl): I-577.

160. Hong M-K, Park S-W, Kim J-J, Lee CW, Park S-J. Comparison of six-month results of coronary stenting versus balloon angioplasty alone in patients with acute myocardial infarction. *Am J Cardiol* 1997; **79:** 1524–27.

161. Siegel RM, Bhaskaran A, Underwood PL et al. Stenting versus optimal balloon angioplasty in direct infarct intervention [abstract]. *Eur Heart J* 1997; 18 (suppl): 125.

162. Spaulding C, Cador R, Benhamda K et al. One-week and six months angiographic controls and one year clinical follow-up of stent implantation during primary angioplasty for acute myocardial infarction [abstract]. *Eur Heart J* 1997; 18 (suppl): 125.

163. Seffenino G, Chierchia S, Fontanelli A et al, on behalf of the RAI registry investigators. Use of stents during emergency coronary angioplasty in patients with high-risk myocardial infarction: in-hospital results from the Italian multicentre registry (RAI) [abstract]. *Eur Heart J* 1997; 18 (suppl): 272.

164. Glatt B, Stratiev V, Guyon P, Chevalier B, Royer T. Two years experience of primary stenting in unselected acute myocardial infarction: one month follow-up [abstract]. *Eur Heart J* 1997; 18 (suppl): 274.

165. Nakagawa Y, Kimura T, Yokoi H, Tamura T, Nosaka M, Nobuyoshi M. Direct angioplasty of non-protected left main coronary artery in acute myocardial infarction, efficacy of stenting [abstract]. *Eur Heart J* 1997; 18 (suppl): 274.

166. Delcán JL, Garcia E, Soriano J et al. Primary coronary stenting in acute myocardial infarction: in hospital results [abstract]. *Eur Heart J* 1997; 18 (suppl): 275.

167. Hausleiter J, Walter H, Pache J, Dirschinger J. 6-month angiographic follow-up of coronary stent placement in patients with acute myocardial infarction [abstract]. *Circulation* 1997; 96 (suppl): I-327.

168. Mahdi NA, Lopez JC, Leon MN, Pathan A, Harrell LC, Palacios IF. Primary stenting in acute myocardial infarction: a comparison of primary PTCA with stent bailout [abstract]. *Circulation* 1997; 96 (suppl): I-327.

169. Mahdi NA, Lopez J, Leon M et al. Comparison of primary coronary stenting to primary balloon angioplasty with stent bailout for the treatment of patients with acute myocardial infarction. *Am J Cardiol* 1998; **81:** 957–63.

170. Le May MR, Labinaz M, Marquis JF et al. Late clinical and angiographic follow-up after stenting in evolving and recent myocardial infarction. *Am Heart J* 1998; **135:** 714–18.

171. Kastrati A, Elezi S, Schühlen H et al. Risk factor analysis for the 30-day outcome after coronary stent implantation in patients with acute myocardial infarction [abstract]. *J Am Coll Cardiol* 1998; 31 (suppl): 233A.

172. Eid-Lidt G, Villavicencio R, Rosas M et al. Coronary stenting in acute myocardial infarction versus "stent-like" coronary balloon angioplasty. *J Am Coll Cardiol* 1998; 31 (suppl): 233A.

173. Lefèvre T, Morice M-C, Karrillon G et al. Coronary stenting in acute myocardial infarction with cardiogenic shock [abstract]. *J Am Coll Cardiol* 1998; 31 (suppl): 95A.

174. Mehta AB, Mardikar HM, Hiregoudar NS, Mathew R, Solanki DR, Sethi RB. Coronary artery stenting in acute myocardial infarction. *Indian Heart J* 1997; **49:** 169–71.

175. Vogt A, Niederer W, Pfafferott C et al, on behalf of the study group of the Arbeitsgemeinschaft Leitentder Kardiologischer Krakenhausärzte (ALKK). Direct percutaneous transluminal coronary angioplasty in acute myocardial infarction:

predictors for short-term outcome and the impact of coronary stenting. *Eur Heart J* 1998; **19:** 917–21.

176. Benzuly KH, O'Neill WW, Gangadharan V et al. Stenting in acute myocardial infarction (STAMI): six month follow-up [abstract]. *J Am Coll Cardiol* 1997; 29 (suppl A): 456A.

177. Benzuly KH, O'Neill WW, Gangadharan V et al. Stenting in acute myocardial infarction (STAMI): bailout, conditional and planned stents [abstract]. *J Am Coll Cardiol* 1997; 29 (suppl A):456A.

178. Monassier J-P, Hamon M, Elias J et al. Early versus late coronary stenting following acute myocardial infarction: results of the STENTIM I Study: (French Registry of Stenting at Acute Myocardial Infarction). *Cathet Cardiovasc Diag* 1997; **42:** 243–48.

179. Stone GW, Brodie BR, Griffin JJ et al, for the Primary Angioplasty in Myocardial Infarction (PAMI) Stent Pilot Trial Investigators. Prospective, multicenter study of the safety and feasibility of primary stenting in acute myocardial infarction: in hospital and 30-day results of the PAMI stent pilot trial. *J Am Coll Cardiol* 1998; **31:** 23–30.

180. Stone GW, Brodie BR, Griffin JJ et al. Improved short-term outcomes of primary stenting compared to primary angioplasty in acute myocardial infarction: the PAMI stent pilot trial [abstract]. *Circulation* 1997; 96 (suppl): I-594.

181. Stone GW. Primary stenting in acute myocardial infarction: the promise and the proof. *Circulation* 1998; **97:** 2482–85.

182. Stone GW, Brodie B, Griffin J et al. A prospective, multicenter trial of primary stenting in acute myocardial infarction – the PAMI Stent Pilot Study [abstract]. *Circulation* 1996; 94 (suppl): I-570.

183. Serruys PW, Garcia-Fernandez E, Kiemeney F et al. Heparin-coated stent in acute myocardial infarction: a pilot study as a preamble to a large randomized trial comparing balloon angioplasty and stenting [abstract]. *Eur Heart J* 1997; 18 (suppl): 272.

184. Grines CL, Morice MC, Mattos L et al. A prospective, multicenter trial using the JJIS heparin-coated stent for reperfusion of acute myocardial infarction [abstract]. *J Am Coll Cardiol* 1997; **29:** 389A.

185. Serruys PW, Grines CL, Stone GW et al. Stent implantation in acute myocardial infarction using a heparin-coated stent: a pilot study as a preamble to a randomized trial comparing balloon angioplasty and stenting. *Int J Cardiovasc Intervent* 1998; **1:** 19–27.

186. Serruys PW, Garcia-Fernandez E, Kiemeney F et al. Stenting in acute MI: a pilot study as preamble to a randomized trial comparing balloon angioplasty and stenting [abstract]. *Circulation* 1997; 96 (suppl): I-326.

187. Rodríguez A, Bernardi V, Fernández M et al, on behalf of the GRAMI Investigators. In-hospital and late results of coronary stents versus conventional balloon angioplasty in acute myocardial infarction (GRAMI Trial). *Am J Cardiol* 1998; **81:** 1286–91.

188. Rodríguez AE, Bernardi VH, Santaera OA et al. Coronary stents improve outcome in acute myocardial infarction: immediate and long term results of the GRAMI Trial [abstract]. *J Am Coll Cardiol* 1998; 31 (suppl): 64A.

189. Rodriguez A, Fernandez M, Bernardi V et al, on behalf of the GRAMI investigators. Coronary stents improved hospital results during coronary angioplasty in acute myocardial infarction: preliminary results of a randomized controlled study (GRAMI Trial) [abstract]. *J Am Coll Cardiol* 1997; 29 (suppl A): 221A.

190. Rodriguez A, Bernardi V, Santaera O, Mauvecin C, Roubin G, Ambrose J, on behalf of the GRAMI investigators. Coronary stents improved hospital outcome in patients undergoing PTCA in acute myocardial infarction: results of a randomized multicenter study (GRAMI trial) [abstract]. *Am J Cardiol* 1997; 80 (suppl 7A): 21S.

191. Saito S, Hosokawa G. Primary Palmaz–Schatz stent implantation for acute myocardial infarction: the final results of Japanese PASTA (Primary Angioplasty vs Stent Implantation in AMI in Japan) trial [abstract]. *Circulation* 1997; 96 (suppl): I-595.

192. Saito S, Hosokawa G, Suzuki S, Nakamura S, for the Japanese PASTA trial study group. Primary stent implantation is superior to balloon angioplasty in acute myocardial infarction – the result of the Japanese PASTA (Primary Angioplasty Versus Stent Implantation in Acute Myocardial Infarction) trial [abstract]. *J Am Coll Cardiol* 1997; 29 (suppl A): 390A.

193. Hoorntje JC, Suryapranata H, de Boer M-J, Zijlstra F, van't Hof AW, van den Brink L. ESCOBAR: primary stenting for acute myocardial infarction: preliminary results of a randomized trial [abstract]. *Circulation* 1996; 94 (suppl): I-570.

194. Suryapranata H, van't Hof AW, Hoorntje JC, de Boer MJ, Zijlstra F. Randomized comparison of coronary stenting with balloon angioplasty in selected patients with acute myocardial infarction. *Circulation* 1998; **97:** 2502–05.

195. Suryapranata H, Hoorntje JCA, de Boer MJ, Zijlstra F. Randomized comparison of primary stenting with primary balloon angioplasty in acute myocardial infarction [abstract]. *Circulation* 1997; 96 (suppl): I-327.

196. Antoniucci D, Santoro GM, Bolognese L et al. Stenting in acute myocardial infarction: preliminary results of the FRESCO study (Florence Randomized Elective Stenting in Acute Coronary Occlusions) [abstract]. *Eur Heart J* 1997; 18 (suppl): 586.

197. Antoniucci D, Santoro GM, Bolognese L et al. Elective stenting in acute myocardial infarction: preliminary results of the Florence randomized elective stenting in acute

coronary occlusions (FRESCO) study [abstract]. *J Am Coll Cardiol* 1997; 29 (suppl A): 456A.

198. Antoniucci D, Santoro GM, Bolognese L, Valenti R, Trapani M, Fazzini PF. Clinical trial comparing primary stenting of the infarct-related artery with optimal primary angioplasty for acute myocardial infarction: results from the Florence Randomized Elective Stenting in Acute Coronary Occlusions (FRESCO) Trial. *J Am Coll Cardiol* 1998; **31:** 1234–39.

199. Stone GW, Brodie B, Griffin J et al. A prospective, multicenter trial of primary stenting in acute myocardial infarction – the PAMI Stent Pilot Study [abstract]. *Circulation* 1996; 94 (suppl): I-570.

200. Serruys PW, Garcia-Fernandez E, Kiemeney F et al. Heparin-coated stent in acute myocardial infarction: a pilot study as a preamble to a large randomized trial comparing balloon angioplasty and stenting [abstract]. *Eur Heart J* 1997; 18 (suppl): 272.

201. Stone GW. Stenting and IIb/IIIa receptor blockade in acute myocardial infarction: an introduction to the CADILLAC Trial. *J Invas Cardiol* 1998; 10 (suppl B): 36B–47B.

202. Nishida Y, Nonaka H, Ueda K et al. In-hospital outcome of primary stenting for acute myocardial infarction using Wiktor coil stent: results from a multicenter randomized PRISAM study [abstract]. *Circulation* 1997; 96 (suppl): I-397.

203. Maillard L, Hamon M, Monassier JP, Raynard P. STENTIM 2- Hospital out-come: elective Wiktor stent implantation in acute myocardial infarction versus balloon angioplasty [abstract]. *Eur Heart J* 1998; 19 (suppl): 59.

204. Horstkotte D, Piper C, Andresen D et al. Stent implantation for acute myocardial infarction: results of a pilot study with 80 consecutive patients [abstract]. *Eur Heart J* 1996; 17 (suppl): 297.

205. Kastrati A, Elez S, Schühlen H et al. Risk factor analysis for the 30-day outcome after coronary stent implantation in patients with acute myocardial infarction [abstract]. *J Am Coll Cardiol* 1998; 31 (suppl): 233A.

206. Califf RM, Fortin DF, Frid DJ et al. Restenosis after coronary angioplasty: an overview. *J Am Coll Cardiol* 1991; **17:** 2B–13B.

207. Bauters C, McFadden EP, Lablanche JM, Quandalle P, Bertrand ME. Restenosis rate after multiple percutaneous transluminal coronary angioplasty procedures at the same site. *Circulation* 1993; **99:** 969–74.

208. Bauters C, Lablanche JM, McFadden EP, Leroyu F, Bertrand ME. Clinical characteristics and angiographic follow-up of patients undergoing early or late dilation for a first restenosis. *J Am Coll Cardiol* 1992; **20:** 845–48.

209. Black AJ, Anderson HV, Roubin GS, Poweklson SW, Douglas JS, King SB. Repeat coronary angioplasty: correlates of a second restenosis. *J Am Coll Cardiol* 1988; **11:** 714–18.

210. Quigley PJ, Hlatky MA, Hinohara T et al. Repeat percutaneous transluminal coronary angioplasty and predictors of recurrent restenosis. *Am J Cardiol* 1989; **63:** 409–13.

211. Williams DO, Gruentzig AR, Kent KM, Detre KM, Kelsey SF, To T. Efficacy of repeat percutaneous transluminal coronary angioplasty for coronary restenosis. *Am J Cardiol* 1984; **53:** 32C–35C.

212. Schatz RA, Baim DS, Leon M et al. Clinical experience with the Palmaz–Schatz coronary stent: initial results of a multicenter study. *Circulation* 1991; **83:** 148–61.

213. de Jaegere PP, Serruys PW, Bertrand M et al. Wiktor stent implantation in patients with restenosis following balloon angioplasty of a native coronary artery. *Am J Cardiol* 1992; **69:** 598–602.

214. Sigwart U, Kaufman U, Goy JJ et al. Prevention of coronary restenosis by stenting. *Eur Heart J* 1988; **9:** 31–37.

215. Levine MJ, Leonard BM, Burke JA et al. Clinical and angiographic results of balloon-expandable intracoronary stents in right coronary stenoses. *J Am Coll Cardiol* 1990; **16:** 332–39.

216. Colombo A, Almagor Y, Maiello L et al. Results of coronary stenting for restenosis [abstract]. *J Am Coll Cardiol* 1994; 25 (suppl): 118A.

217. Savage MP, Fischman DL, Schatz RA et al. Long-term angiographic and clinical outcome of a balloon-expandable stent in the native coronary circulation. *J Am Coll Cardiol* 1994; **24:** 1207–12.

218. de Jaegere P, Serruys PW, Bertrand M et al. Angiographic predictors of recurrence of restenosis after Wiktor stent implantation in native coronary arteries. *Am J Cardiol* 1993; **72:** 165–70.

219. Moscucci M, Piana RN, Kuntz RE et al. Effect of prior coronary restenosis on the risk of subsequent restenosis after stent replacement or directional atherectomy. *Am J Cardiol* 1994; **73:** 1147–53.

220. Mittal S, Weiss D, Hirshfeld JW, Kolansky DM, Herrmann HC. Comparison of outcome after stenting for de novo versus restenotic narrowings in native coronary arteries. *Am J Cardiol* 1997; **80:** 711–15.

221. Debbas NMG, Sigwart U, Eeckhout E et al. Intracoronary stenting for restenosis: long-term follow-up: a single center experience. *J Invas Cardiol* 1996; **8:** 241–48.

222. Rocha-Singh K, Morris N, Wong SC, Schatz R, Teirstein P. Coronary stenting for treatment of ostial stenoses of native coronary arteries or aortocoronary saphenous venous grafts. *Am J Cardiol* 1995; **75:** 26–29.

223. Rechavia E, Litvack F, Macko G, Eigler N. Stent implantation of saphenous vein graft aorto-osteal lesions in patients with unstable ischemic syndromes: immediate angiographic results and long-term clinical outcome. *J Am Coll Cardiol* 1995; **25:** 866–70.

224. Zampieri P, Colombo A, Almagor Y, Mairello L, Finci L. Results of coronary stenting of ostial lesions. *Am J Cardiol* 1994; **73**: 901–03.

225. Wong SC, Hong M, Popma J et al. Stent placement for the treatment of aorto-osteal saphenous vein graft lesions [abstract]. *J Am Coll Cardiol* 1994; 23 (suppl): 118A.

226. Fenton S, Fischman D, Savage M et al. Does stent implantation in osteal saphenous vein graft lesions reduce restenosis [abstract]? *J Am Coll Cardiol* 1994; 23 (suppl): 118A.

227. Wong SC, Popma J, Hong M et al. Procedural results and long term clinical outcomes in aorto-osteal saphenous vein graft lesions after new device angioplasty [abstract]. *J Am Coll Cardiol* 1994; 25 (suppl): 394A.

228. Jain SP, Liu MW, Babu R et al. Balloon vs debulking devices vs stenting for right coronary osteal disease: acute and long term results [abstract]. *Circulation* 1996; 94 (suppl): I-248.

229. De Cesare NB, Bartorelli AL, Galli S et al. Treatment of osteal lesions of the left anterior descending coronary artery with Palmaz-Schatz coronary stent. *Am Heart J* 1996; **132**: 716–20.

230. Conley MJ, Ely RL, Kisslo J et al. The prognostic spectrum of left main stenosis. *Circulation* 1978; **57**: 947–52.

231. Chairman BR, Fisher LD, Bourassa MG et al. Effect of coronary bypass surgery on survival patterns in patients with left main coronary artery disease. Report of the Collaborative Study in Coronary Artery Surgery (CASS). *Am J Cardiol* 1981; **48**: 765–77.

232. Takaro T, Peduzzi P, Detre KM et al. Survival in subgroups with left main coronary artery disease: VA cooperative Study of Surgery for Coronary Artery Disease. *Circulation* 1982; **66**: 14–22.

233. O'Keefe JH, Hartzler GO, Rutherford BD et al. Left main coronary angioplasty: early and late results of 127 acute and elective procedures. *Am J Cardiol* 1989; **64**: 144–47.

234. Hartzler GO, Rutherford BD, McConohay DR, Johnson WL, Giorgi LV. "High-risk" percutaneous transluminal coronary angioplasty. *Am J Cardiol* 1988; 61 (suppl): 33G–37G.

235. Miketic S, Tebbe U, Carlsson J, Engel HJ, Glunz HG, Neuhaus KL, for the Arbeitsgemeinschaft Leitender Kardiologischer Krankenhausärzte (ALKK) Study Group. Percutaneous transluminal coronary angioplasty of left main stenosis: results of the German PTCA registry [abstract]. *Eur Heart J* 1998; 19 (suppl): 628.

236. Vogel JH, Ruiz CE, Jahnke EJ et al. Percutaneous (non-surgical) supported angioplasty in unprotected left main disease and severe left ventricular dysfunction. *Clin Cardiol* 1989; **2**: 297–300.

237. Turi ZG, Rezkella S, Campbell CA et al. Left main percutaneous transluminal angioplasty with the autoperfusion catheter in an animal model. *Cathet Cardiovasc Diagn* 1990; **21:** 45–50.

238. Vijayanagar R, Bognolo DA, Eckstein PF et al. The role of intra-aortic balloon pump in the management of patients with main left coronary artery disease. *Cathet Cardiovasc Diagn* 1981; **7:** 397–401.

239. Tommaso CL, Vogel JHK, Vogel RA. Coronary angioplasty in high-risk patients with left main coronary stenosis: results from the national registry of elective supported angioplasty. *Cathet Cardiovasc Diagn* 1992; **25:** 169–73.

240. Ryan TJ, Faxon DP, Gunnar RM et al. Guidelines for percutaneous transluminal coronary angioplasty. A report of the American College of Cardiology/American Heart Association Task Force on assessment of diagnostic and therapeutic cardiovascular procedures (subcommittee on percutaneous transluminal coronary angioplasty). *Circulation* 1988; **78:** 486–502.

241. Laham RJ, Carrozza JP, Baim DS. Treatment of unprotected left main stenoses with Palmaz–Schatz stenting. *Cathet Cardiovasc Diagn* 1996; **37:** 77–80.

242. Chauhan A, Zubaid M, Ricci DR et al. Left main intervention revisited: early and late outcome of PTCA and stenting. *Cathet Cardiovasc Diagn* 1997; **41:** 21–29.

243. De Gregorio J, Kobayashi N, Kobayashi Y et al. The unprotected left main: is stenting a viable alternative? Short-term results and long-term follow-up [abstract]. *Eur Heart J* 1998; 19 (suppl): 628.

244. Fajadet J, Brunel P, Jordan C, Cassagneau B, Marco J. Is stenting of left main coronary artery a reasonable procedure [abstract]. *Circulation* 1995; 92 (suppl): I-74.

245. Fajadet J, Brunel P, Jordan C et al. Stenting of unprotected left main coronary stenosis without coumadin. *J Am Coll Cardiol* 1996; 27 (suppl A): 277A.

246. Hausleiter J, Dirschinger J, Schühlen H, Kreis A, Elezi S. Left main stenting [abstract]. *Circulation* 1996; 94 (suppl): I-331–I-332.

247. Karam C, Jordan C, Fajadet J, Cassagneau B, Laurent J-P, Marco J. Six-month follow-up of unprotected left main coronary artery stenting [abstract]. *Circulation* 1996; 94 (suppl): I-672.

248. Lopez JJ, Ho KKL, Stoler RC et al. Percutaneous treatment of protected and unprotected left main coronary stenosis with new devices: immediate angiographic results and intermediate-term follow-up. *J Am Coll Cardiol* 1997; **29:** 345–52.

249. Amin FR, Kelly PA, Kurbaan AS, Clague JR, Sigwart U. Stenting for unprotected and protected left main disease: a comparison of short- and long-term outcome. *J Interven Cardiol* 1997; **10:** 401–07.

250. Macaya C, Alfonso F, Iniguez A, Goicolea J, Hernandez R, Zarco P. Stenting for

elastic recoil during angioplasty of the left main coronary artery. *Am J Cardiol* 1992; **70:** 105–07.

251. Sathe S, Sebastian M, Vohra J, Valentine P. Bailout stenting for left main coronary artery occlusion during diagnostic angiography. *Cathet Cardiovasc Diagn* 1994; **31:** 70–72.

252. Garcia-Robvles JA, Garcia E, Rico M, Esteban E, Perez de Prado A, Delcan JL. Emergency coronary stenting for acute occlusive dissection of the left main coronary artery. *Cathet Cardiovasc Diagn* 1993; **30:** 227–29.

253. Park S-J, Park S-W, Hong M-K et al. Stenting of unprotected left main coronary artery stenoses: immediate and late outcomes. *J Am Coll Cardiol* 1998; **31:** 37–42.

254. Laruelle CJJ, Brueren GBR, Ernst SMPG et al. Stenting of "unprotected" left main coronary artery stenoses: early and late results. *Heart* 1998; **79:** 148–52.

255. Romero M, Suárez de Lezo J, Medina A et al. Elective stent treatment of unprotected left main coronary stenosis [abstract]. *Eur Heart J* 1998; 19 (suppl): 627.

256. Barragan P, Silvestri M, Simeoni JB et al. Stenting in unprotected left main coronary artery: immediate and follow-up results [abstract]. *Circulation* 1996; 94 (suppl): I-672.

257. Tamura T, Nobuyoshi M, Nosaka H et al. Palmaz-Schatz stenting in unprotected and protected left main coronary artery: immediate and follow-up results [abstract]. *Circulation* 1996; 94 (suppl): I-671.

258. Tamura T, Yokoi H, Nakagawa Y et al. Palmaz–Schatz stenting in unprotected and protected left main coronary artery: immediate and follow-up results [abstract]. *Eur Heart J* 1997; 18 (suppl): 387.

259. Silvestri M, Barragan P, Roquebert PO et al. Unprotected left main coronary artery stenting: immediate and follow-up results [abstract]. *Eur Heart J* 1997; 18 (suppl): 27.

260. Ellis SG, Moses J, White HJ et al. Contemporary percutaneous treatment of unprotected left main stenosis – a preliminary report of the ULTIMA (unprotected left main trunk intervention multicenter assessment) registry. *Circulation* 1996; 94 (suppl): I-671.

261. Meier B, Gruentzig AR, King SB III et al. Risk of side branch occlusion during coronary angioplasty. *Am J Cardiol* 1984; **53:** 10–14.

262. Safian R, Schreiber T, Baim D. Specific indications for directional coronary atherectomy: origin left anterior descending coronary artery and bifurcation lesions. *Am J Cardiol* 1993; 72 (suppl E); 35E–41E.

263. Lewis BE, Leya FS, Johnson SA et al, for the CAVEAT Investigators. Outcome of angioplasty (PTCA) and atherectomy (DCA) for bifurcation and non bifurcation lesions in CAVEAT [abstract]. *Circulation* 1993; 88 (suppl): I-601.

264. Bittl JA, Sanborn TA, Tcheng JE, Siegel RM, Ellis SG. Clinical success, complications and restenosis rates with eximer laser coronary angioplasty: the Percutaneous Eximer Coronary Angioplasty Registry. *Am J Cardiol* 1992; **70:** 1533–39.

265. Whitlow PL, Cowley M, Bass T, Warth D. Risk of high speed rotational atherectomy in bifurcation lesions [abstract]. *J Am Coll Cardiol* 1993; 21 (suppl): 445A.

266. Warth DC, Leon MB, O'Neill W, Zacca N, Polissar NL, Buchbinder M. Rotational atherectomy multicenter registry: acute results, complications and 6-month angiographic follow-up in 709 patients. *J Am Coll Cardiol* 1994; **24:** 641–48.

267. Meier B. Kissing balloon coronary angioplasty. *Am J Cardiol* 1984; **54:** 918–20.

268. Fischman DL, Savage MP, Leon MB et al. Fate of lesion-related side branches after coronary artery stenting. *J Am Coll Cardiol* 1993; **22:** 1641–43.

269. Aputo RP, Chafizedeh ER, Stoler RC et al. "Stent Jail" – a minimum security prison. *J Invas Cardiol* 1996; **8:** 39.

270. Erminia M, Sklar MA, Russo RJ, Claire D, Schatz RA, Teirstein PS. Escape from stent jail: an *in vitro* model [abstract]. *Circulation* 1995; 92 (suppl): I-688.

271. Nakamura S, Hall P, Maiello L, Colombo A. Techniques for Palmaz–Schatz stent deployment in lesions with a large side branch. *Cathet Cardiovasc Diagn* 1995; **34:** 353–61.

272. Colombo A, Gaglione A, Nakamura S. "Kissing" stents for bifurcation coronary lesion. *Cathet Cardiovac Diagn* 1993; **30:** 327–30.

273. Colombo A, Maillo L, Itoh A et al. Coronary stenting of bifurcation lesions: immediate and follow-up results [abstract]. *J Am Coll Cardiol* 1996; 27 (suppl): 277A.

274. Fort S, Lazzam C, Schwartz L. Coronary "Y" stenting: a technique for angioplasty of bifurcation stenoses. *Can J Cardiol* 1996; **12:** 678–82.

275. Teirstein PS. Kissing Palmaz–Schatz stents for coronary bifurcation stenoses. *Cathet Cardiovasc Diagn* 1996; **37:** 311–13.

276. Khoja A, Özbek C, Bay W, Heisel A. Trouser-like stenting: a new technique for bifurcation lesions. *Cathet Cardiovasc Diagn* 1997; **41:** 192–96.

277. Carlson TA, Guarneri EM, Stevens KM, Norman SL, Schatz RA. "T stenting": the answer to bifurcation lesions? [abstract]. *Circulation* 1996; 94 (suppl): I-86.

278. Carrie D, Karouny E, Chouairi S, Puel J. "T"-shaped stent placement: a technique for the treatment of dissected bifurcation lesions. *Cathet Cardiovasc Diagn* 1996; **37:** 311–13.

279. Wong P, Tse KK, Chan W, Ko P, Tai YT. Treatment of bifurcation stenosis with the Multi-Link coronary stent. *J Invasive Cardiol* 1998; **10:** 34–41.

192

280. Kobayashi Y, Colombo A, Akiyama T, Reimers B, Martini G, di Mario C. Modified "T" stenting: a technique for kissing stents in bifurcational coronary lesion. *Cathet Cardiovasc Diagn* 1998; **43:** 323–26.

281. Foley DP, Serruys PW. Bifurcation lesion stenting. *Thoraxcenter J* 1996; **8:** 32–36.

282. Chevalier B, Glatt B. Kissing stenting in bifurcation lesions [abstract]. *Eur Heart J* 1996; 17 (suppl): 218.

283. Sugioka J, Mitudo K, Doi O et al. Stenting of bifurcadion lesions with the Wiktor stent. *J Invas Cardiol* 1998; **10:** 181–86.

284. di Mario C, Colombo A. Trousers-stents: how to choose the right size and shape? *Cathet Cardiovasc Diagn* 1997; **41:** 197–99.

285. Lefèvre T, Louvard Y, Morice MC et al. Should we stent bifurcation lesions? A single centre prospective study [abstract]. *Eur Heart J* 1997; 18 (suppl): 26.

286. Carrié D, Dambrin G, Berdagué P et al. Clinical and angiographic follow-up after coronary stenting of bifurcation lesions with the Wiktor stent [abstract]. *Eur Heart J* 1997; 18 (suppl): 386.

287. Polachek P. Relation of myocardial bridges and loops on the coronary arteries to coronary occlusions. *Am Heart J* 1961; **61:** 44–52.

288. Kramer JR, Kitazume H, Proudfoot WL, Sones FM. Clinical significance of isolated coronary bridges: benign and frequent condition involving the left anterior descending artery. *Am Heart J* 1982; **103:** 283–8.

289. Ge J, Erbel R, Rupprecht H-J et al. Comparison of intravascular ultrasound and angiography in the assessment of myocardial bridging. *Circulation* 1994; **89:** 1725–32.

290. Feld H, Guadanino V, Shani J et al. Exercise-induced ventricular tachycardia in association with a myocardial bridge. *Chest* 1991; **99:** 1295–6.

291. Julliere Y, Berder V, Suty-Selton C et al. Isolated myocardial bridges with angiographic milking of the left anterior descending coronary artery: A long-term follow-up study. *Am Heart J* 1995; **129:** 663–5.

292. Nobel J, Bourassa MG, Petitclerc R, Dydra I. Myocardial bridging and milking effect of the left anterior descending coronary artery: normal variant or obstruction? *Am J Cardiol* 1976; **37:** 993–9.

293. Ciampricotti R, El Gamal M. Vasospastic coronary occlusion associated with a myocardial bridge. *Cathet Cardiovasc Diagn* 1988; **14:** 118–20.

294. Rossi L, Dander B, Nidasio GP et al. Myocardial bridges and ischemic heart disease. *Eur Heart J* 1980; **1:** 239–45.

295. McCabe MJ, Weston CF, Frases AG. Acute myocardial infarction related to smoke inhalation and muscle bridging. *Postgraduate Med J* 1992; **68:** 758–61.

193

296. Vasan RS, Bahl VK, Rajani M. Myocardial infarction associated with a myocardial bridge. *Int J Cardiol* 1989; **25:** 240–1.

297. Feldman AM, Baughman KL. Myocardial infarction associated with a myocardial bridge. *Am Heart J* 1986; **111:** 784–7.

298. Endo M, Lee YW, Hayashi H, Wada J. Angiographic evidence of myocardial squeezing accompanying tachyarrythmia as a possible cause of myocardial infarction. *Chest* 1978; **73:** 431–3.

299. Shotar A, Bussutil A. Myocardial bars and bridges and sudden death. *Forensic Sci Int* 1994; **68:** 143–7.

300. Bestetti RB, Costa RS, Oliviera JS. Can isolated myocardial bridging of the left anterior descending artery be associated with sudden death during exercise? *Acta Cardiol* 1991; **46:** 27–30.

301. Iverson S, Hake U, Oelert H et al. Surgical treatment of myocardial bridging causing coronary artery obstruction. *Scand J Thoracic Cardiovasc Surg* 1992; **26:** 107–11.

302. Sueda T, Matsuura Y, Okomoto M et al. Surgical repair of Wolff-Parkinson-White syndrome complicated with myocardial bridging. *Ann Thorac Surg* 1991; **51:** 119–21.

303. Singhi SK, Mannino SC, Agster B, Barmada B. Myocardial bridging requiring debridging and revascularizaiton: a case report and review of the literature. *J Invas Cardiol* 1991; **3:** 250–4.

304. Grondin P, Bourassa MG, Noble J et al. Successful course after supra-arterial myotomy for myocardial bridging and milking effect of the left anterior descending artery. *Ann Thorac Surg* 1977; **24:** 423–7.

305. Farqui A, Moloy W, Felner JM et al. Symptomatic myocardial bridging of a coronary artery. *Am J Cardiol* 1978; **41:** 1305–11.

306. Laifer LI, Weiner BH. Percutaneous transluminal coronary angioplasty of a coronary artery stenosis at the site of myocardial bridging. *Cardiology* 1991; **79:** 245–8.

307. Cohen HM, Juska J, Kleiman JK. PTCA of complex athersclerotic lesion at the site of LAD myocardial bridging. *Cathet Cardiovasc Diagn* 1996; **37:** 272–6.

308. Colleran JA, Tierney JP, Prokopchak R et al. Angiographic presence of myocardial bridge after successful percutaneous transluminal coronary angioplasty. *Am Heart J* 1996; **131:** 196–208.

309. Matevosov AL, Babunashvili AM. Transcutaneous transluminal angioplasty of proximal coronary artery stenosis in the presence of associated "myocardial bridge" (description of 5 cases). *Kardiologia* 1993; **33:** 88–91.

310. Cappelletti A, Margonato A, Chierchia S. Coronary angioplasty in the presence of a myocardial bridge: a clinical case. *Cardiologia* 1991; **36:** 477–80.

311. Stables RH, Knight CJ, Sigwart U et al. Coronary stenting in the management of myocardial ischemia caused by muscle bridging. *Br Heart J* 1995; **74:** 90–92.

312. Akilli A, Kultursay H, Akin M et al. Stenting of myocardial bridging. *J Invas Cardiol* 1997; **9:** 529–33.

313. Mahon NG, Sugrue DD. Treatment of a long segment of symptomatic myocardial bridging with multiple coronary stents. *J Invas Cardio* 1997; **9:** 484–7.

314. Schwarz ER, Haager PK, Radke PW et al. Long-term effects of stent implantation in patients with symptomatic myocardial bridges [abstract]. *J Am Coll Cardiol* 1998; 31 (suppl): 234a.

315. Keogh AM, Valantine HA, Hunt SA et al. Impact of proximal or midvessel discrete coronary artery stenosis on survival after heart transplantation. *J Heart Lung Transplant* 1992; **11:** 892–901.

316. Gao SZ, Schroeder JS, Hunt SA, Stinson EB. Retransplantation for severe accelerated coronary artery disease in heart transplant recipients. *Am J Cardiol* 1988; **62:** 876–81.

317. Christensen BV, Meyer SM, Iacarella CI, Kubo SH, Wilson RF. Coronary angioplasty in heart transplant recipients: a quantitative angiographic long-term follow-up study. *J Heart Lung Transplant* 1994; **13:** 212–20.

318. Halle AA, Disciascio G, Massin EK et al. Coronary angioplasty, atherectomy and bypass surgery in cardiac transplant recipients. *J Am Coll Cardiol* 1995; **26:** 120–8.

319. Swan JW, Norell M, Yacoub M, Mitchell AG, Ilsley C. Coronary angioplasty in cardiac transplant recipients. *Eur Heart J* 1993; **14:** 64–70.

320. Seydoux C, Berguer DG, Eeckhout E et al. Coronary stenting for coronary artery narrowing in a heart transplant recipient. *Transpl Int* 1996; **9:** 433–6.

321. Foster MT, Atkinson JB, Yeoh TK, Fischell TA. Histopathology of restenosis after stenting of narrowed coronary arteries after cardiac transplantation during the teenage years. *Am J Cardiol* 1997; **80:** 389–93.

322. Heublein B, Pethig K, Maass C, Wahler T, Haverich A. Coronary artery stenting in cardiac allograft vascular disease. *Am Heart J* 1997; **134:** 930–8.

323. Wong PMT, Piamsomboon C, Mathur A et al. Efficacy of coronary stenting in the management of cardiac allograft vasculopathy. *Am J Cardiol* 1998; **82:** 239–41.

324. Wong PMT, Piamsomboon C, Mathur A et al. Do stents reduce restenosis in cardiac allograft vasculopathy? [abstract]. *Circulation* 1997; 96 (suppl): I-709.

5. STENT GUIDANCE AND ADJUNCTIVE APPROACHES

Coronary angiography

Coronary angiography has been the mainstay for the guidance of not only intracoronary stenting procedures but also all coronary interventional procedures. Visual estimation or "eyeballing" of dimensions from the angiogram has been shown notoriously inaccurate in a limited number of studies, but proof of point comes mostly from the personal experiences of the interventionalists.[1] In particular, the presence of minor residual narrowings (<20% residual stenosis) are often overlooked with visual assessment. A precise and accurate delineation of angiographic contours can be provided by algorithms widely available on-line in digital angiographic systems. The accuracy and reproducibility of such systems have been repeatedly shown.[2-4] Off-line quantitative angiographic analysis has been developed for clinical trials. The technique has been validated using precisely matched phantoms, either ex vivo[5,6] or positioned to create pseudo-stenoses in vivo,[7] and in stented pig coronary vessels.[8] By use of automated edge detection algorithms, the goal of treatment is a complete absence of residual stenosis or the presence of a "negative diameter stenosis" within the stent when visualized in multiple views. In most cases, the detection of residual in-stent narrowing is possible with quantitative coronary angiography, and these systems can therefore provide a relatively inexpensive means for the guidance and the optimization of coronary stent implantation.

Angiography has several limitations, however. Angiographic techniques determine only lumen size and not vessel size, and therefore severe and diffuse involvement of an entire artery may not be recognized, and the severity of a lesion may be substantially underestimated.[9-12] These limitations are particularly significant in coronary stent implantation, because in diffusely diseased vessels the sole use of angiography carries the risk of inappropriate sizing of the stent on a falsely normal reference segment. With intravascular ultrasound (IVUS) it is relatively easy to identify the true lumen dimensions. After stenting, angiography typically overestimates the increase in lumen area after stent deployment since it does not distinguish stent diameter and lumen diameter in patients with suboptimum stent expansion.[13-16] The discrepancy between IVUS-determined diameter and that determined angiographically decreases with progressively higher inflation pressures.[17,18] In addition, angiographic techniques do not offer much information on stent–strut contact with the vessel wall, the degree of stent symmetry, or the adequacy of stent expansion. Moreover, detailed information on complicating marginal dissections at the proximal inflow or distal outflow of stented segments cannot be obtained with current quantitative angiography algorithms. The full extent of intimal dissections and their subsequent management may be better defined with IVUS than with angiography. Hoyne and colleagues[19] reported that angiographically visualized dissections suggested a much larger cross-sectional lumen than that measured with IVUS, and that coronary dissections and intimal flaps were more often identified with ultrasound. In a provocative report by Itoh and colleagues,[20] it has been shown that the correlation between angiographically determined minimum luminal diameter (MLD) and IVUS MLD varies widely depending on the stent design, with 'less strut, less metal' stents showing a particularly poor correlation under IVUS.[20] This suggests that information obtained by IVUS may be more appropriate for the use of particular stent types. Moderately radio-opaque stents, like the Wallstent, might be adequately assessed by angiographic means alone. The reliability of quantitative coronary angiography is expected to improve with the introduction of the gradient field transform algorithm for the tracking of dissections and complex lesions,[21] and with the application of dynamic algorithms with adaptive weighting of the first and second derivatives to address the overestimation of small lumen diameters and the underestimation of large luminal diameters (and thus the underestimation of acute luminal gain and recoil).[22] Whether more detailed information on pre-stent lesion morphology and post-stent characteristics will translate into improved short-term and long-term outcomes after stenting is not yet known, and is the focus of several randomized trials of angiographic versus IVUS-guided stent implantation. Results of the SIPS trial[23-25] and a multicentre French trial[26-28] suggest that the additional information provided by IVUS guidance does not significantly reduce the need for target vessel revascularization or the restenosis rate at 6 months follow-up.

Role of intravascular ultrasound

Without a doubt, the amount of information gained by intravascular ultrasound (IVUS) far exceeds that of angiographic measurements. Intracoronary measurements enable visualisation of a full 360° circumference, and pre-intervention IVUS provides information on lesion morphology and the extent of atherosclerotic disease. Pre-intervention IVUS also allows direct measurements of inner dimensions, including minimal and maximal diameter and cross-sectional area, which may assist in device selection and balloon sizing. Additional information that may be obtained with IVUS before stent implantation include an assessment of the adequacy of balloon angioplasty, identification or exclusion of thrombus, and determination of stent size. Post-stent IVUS can be used to identify the adequacy of lesion coverage by the stent and plaque prolapse, and to assess the parameters for optimal stent implantation. Vessel injury, in the form of edge tears at the ends of the stent, is frequently observed with IVUS (around 13% of cases) but cannot be visualized with angiography.[29,30] Whether the additional information obtained with IVUS, which complements angiographic findings, will have a clinical impact, and whether the benefit of this additional information will outweigh the additional cost of the procedure, is not yet known.

The use of IVUS in coronary stenting was heralded by provocative reports from Antonio Colombo and his group from Milan. Initial IVUS observations by that group showed that the "traditional" stent-deployment techniques resulted in an acceptable angiographic appearance, but that around 80% of stents were under-expanded by use of the following criteria: minimal intra-stent cross-sectional area less than 70% of balloon cross-sectional area; and balloon size 0.5 mm larger than the reference vessel diameter.[13,14] They also showed that the use of larger balloons and higher pressures resulted in increased cross-sectional areas. These observations led to the hypothesis that stent thrombosis was more likely due to stent under-expansion than to a property inherent to the stent itself, because the under-expanded stent struts served as a nidus for thrombus formation. This hypothesis was later tested in a prospective clinical trial that began in 1993.[31] In that observational study, 334 consecutive patients underwent Palmaz–Schatz stent implantation. Routine high-pressure balloon angioplasty was done, and IVUS was used to confirm and document optimal stent deployment. Postprocedural treatment consisted of antiplatelet agents alone. At 1 month, the incidence of stent thrombosis was 0.9%. At the time of the report from Colombo's group, both low and high-pressure balloon stent deployment was being done with oversized balloons. The approach outlined by these investigators stressed the achievement of a vessel lumen of uniform calibre in the reference and stented segments, with high-pressure dilatation using a minimally compliant or a non-compliant balloon that matches the size of an angiographically normal segment.

The report of Colombo and colleagues[31] suggested two novel elements in a strategy for stent implantation: high-pressure in-stent dilatation and ultrasound guidance. The result was "optimized" stent implantation, which abolished the need for postprocedural anticoagulation. In that series, patients who did not meet the ultrasound criteria despite high pressure balloon dilatation were subsequently anticoagulated with coumadin. However, it was not clear from the study of Colombo and colleagues[31] whether high-pressure balloon inflation without ultrasound would reduce the risk of subacute stent thrombosis. A similar strategy was used in the multicentre MUSIC (Multicentre Ultrasound Stenting In Coronaries) study,[32] which was designed to validate the feasibility of IVUS-guided stenting without subsequent anticoagulation in vessels greater than 3.0 mm in diameter, and to validate the effect of IVUS-guided stenting on the 6-months restenosis rate. IVUS criteria to define optimum stent deployment were predetermined for use in that study. These criteria included complete stent apposition, optimum stent expansion (in-stent lumen area of proximal stent entrance ≥90% of proximal reference lumen area and minimum stent area [MSA] ≥90% of the average of the proximal and distal reference segments, or MSA ≥100% of the reference segment with the smallest lumen area [80% and 90% respectively, if the MSA is ≥9.0 mm^2]) and symmetric stent expansion (ratio of minimum lumen diameter to maximum lumen diameter ≥0.7). These criteria have since become generally accepted as the IVUS standards for optimum stent deployment. A total of 161 patients with stable angina and a de-novo coronary artery lesion were enrolled, and 155 of these had successful stent implantation with IVUS assessment. In 81% of these patients the criteria for optimum stent deployment were met, and these patients were treated with aspirin only. Those patients who did not meet the criteria were treated with either aspirin alone or with aspirin and a vitamin K antagonist. An overall subacute thrombosis rate of 1.3% was reported in this study. Bypass surgery was necessary in 1.3% of cases and repeat angioplasty was necessary in 4.6% of cases. The 6-months restenosis rate of 9.7% is the lowest reported in the literature to date. Although it is tempting to conclude from these results that the use of IVUS-guided stent implantation may improve long-term angiographic and clinical results, these data must be further scrutinized. Between 1991 and 1997, the results of four trials of the same stent in vessels of similar size, and in patients with comparable baseline demographic characteristics, have been analysed by one central laboratory (Cardialysis, Rotterdam, Netherlands).[32-35] Meta-analysis of the angiographic results confirmed the "bigger is better" hypothesis, which maintains that a larger lumen post-procedure results in a better long-term outcome (figure 5.1). Thus, the fact that the patients in the MUSIC trial had the lowest restenosis rate is probably related to the larger MLD post-procedure, and is not a direct result of the use of IVUS guidance.

The results of a non-randomized prospective comparison of IVUS and angiography guided Palmaz–Schatz stent implantation were reported by Blasini and colleagues.[36] In their study, 125 consecutive patients underwent IVUS-guided stent implantation, of whom 64 fulfilled the IVUS criteria for optimal stent implantation. A further 125 patients received stents under angiographic guidance. The IVUS group of patients showed a significantly lower restenosis rate of 21%, compared with 30% in the control group (p=0.033). Patients that met the IVUS criteria for optimum stent implantation had a significantly lower restenosis rate than those that did not (14% vs 28%, p=0.038), although they also had a significantly larger MLD immediately after stent implantation, which may explain that finding.

The necessity for ultrasound guidance was questioned by several observational

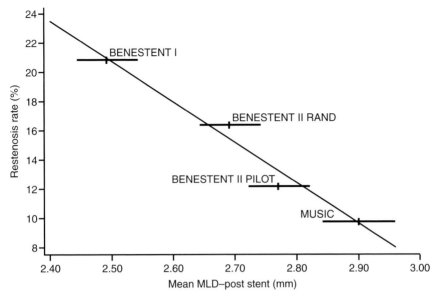

Figure 5.1: *Progressively decreasing restenosis rate with increasing minimal luminal diameter following implantation of Palmaz-Schatz stents. (From Serruys PW, Kootstra J, Melkert R, de Jaegere P, van den Brand M, Morel M. Peri-procedural QCA following Palmaz-Schatz stent implantation predicts restenosis rate at 6 months: result of a meta-analysis of BENESTENT-I, BENESTENT-II Pilot, BENESTENT-II and MUSIC [abstract]. J Am Coll Cardiol 1998; 31 (suppl): 64A).*

trials that adopted the technique described by Colombo's group but utilized angiography instead of ultrasound to guide optimal stent implantation. A large French trial[37] has reported the 30-day clinical outcome of a prospective registry of 2900 patients in whom successful coronary artery stenting was done without coumadin anticoagulation. In that trial, angiographically guided stent implantation used relatively high pressure in-stent post-dilatation, with 82% of the patients receiving Palmaz–Schatz stents. Postprocedural treatment included aspirin and ticlopidine. Low-molecular-weight heparin treatment was progressively reduced in four consecutive stages from 1-month treatment to none. Overall, subacute stent thrombosis occurred in 1.8% of patients, indicating that IVUS was not necessary to reduce the rate of subacute occlusion. Using a regimen of aspirin, ticlopidine, and periprocedural dextran therapy without IVUS guidance, Lablanche and colleagues[38] reported their results of stent implantation in 529 consecutive patients. Palmaz–Schatz, Wiktor, Gianturco–Roubin, and AVE stents were implanted as bailout therapy in cases of failed angioplasty, of suboptimal results after angioplasty, and electively. Stent thrombosis occurred in 5.4% of the patients stented as a bailout procedure and in 1.8% of patients stented after a suboptimal result, with no thrombotic events occurring in those treated electively. In 1.8% of the patients, ticlopidine treatment had to be stopped prematurely because of the development of adverse effects.

A report by Goods and colleagues[39] showed that the high-pressure stent dilatation technique introduced by Colombo's group can be applied to the implantation of coil stents. IVUS was not used to guide stent deployment. A post-stent protocol of aspirin and ticlopidine was used in 264 patients with angiographically determined successful stent implantation. During the 30-days follow-up, stent thrombosis occurred in only 0.9% of patients, indicating that without IVUS, patients receiving the balloon expandable coil stent with optimal angiographic results can be managed safely with a combination of aspirin and ticlopidine without anticoagulation.

At present, the issue of the routine use of IVUS for the guidance of stenting procedures has divided the interventional cardiology community. The favourable results of observational trials, in which high-pressure balloon optimization of stent implantation was done without adjunctive IVUS examination, has led many to conclude that IVUS is not essential for a favourable post-stent outcome. The supporters of routine IVUS contend that IVUS is necessary before stent implantation to give information on the plaque quality and therefore on the compliance of the lesion, so that the appropriate device is selected.[40,41] They also maintain that when examined with ultrasound, echo-free spaces, oblique strut position, and stent asymmetry are commonly seen in stents implanted with high pressure balloon post-treatment,[42] with more than 40% of stents with an acceptable angiographic result after high-pressure expansion still requiring additional dilatation with higher pressures or a larger balloon for ultrasound "optimization".[31] These findings are presented as arguments against the use of a "blind" angiography-only approach. The basis of the current controversy is whether optimum stent deployment should be defined based on clinical outcome or on IVUS confirmation. The results of the SIPS and the multicentre French trials show that in a select subset of patients, the routine use of IVUS does not improve the clinical outcome. If the results of the AVID and OPTICUS trials corroborate these findings, then the controversy should end. Until these results are available, the use of IVUS for routine stent deployment should be discouraged. IVUS is expensive, it increases the catheterization laboratory time, and it is not without risk. In addition, the IVUS-defined criteria for optimum stent deployment, touted by supporters of the routine use of the technique, are arbitrary and have not been tested in a controlled manner. This may account in part for the similarity in clinical outcome between the two groups in the SIPS and the French trials, and in the early reports of the AVID trial.[43]

Although the available results suggest that there may be no benefit in the routine use of IVUS guidance for stent implantation, certain lesion subsets may benefit from the use of IVUS to guide treatment. In this regard, Antonio Columbo's group has once again challenged the dogmas of stent implantation, and introduced the concept of "spot stenting". The tenets of conventional stent implantation dictate that stent placement should fully cover the lesion from a proximal disease-free segment to a distal disease-free segment. Applying this principle to long lesions requires the use of long or multiple stents, both of which have been implicated as contributing factors in restenosis. This is of particular importance in small vessels, for which evidence shows that there is no benefit to stent implantation over balloon angioplasty alone. The strategy of IVUS-guided spot stenting described by Colombo's group is a strategy of provisional stenting modified to allow its application to long lesions and to small vessels. In that group's approach, patients with lesions longer than 15 mm or in vessels less than 3.0 mm in diameter are treated first with an angiographically oversized balloon. IVUS assessment is then done, and if predetermined IVUS criteria are met (achievement of a lumen cross-sectional area $\geq$ 50% of the vessel cross-sectional area at the lesion site, or a true minimum cross-sectional area ≥ 5.5 mm^2) the procedure is terminated. If the IVUS criteria are not met, further balloon treatment is done with a larger balloon or at higher pressures, followed by repeat IVUS examination. If at this stage the IVUS criteria are met, then the procedure is terminated. If not, stent implantation is done focally at the site where the IVUS criteria are not met. If stent implantation is to be done, then the shortest stent length necessary to obtain optimum results is chosen. Stents are expanded with a balloon that is sized according to IVUS-determined media to media diameter, to achieve a minimum luminal cross-sectional area greater than 60% of the vessel cross-sectional area at the lesion site or greater than 60% of the average reference vessel area (average between distal and proximal reference cross-sectional area). This approach is based on the premise that IVUS guidance will: 1) maximize the probability of achieving prespecified criteria of lumen enlargement with balloon angioplasty alone, thereby removing the need for stenting; and 2) allow the identification of the segment or segments where the lumen is not optimum so that a stent can be focally implanted at that site. Early experience with this approach shows that it is superior to traditional angioplasty and may be better than traditional stenting where the lesion is covered from normal segment to normal segment. More data on this technique are needed to validate the approach.

Doppler flow

Coronary flow reserve (CFR) is defined as the ratio of hyperaemic to baseline coronary flow velocity. Values greater than 2 are normal, but values less than 2 suggest the presence of a functionally significant epicardial obstruction. Hyperaemia is induced in the catheterization laboratory by the intravenous or intracoronary administration of one of several pharmacological agents. CFR can now be measured using a steerable guidewire with a tip-mounted piezoelectric crystal. Ultrasound doppler signals are transmitted from the tip of the wire to the processor, where they are converted to the spectral display seen on the monitor. CFR measurements are used primarily to assess the physiological significance of a stenosis and the functional status of the distal microvascular bed before and after coronary interventions. The role of Doppler-flow assessment in interventional procedures is currently being assessed in several institutions. It has been shown that CFR is commonly not normalized after percutaneous transluminal coronary angioplasty (PTCA), although reports suggest that CFR may be normalized after stent implantation.[44] Several studies suggest that doppler techniques may be used to identify angiographically indiscernible residual disease or non-flow limiting dissection after angioplasty.[45-47] The Doppler wire itself can be used as an alternative to a conventional PTCA guidewire.[48] Thus doppler-flow measurements may be ideally suited to identify suboptimal results after PTCA to assess the need for stenting or other interventions. It has also been proposed that doppler techniques may be used to assess for optimum stent deployment, with the goal of generating laminar blood flow through the stent.[49] Further potential applications of doppler technology to coronary stenting are currently under investigation.

Angioscopy

The use of angioscopy has been described for the identification of incomplete stent apposition and residual dissection.[50] It has been shown, however, that IVUS is superior to angioscopy for the assessment of stent expansion, stent symmetry, and indicators of optimum implantation.[51] A role for angioscopy has been proposed for the evaluation of thrombus after transluminal extractional atherectomy (TEC) or intracoronary thrombolysis before stent implantation[52] and for interventions in saphenous vein bypass grafts.[53]

Debulking devices

There have been several hypotheses advanced to explain the observation that the restenosis rates for stented complex lesions is much higher than the rates in more simple "BENESTENT-like" lesions. One suggestion is that suboptimal results of stent placement in complex lesions may be a consequence of the presence of a large plaque burden, with or without severe calcification, which can transform the usually muscular elastic coronary artery into a rigid conduit. The rigid vessel and plaque burden, with or without calcification, may limit complete stent expansion and may contribute to late lumen loss.[54,55] In an attempt to reduce the restenosis rates in this lesion subset, various devices are being tested for the synergistic combination of debulking before coronary stenting.

Directional coronary atherectomy (DCA)

Directional coronary atherectomy (DCA) is effective in the removal of fibrotic non-calcified plaque, thus making the rigid diseased arterial wall more amenable to balloon dilatation and optimum stent deployment.[56-58] DCA followed by coronary stenting is feasible and results in a larger lumen immediately after the procedure than DCA followed by PTCA.[59-62] Whether this will result in a better long-term outcome ("bigger is better" contention[67]), or whether a device-specific effect will adversely affect the results, has yet to be seen. Results from small observational trials appear promising, with target lesion revascularization rates at 6 months of around 7%.[63-66] The application of DCA before stenting is currently limited by the large profile of the atherectomy device, its inability to cut calcified plaque, and its poor trackability.

Rotational atherectomy

In heavily calcified lesions, incomplete and asymmetric stent expansion occurs in up to 50% of cases.[54] Since optimum stent expansion is a crucial factor both for reducing the incidence of subacute stent thrombosis and for reducing the probability of restenosis ("bigger is better" concept[67]), the aim of debulking strategies is to eliminate fibro-calcific lesions to change vessel compliance, to increase the early gain in MLD, and thereby to allow stent delivery and expansion. Rotational atherectomy is the preferred strategy for the ablation of calcified plaque,[68] and by using a Rotablator intimal disruption is minimized, thereby reducing the risk of dissection seen with routine balloon dilatation. Rotablator atherectomy followed by Palmaz–Schatz stenting is superior to a Rotablator/PTCA combination, resulting in larger postprocedural lumen[69-73] and a lower residual stenosis as assessed by IVUS.[71-73] Rotational atherectomy followed by stent implantation also results in a relatively low incidence of angiographic restenosis (10–18%) when compared with results usually seen with other strategies in this calcified and complex lesion subset.[65,72-74]

There are, however, some complications which are specific to rotational atherectomy. Rotablator-induced no-reflow or slow flow can occur, which can be minimized by keeping burr runs short (<20 seconds). When slow flow occurs, it can be treated by intracoronary nitroglycerin, verapamil or both. Transient heart block can occur with rotational atherectomy, warranting prophylactic insertion of a temporary pacemaker, particularly in right coronary and dominant circumflex lesions. Vessel perforation can occur, most commonly in highly angulated lesions, where guidewire bias can direct the burr to the disease-free wall. Despite these risks, the periprocedural complication rate has been acceptably low in the above series. One small randomized clinical trial that compared stand-alone stenting with rotablation followed by stenting in 150 patients with native coronary disease (both calcified and non-calcified lesions) has recently been completed, although final results are not yet available.[75] Large randomized trials are needed to verify the encouraging initial findings, to confirm the low complication rates of observational series, and to find out whether the Rotablator and stent devices are truly synergistic.

Transluminal extraction atherectomy (TEC)

TEC has been used in stent implantation in high risk (totally occluded, thrombus containing, or degenerated) saphenous vein grafts, with very favourable results.[52,76-80] The rationale for this combined approach is based on the idea that TEC will partially remove plaque and thrombus, thereby reducing the potential for distal embolization, while stenting will reduce the incidence of restenosis. Only with a larger body of supportive data can firm conclusions be made about the benefits of this relatively new strategy over more conventional therapies.

Eximer laser coronary angioplasty (ELCA)

Limited data are available for the combination strategy of ELCA followed by coronary stenting. Results from the Washington Hospital Center, however, suggest that high-risk saphenous vein graft lesions can be successfully treated using this approach, with favourable long-term results.[77,80] The recent introduction of smaller catheters, and eccentric lasers with higher fluency, promise to improve the capability of debulking and to improve the success of this approach. A unique approach to the use of ELCA as adjunctive therapy to coronary stenting has recently been reported.[81] In this situation, laser angioplasty was done inside a stent that was suboptimally expanded due to a non-dilatable non-calcified plaque. After the laser treatment, additional balloon dilatation resulted in full stent expansion and led to a good final result.

In summary, preliminary, non-randomized, observational experience with these devices has shown the feasibility, safety and favourable short-term and long-term outcome for patients undergoing debulking before stenting. The increased procedure time and the additional costs incurred by the use of these devices must be considered, however, and these approaches must be applied in selected subsets of patients for whom debulking or stenting as a stand-alone strategy would be associated with a high acute or long-term failure rate. Recently, Moses and Moussa[65] have proposed the following clinically relevant algorithm for the application of these synergistic therapies.

(1) Directional atherectomy prior to stenting. Non-calcified lesions technically accessible to both DCA and stenting located in vessels greater than 2.5 mm in diameter and with any of the following characteristics: aorto-ostial lesions, bifurcation lesions, lesions that need two or more stents, chronic total occlusions.

(2) Rotablation prior to stenting. Calcified (moderate to severe calcifications) lesions accessible to both rotablation and stenting located in native coronary arteries greater than 2.5 mm in diameter.

(3) Transluminal extraction atherectomy prior to stenting. Lesions accessible to both TEC and stenting, located in saphenous vein grafts with large plaque burden or thrombus.

(4) Eximer laser coronary angioplasty prior to stenting Long non-calcified lesions, located in small vessels (2.5–3.0 mm) and accessible to both ELCA and stenting.

Until the results of large randomized trials are available, the recommendations of Moses and Moussa provide a useful guide for the use of these devices in the setting of coronary stenting.

References

1. Zir LM, Miller SW, Dinsmore RE. Intraobserver variability in coronary angiography. *Circulation* 1976; **53**: 627–32.

2. Di Mario C, Haase J, den Boer A, Reiber JHC, Serruys PW. Edge detection versus densitometry in the quantitative assessment of stenosis phantoms: an in vivo comparison in porcine coronary arteries. *Am Heart J* 1992; **124**: 1181–89.

3. Foley DP, Escaned J, Strauss BH et al. Quantitative coronary angiography in interventional cardiology: application to scientific research and clinical practice. *Progr Cardiovasc Dis* 1994; **36**: 363–84.

4. Keane D, Haase J, Slager C et al. Comparative validation of quantitative coronary angiographic systems: results and implications from a multicenter study using standardized approach. *Circulation* 1995; **91**: 2402–12.

5. Spears JR, Sandor T, Als AV et al. Computerized image anlaysis for quantitative measurement of vessel diameter from cineangiograms. *Circulation* 1983; **68**: 453–61.

6. Weisel J, Grunwald AM, Tobiasz Z et al. Quantitation of absolute area of a coronary arterial stenosis: experimental validation with a preparation in vivo. *Circulation* 1986; **74**: 1099–106.

7. Mancini GBJ, Simon SB, McGillem MJ et al. Automated quantitative coronary angiography: morphometric and physiologic validation in vivo of a rapid digital angiographic method. *Circulation* 1987; **75**: 452–60.

8. Kjelsberg MA, Seifert P, Edelman ER, Rogers C. Design-dependent variations in coronary stent stenosis measured as precisely by angiography as by histology. *J Invas Cardiol* 1998; **10**: 142–50.

9. Arnett EN, Isner JM, Redwood DR et al. Coronary artery narrowing in coronary heart disease: comparison of cinangiographic and necropsy findings. *Ann Intern Med* 1979; **91**: 350–56.

10. Grondin CM, Dyrda I, Pasternac A, Campeau L, Bourassa MG, Lespérance J. Discrepancies between cinangiographic and postmortem findings in patients with coronary artery disease and recent myocardial revascularization. *Circulation* 1974; **49**: 703–08.

11. Schwartz JN, Kong Y, Hackel DB, Bartel AG. Comparison of angiographic and postmortem findings in patients with coronary artery disease. *Am J Cardiol* 1975; **36**: 174–78.

12. Yamagishi M, Miyatake K, Tamai J, Nakatani S, Koyama J, Nissen SE. Intravascular ultrasound detection of atherosclerosis at the site of focal vasospasm in angiographically normal or minimally narrowed coronary segments. *J Am Coll Cardiol* 1994; **23**: 352–57.

13. Goldberg SL, Colombo A, Nakamura S, Almagor Y, Maiello L, Tobis J. Benefit of intracoronary ultrasound in the deployment of Palmaz–Schatz stents. *J Am Coll Cardiol* 1994; **24**: 996–1003.

14. Nakamura S, Colombo A, Gaglione S et al. Intracoronary ultrasound observations during stent implantation. *Circulation* 1994; **89**: 2026–34.

15. Mudra H, Klauss V, Blasini R et al. Ultrasound guidance of Palmaz–Schatz intracoronary stenting with a combined intravascular balloon catheter. *Circulation* 1994; **90**: 1252–61.

16. Hoffmann R, Mintz GS, Popma JJ et al. Overestimation of acute lumen gain and late lumen loss by quantitative coronary angiography (compared with intravascular ultrasound) in stented lesions. *Am J Cardiol* 1997; **80**: 1277–81.

17. Blasini R, Schuhlen H, Mudra H et al. Angiographic overestimation of lumen size after coronary stent placement: impact of high pressure dilatation [abstract]. *Circulation* 1995; 92 (Suppl): I-223.

18. Blasini R, Neumann F-J, Schmitt C, Bökenkamp J, Schömig A. Comparison of angiography and intravascular ultrasound for the assessment of lumen size after coronary stent placement: impact of dilation pressures. *Cathet Cardiovasc Diagn* 1997; **42**: 113–19.

19. Hoyne J, Mahon DJ, Tobis JM. Intravascular ultrasound imaging. *Trends Cardiovasc Med* 1991; **1**: 305–11.

20. Itoh A, Hall P, Moussa I et al. Comparison of quantitative angiography and intravascular ultrasound after coronary stent implantation with 6 different stents [abstract]. *Circulation* 1996; 94 (suppl): I-263.

21. van der Zwet PMJ, Reiber JHC. A new approach for the quantification of complex lesion morphology. The gradient field transform: basic principles and validation results. *J Am Coll Cardiol* 1994; **24**: 216–24.

22. Keane D, Gronenschild E, Slager CJ, Ozaki Y, Haase J, Serruys PW. In vivo validation of an experimental adaptive quantitative coronary angiography algorithm to circumvent overestimation of small lumen diameters. *Cath Cardiovasc Diag* 1995; **36**: 17–24.

23. Hodgson JMcB, Frey AW, Roskamm H. Net gain after six month angiographic follow-up is greater when IVUS is used to guide initial interventions: chronic SIPS trial results [abstract]. *Am J Cardiol* 1997; 80 (suppl 7A):17S.

24. Hodgson JMcB, Frey AW, Müller C, Roskamm H. Comparison of acute procedure cost and equipment utilization with strategies of ICUS guided *vs* angiographic guided PTCA and stenting: preliminary results of the Strategy of ICUS-guided PTCA and Stenting (SIPS) study [abstract]. *Circulation* 1996; 94 (suppl): I–235.

25. Frey AW, Roskamm H, Hodgson JMcB. IVUS-guided stenting: does acute angiography predict long term outcome? Insights from the strategy of IVUS-guided PTCA and stenting (SIPS) trial [abstract]. *Circulation* 1997; 96 (suppl): I–222.

26. Schiele F, Meneveau N, Vuillemont A et al. Restenosis after intracoronary ultrasound-guided stent deployment; a randomized multicentric study: results on the 6 month angiographic restenosis rate [abstract]. *J Am Coll Cardiol* 1998; 31 (suppl):103A.

27. Schiele FJ, Meneveau NF, Vuillemont AR et al. A randomized study of angiography versus ultrasound-guided stent implantation: immediate and 6-month results [abstract]. *Circulation* 1997; 96 (suppl): I–222.

28. Schiele F, Meneveau N, Vuillemont A et al. Impact of Intravascular ultrasound guidance in stent deployment on 6-month restnosis rate: a multicenter, randomized study comparing two strategies — with and without intravascular ultrasound guidance. *J Am Coll Cardiol* 1998; **32**: 320–28.

29. Schwarzacher SP, Metz JA, Yock PG, Fitzgerald PJ. Vessel tearing at the edge of intracoronary stents detected with intravascular ultrasound imaging. *Cathet Cardiovasc Diagn* 1997; **40**: 152–55.

30. Metz JA, Mooney MR, Walter PD et al. Significance of edge tears in coronary stenting: initial observations from the STRUT registry [abstract]. *Circulation* 1995; 92 (suppl): I-546.

31. Colombo A, Hall P, Nakamura S et al. Intracoronary stenting without anticoagulation accomplished with intravascular ultrasound guidance. *Circulation* 1995; **91**: 1676–88.

32. de Jaegere P, Mudra H, Figulla H et al. Intravascular ultrasound-guided optimized stent deployment: immediate and 6 months clinical and angiographic results from the Multicenter Ultrasound Stenting in Coronaries study (MUSIC study). *Eur Heart J* 1998; **19**: 1214-23.

33. Serruys PW, de Jaegere P, Kiemeneij F et al, for the Benestent Study Group. A comparison of balloon-expandable-stent implantation with balloon angioplasty in patients with coronary artery disease. *N Engl J Med* 1994; **331**: 489–95.

34. Serruys PW, Emanuelsson H, van der Giessen W et al, on behalf of the BENESTENT II Study Group. Heparin coated Palmaz-Schatz stents in human coronary arteries. Early outcome of the BENESTENT II Pilot Study. *Circulation* 1996; **93**: 412–22.

35. Serruys PW, Sousa E, Belardi J et al. BENESTENT-II Trial: subgroup analysis of patients assigned either to angiographic and clinical follow-up or clinical follow-up alone [abstract]. *Circulation* 1997; 96 (suppl): I-653.

36. Blasini R, Neumann F-J, Schmitt C, Walter H, Schömig A. Restenosis rate after intravascular ultrasound-guided coronary stent implantation. *Cathet Cardiovasc Diagn* 1998; **44**: 380–86.

37. Karrillon GJ, Morice MC, Benveniste E et al. Intracoronary stent implantation without ultrasound guidance with replacement of conventional anticoagulation therapy by antiplatelet therapy: 30-day clinical outcome of the French Multicenter Registry. *Circulation* 1996; **94**:1519–27.

38. Lablanche J-M, McFadden EP, Bonnet J-L et al. Combined antiplatelet therapy with ticlopidine and aspirin: a simplified approach to intracoronary stent management. *Eur Heart J* 1996; **17**: 1373–80.

39. Goods CM, Al-Shaibi KF, Yadav SS et al. Utilization of the coronary balloon-expandable coil stent without anticoagulation or intravascular ultrasound. *Circulation* 1996; **93**: 1803–08.

40. Moussa I, Di Mario C, Francesco LD et al. Stents don't require systemic anticoagulation…but the technique (and results) must be optimal. *J Invas Cardiol* 1996; 8 (suppl E): 3E–7E.

41. Moussa I, Di Mario C, Francesco LD et al. Subacute stent thrombosis in the era of intravascular ultrasound-guided coronary stenting without anticoagulation: frequency, predictors and clinical outcome. *J Am Coll Cardiol* 1997; **29**: 6–12.

42. Görge G, Haude M, Ge J et al. Intravascular ultrasound after low and high inflation pressure coronary stent implantation. *J Am Coll Cardiol* 1995; **26**: 725–30.

43. Russo RJ, Teirstein PS, for the AVID Investigators. Angiography versus intravascular ultrasound-directed stent placement [abstract]. *Circulation* 1996; 94 (suppl): I-263.

44. Bowers TR, Safian RD, Stewart RE, Shoukfeh MM, Benzuly KH, O'Neill WW. Normalization of coronary flow reserve immediately after stenting but not after PTCA. *J Am Coll Cardiol* 1996; 27 (suppl): 19A.

45. Kern MJ, Aguirre FV, Donohue TJ, Bach RG, Caracciolo EA, Wolford TL. Impact of residual lumen narrowing on coronary flow after angioplasty and stent: intravascular ultrasound Doppler and imaging data in support of physiological-guided coronary angioplasty [abstract]. *Circulation* 1995; 92 (suppl): I-263.

46. Verna E, Gil R, Di Mario C, Sunamura M, Gurne O, Porenta G, on behalf of the DEBATE Study Group. Does coronary stenting following balloon angioplasty improve distal coronary flow reserve? [abstract]. *Circulation* 1995; 92 (suppl): I-536.

47. Haude M, Baumgart D, Caspari G, Erbel R. Does adjunct coronary stenting in comparison to balloon angioplasty have an impact on Doppler flow velocity parameters? [abstract]. *Circulation* 1995; 92 (suppl): I-546.

48. DEBATE Study Group. Doppler guide wire as a primary guide wire for PTCA. Feasibility, safety and continuous monitoring of the results [abstract]. *Circulation* 1995; 92 (suppl): I-263.

49. Schwartz RS. Characteristics of an ideal stent based upon restenosis pathology. *J Invas Cardiol* 1996; 8: 386–87.

50. Teirstein P, Schatz R, Wong C, Rocha-Singh K. Coronary stenting with angioscopic guidance. *Am J Cardiol* 1995: 75: 344–47.

51. Shaknovich A, Lieberman S, Kreps E et al. Qualitative comparison of intravascular ultrasound and angioscopy with angiographic assessment of Palmaz–Schatz (PS) coronary stents [abstract]. *J Am Coll Cardiol* 1994; 23 (suppl): 72A.

52. Kaplan BM, Safian RD, Grines CL et al. Usefulness of adjunctive angioscopy and extraction atherectomy before stent implantation in high-risk aortocoronary saphenous vein grafts. *Am J Cardiol* 1995; 76: 822–24.

53. Annex BH, Ajluni SC, Larkin TJ, O'Neill WW, Safain RD. Angioscopic guided interventions in a saphenous vein bypass graft. *Cathet Cardiovasc Diagn* 1994; 31: 330–33.

54. Fitzgerald P, STRUT registry investigators. Lesion composition impacts size and symmetry of stent expansion: Initial report from the strut registry [abstract]. *J Am Coll Cardiol* 1995; 25 (suppl): 49A.

55. Moussa I, Di Mario C, Moses J et al. The impact of preintervention plaque area as determined by intravascular ultrasound on luminal renarrowing following coronary stenting [abstract]. *Circulation* 1996; 94 (suppl): I-528.

56. Safian RD, Gelbfish JS, Erny RE et al. Coronary atherectomy: clinical, angiographic, and histological findings and observations regarding potential mechanisms. *Circulation* 1990; 82: 69-79.

57. Suneja R, Nair R, Reddy K et al. Mechanisms of angiographically successful directional coronary atherectomy: evaluation by intracoronary ultrasound and comparison with transluminal coronary angioplasty. *Am Heart J* 1993; 126: 507–14.

58. Ibrahim A, Kronenberg M, Boor P et al. Atherectomy and angioplasty improve compliance and reduce thickness of iliac arteries — an *in vitro* ultrasound study [abstract]. *Circulation* 1994; 90 (suppl): I-534.

59. Kiesz RS, Rozek MM, Mego DM et al. Device synergy: directional atherectomy and stenting significantly decreases residual stenosis. *Eur Heart J* 1996; 17 (suppl): 175.

60. Mintz G, Pichard A, Dussalilant G et al. Acute results of adjunct stents following directional coronary atherectomy [abstract]. *Circulation* 1995; 92 (suppl): I-328.

61. Bramucci E, Angoli L, Merlini PA et al. Acute results of adjunct stent following directional coronary atherectomy [abstract]. *Eur Heart J* 1997; 18 (suppl): 119.

62. Moussa I, Moses J, Di Mario C et al. Results of the pilot phase of stenting after optimal lesion debulking: the SOLD trial [abstract]. *Eur Heart J* 1997; 18 (suppl): 119.

63. Moussa I, Moses JW, Strain JE et al. Angiographic and clinical outcome of patients undergoing "Stenting after Optimal Lesion Debulking": the "SOLD" pilot study [abstract]. *Circulation* 1997; 96 (suppl): I-81.

64. Bramucci E, Angoli L, Merlini PA et al. Acute results of adjunct stent following directional coronary atherectomy [abstract]. *J Am Coll Cardiol* 1997; 29 (suppl): 415A.

65. Moses J, Moussa I. Debulking prior to coronary stenting: a promising synergy in catheter-based coronary interventions. *J Invas Cardiol* 1998; 10 (suppl) B: 48B-52B.

66. Bramucci E, Angoli L, Merlini PA et al. Acute and long-term results of adjunctive stent implantation following directional coronary atherectomy [abstract]. *Circulation* 1997; 96 (suppl): I-80.

67. Kuntz RE, Gibson CM, Nobuyoshi M, Baim DS. Generalized model of restenosis after conventional balloon angioplasty, stenting and directional atherectomy. *J Am Coll Cardiol* 1993; 21: 15–25.

68. O'Neill W. Mechanical rotational atherectomy. *Am J Cardiol* 1992; 69 (suppl F):12F–18F.

69. Dussaillant GR, Mintz GS, Pichard AD et al. The optimal strategy for treating calcified lesions in large vessels: comparison of intravascular ultrasound results of rotational atherectomy + adjunctive PTCA, DCA, or stents. *J Am Coll Cardiol* 1996; 27 (suppl): 153A.

70. Hoffman R, Mintz GS, Kent KM et al. Comparitive early and nine-month results of rotational atherectomy, stents, and the combination of both for calcified lesions in large coronary arteries. *Am J Cardiol* 1998; 81: 552–57.

71. Mintz G, Dussalilant G, Wong SC et al. Rotational atherectomy followed by adjunct stents: the preferred therapy for calcified lesions in large vessels? [abstract]. *Circulation* 1995; 92 (suppl): I-329.

72. Hoffmann R, Mintz GS, Kent KM et al. The optimal therapy for calcified lesions in large coronary vessels: comparitive acute and follow-up results of rotational atherectomy, stents and the combination [abstract]. *Eur Heart J* 1997; 18 (suppl): 120.

73. Abizaid A, Mehran R, Mintz GS et al. Adjunct stent therapy improves procedural results and late clinical outcomes in patients after rotational atherectomy [abstract]. *Eur Heart J* 1997; 18 (suppl): 120.

74. Carstens JS, Buchbinder M. Rotastenting: latest clinical update including technique and results. *J Interven Cardiol* 1997; **10**: 237–39.

75. Niazi KA, Patel AA, Nozha F et al. A prospective randomized study of the effects of debulking on restenosis (Edres trial) [abstract]. *Circulation* 1997; 96 (suppl): I-709.

76. Hong MK, Pichard A, Kent KM et al. Assessing a strategy of stand-alone extraction atherectomy followed by staged stent placement in degenerated saphenous vein graft lesions [abstract]. *J Am Coll Cardiol* 1995; 25 (suppl): 394A.

77. Hong MK, Wong SC, Popma JJ et al. Favorable results of debulking followed by immediate adjunct stent therapy for high risk saphenous vein graft lesions [abstract]. *J Am Coll Cardiol* 1996; 27 (suppl): 179A.

78. Labib A. TEC before stenting in acute myocardial infarction. *J Invas Cardiol* 1996; **8**: 235–38.

79. Braden GA, Xenopoulos NP, Young T, Utley L, Kutcher MA, Applegate RJ. Transluminal extraction catheter atherectomy followed by immediate stenting in treatment of saphenous vein grafts. *J Am Coll Cardiol* 1997; **30**: 657–63.

80. Hong MK, Satler LF, Kent KM et al. Six-month results of debulking followed by immediate stent therapy for high risk saphenous vein graft lesions. *J Am Coll Cardiol* 1997; 29 (suppl): 17A.

81. Goldberg SL, Colombo A, Akiyama T. Stent under-expansion refractory to balloon dilatation: a novel solution with excimer laser. *J Invas Cardiol* 1998; **10**: 269–73.

6. COMPLICATIONS OF CORONARY STENTING

Subacute stent thrombosis

The problem

Despite a high rate of procedural success, the early experience with stenting was confounded by an unacceptably high (circa 25%) rate of stent thrombosis[1,2] (table 6.1). Although increased operator experience and knowledge of the indications for stent implantation have contributed to a decrease in the rate of stent thrombosis, two pivotal changes in clinical practice have had the greatest effect on the incidence of this complication: the implementation of high-pressure balloon expansion of stents, and the simultaneous finding of the benefits of enhanced antiplatelet therapy. With these improvements in stent deployment and

Table 6.1 Subacute stent thrombosis

Indication	No. of series	Time frame	No. of patients	% Subacute thrombosis (range)
With oral anticoagulation				
Emergency placement	21	1988–94	1928	10.1 (1.9–36.1)
Elective placement	10	1991–94	1775	4.5 (0.5–5.4)
Randomized trials	3	1994	597	3.7 (3.4–4.5)
Saphenous vein graft	12	1989–94	1016	2.2 (0–10.1)
Without oral anticoagulation				
Various	24	1994–95	2630	1.3 (0–6)

Data from Mak K-H, Belli G, Ellis SG, Moliterno DJ. Subacute stent thrombosis; evolving issues and current concepts. J Am Coll Cardiol 1996; **27**: 494–503.

periprocedural management, recent studies have reported thrombosis rates of less than 2% when stents are implanted electively[3–5] and 5% in the treatment of abrupt closure.[5] Although the rates are low compared with the results from the early series, stent thrombosis is a disastrous complication that carries with it a high risk of ischaemic sequelae. The pooled data from several trials show rates of myocardial infarction and death of 61% and 12%, respectively.[6] These devastating outcomes have encouraged continued attempts to solve stent thrombosis.

Acute stent thrombosis occurs within hours of the stenting procedure and is almost always due to incomplete stent expansion and vessel dissection. Patients are still hospitalized, and therefore diagnosis and treatment are usually rapid. With routine high-pressure balloon expansion acute thrombosis is rare, complicating less than 1% of stent procedures.[6] Subacute thrombosis, on the other hand, is a more common occurrence with a less easily defined aetiology. It can occur up to 30 days after the stent procedure, with the modal presentation being between days 5 and 6 for both the Wiktor and the Palmaz–Schatz stent.[7–9] In their experience with the Palmaz–Schatz stent used as a bailout device, Schömig and colleagues[10] observed that 43% of patients with subacute stent thrombosis present within the first week, and 80% present in the first 2 weeks.[10] Therefore, patients with subacute occlusion have commonly been discharged from hospital, and ischaemic sequelae and death are common.

Factors affecting stent thrombosis

Device related
The presence of foreign material within the vascular system increases the risk of thrombosis through several interrelated mechanisms. These can be broadly classified as surface interactions and rheological factors.

Surface interactions
Stent implantation initiates an complex interaction between the blood components and the metallic surface of the stent. Endothelialization of implanted stents is a relatively slow process that is only completed 2 to 3 months after implantation.[11,12] The clinical observation that the risk for thrombotic occlusion is maximum in the first 2 weeks after stenting illustrates that passivation of the stented surface can occur despite only partial endothelial coverage. Adsorption of the plasma proteins to the surface of the stent, to form a monolayer, occurs immediately upon stent deployment.[13] The nature of the component proteins forming this monolayer is determined by the concentration of the various constituents in the plasma and the affinity of each of the proteins for the metal surface. Protein collisions, with subsequent adsorption to the stent surface, are most likely to be dominated by albumin, since this is the most abundant plasma

protein and therefore displays a competitive advantage. However, other proteins like fibrinogen, compliment factors, fibronectin, and high molecular weight kininogen have a higher affinity for the metal surface and will soon displace the preadsorbed albumin from the stent (the Vroman effect).[14] The composition of the stent and the character of its surface can influence its ability to adsorb selectively and conformationally change plasma proteins. The adsorption of these proteins influences the subsequent interaction with the cellular components of circulating blood. In stented segments, circulating platelets can adhere not only to the exposed collagen of the underlying damaged vessel wall, but also to the protein adsorbed to the stent surface. Adherence of the platelets results in their activation, the release of chemo-attractant molecules from their granules, and the subsequent formation of a platelet aggregate.

The coagulation cascade also plays an important role in stent thrombosis. Activation of the coagulation sequence results in the formation of a fibrin clot by the enzymatic cleavage of fibrinogen to fibrin by thrombin. The coagulation cascade can be initiated through both the extrinsic and the intrinsic pathway. The extrinsic pathway is initiated by the contact of factor VII with thromboplastin released by the injured vessel. The intrinsic pathway is triggered by the adsorption of factor XII to the foreign surface and its conversion to factor XIIa.

The characteristics of the stent itself have been shown to influence the adsorption of proteins to the surface, the subsequent activation of circulating platelets, and the proclivity for thrombosis.[15] Results of in-vitro experiments suggest that metals that possess a higher surface potential cause pronounced attraction of negatively charged platelets and plasma proteins.[16,17] A rough surface texture has also been thought to promote stent thrombosis.[18] In a rabbit model, stent surface charge was not seen to contribute to thrombogenicity, but surface texture was an important factor in determining the biocompatibility of coated Palmaz–Schatz stents,[19] perhaps by providing more surface area to circulating blood components. In this regard, electrochemical polishing of stainless-steel devices has been shown to result in a less thrombogenic surface.[20,21] The rapidity of the binding of fibrinogen and platelets to stainless-steel surfaces on contact with blood has prompted the search for a more biocompatible alternative to stainless steel. Initial evaluation of stents made of tantalum suggested that they were less thrombogenic than stainless steel.[22,23] However, in both the baboon arteriovenous shunt model and the pig coronay model, controlled evaluation 2 hours after implantation led to the conclusion that there was no difference in the thrombogenicity of tantalum and stainless steel coil stents.[24] A comparison between stainless steel and nitinol slotted-tube stents in the rabbit carotid artery model showed that stainless steel was more thrombogenic and caused more extensive vascular injury than nitinol.[25,26] Platinum and gold coatings are currently being considered for coronary stents. These metals are particularly resistant to corrosion and may be less thrombogenic than their stainless steel counterparts. Gold also has the added advantage of antibacterial properties, and may exhibit antiproliferative effects.[19]

Interest in the use of polymers is mounting, either as the sole material of stent construction, as a component of polymer–metal composite stents, or as a surface coating for metal stents, as a means to decrease the thrombogenicity of implanted devices. Many different biodegradable and inert synthetic polymers have been tested in animal models as the sole component of coronary stents, including polyethylene terephthalate (Dacron),[27,28] polyhydroxybutyrate valerate,[29] poly-L-lactic acid,[30] polyglycolic acid,[31,32] and a co-polymer of polyglycolic and polylactic acid.[33] Although at times contradictory, the results of the use of these polymeric stents in animal models have been disappointing overall. The inconsistency of the results has made it apparent that the reaction to the polymeric materials differs not only across species, but also in different vascular beds within the same animal, making a direct extrapolation of the results to the human condition extremely difficult.

A polymer–metal composite stent design has recently been described.[34] The device is an ACS locking stent backbone between a poly-L-lactic acid/ e-polycaprolactone laminate. The stent is designed to provide mechanical hoop strength and to be a platform for local drug delivery through impregnation of the bioabsorbable polymer. This stent design is currently in the research and development stage.

Although data are limited, the results of several studies have indicated that the use of long stents may increase the risk of stent thrombosis. The use of a 20 mm long coil stent as opposed to a stent 12 mm in length was associated with a higher incidence of stent thrombosis in a recently reported observational study that included 288 patients stented for various indications[35] (9.4% versus 3.1%, p < 0.3). Similar results were reported in 115 patients treated for acute or threatened vessel closure with 20 mm and 12 mm coil stents, with a 10% incidence of stent thrombosis in the long stent group compared with 0% in the group receiving the short stent.[36] The presence of more metal, providing a greater thrombogenic surface in the longer stents, has been proposed as one factor contributing to a higher incidence of thrombosis, although other factors such as the indication for the use of the longer stent must also be considered. Long stents are usually chosen for the treatment of long or spiral dissections, and for long, tortuous, and ulcerated lesions. It may be that the characteristics of the lesion itself contribute more to the thrombogenicity of the stented site than does the metal of the stent.

Whether the implantation of multiple stents carries with it an increased risk of thrombosis over single stent implantation is still open to question. Three early investigations have shown the placement of multiple stents to significantly increase the incidence of thrombosis,[37–40] but several other trials have not shown a difference in the results using single and multiple stents.[8,41–46] A recently reported observational trial, comparing the clinical outcome after single and multiple stent implantation with high-pressure post-stent balloon dilatation technique, also did not show a difference with optimum multiple stent deployment.[47] By contrast, the report of an observational trial that assessed the outcome between patients treated with one or two stents and those treated with three or more found that the patients receiving more than two stents showed a significantly higher rate of restenosis and need for target vessel revascularization due to subacute thrombosis and late restenosis.[48] Whereas intuitively one may think that multiple stent deployment will present a greater thrombogenic surface, it has been proposed that technical difficulties with the placement of single short stents may result in suboptimal final results and a greater likelihood of persistent dissections, which may counter the thrombogenic effects of the presence of more metal. Clearly, further trials are necessary to address this important controversy.

Rheological factors

The nature of the flow in a vessel determines the degree to which blood elements interact with the structures on the vessel wall. Under laminar flow conditions, blood moves in a well-defined, streamlined fashion, with mass transfer of materials occurring by diffusion through the fluid. The presence of a stent in a vessel has been shown in an animal model to induce significant changes in blood flow and arterial pulsatility.[49] There are substantial differences in haemodynamic and wall rheological characteristics of implanted stents of different designs,[49] and the "hydrodynamic compatibility" of a stent, is now recognized as an important feature of ideal stent design. In-vitro assessment of fluid dynamics in a stented artery model has shown that immediately before and behind the expanded stent wires was a region of very low velocity flow, while maximum turbulence was seen directly over the stent struts.[50] These stagnant flow areas are the site of fibrin and platelet deposition. Enhanced shear stress can act as a platelet agonist, causing aggregation.[51] As the ratio of the distance between stent struts and the profile of the stent is reduced (the pitch to height ratio of coil stents), the peri-strut stagnation and maximum turbulence of the flow increase.[52] These findings suggest that a stent designed with optimum strut spacing and thin stent struts would result in less disturbed flow when deployed. These results may also account for the empirical findings of Colombo's group concerning optimum apposition of the stent to the vessel wall with high-pressure balloon inflation. A poorly deployed stent would have a smaller fraction of the stent strut embedded and would thus present a higher profile to the flowing blood (a lower pitch to height ratio). The greater amount of exposed metal in this circumstance would perhaps contribute to the observed high thrombotic potential.

There is further evidence that stent design and configuration can influence stent thrombosis. With deployment techniques held constant, in-vitro studies have shown that increases in flow velocity and turbulence are highest with wire loop stents, and that single articulation slotted-tube stents actually reduced both flow velocity and turbulence. Helically wound wire stents resulted in changes intermediate between the two other designs.[52] These findings have been supported by findings in an animal model in which a significantly higher incidence of stent thrombosis was seen in arterial segments stented with a corrugated ring stent compared with a slotted-tube device.[15] A small retrospective trial failed to show any differences between the Palmaz-Schatz, Wiktor, or Gianturco Roubin stents with respect to stent thrombosis, although the retrospective nature and the small size of this trial limits its interpretation.[54]

Two small randomised trials have been reported comparing stents of two different designs.[53,55] No differences were seen in the incidence of thrombosis, but the trials were not powered to show small differences in the (already low) incidence. Larger randomised trials are needed to conclusively show that stent configuration affects device thrombogenicity in clinical applications.

Patient-related factors
Vessel characteristics

The anatomical location of coronary lesions and their characteristics are important determinants of their propensity to thrombose after coronary stenting. These characteristics may be independent of the lesion (eg, reference vessel diameter), may be the indication for stent placement (eg, bailout), or may be a result of the intervention (eg, presence of thrombus before stent placement).

Vessel size. An increase thrombotic risk when stents were deployed in small-calibre vessels ($<$ 3 mm) was seen early in the clinical use of coronary stents,[1] which led to the exclusion of patients with lesions in small vessels from many of the later stent trials. This finding was supported by several subsequent observational studies.[35,36,41] Thrombosis rates of 9.5% have been reported for vessels stented with a 2.5 mm device,[35] and rates as high as 25% have been reported for stented vessels with a diameter of 2.0 mm.[41] Results of more recent studies, using higher balloon-pressure inflation to optimize stent delivery, are more encouraging. With the use of a Gianturco–Roubin Flex-Stent in bailout situations after failed angioplasty, a thrombosis rate of below 5% was reported.[56] Better results were seen with stent placement for elective situations in small vessels.[57–61] Despite this improvement, vessel size of less than 3.0 mm remains an important predictor of stent thrombosis, probably because of the presence of relatively more metal per lumen area and less flow in smaller vessels.

Lesion characteristics. Several reports assessing the predictors of stent thrombosis with multivariate analysis have identified lesion characteristics that are independent predictors of higher risk of stent thrombosis. The characteristics that were predictive of post-stent thrombosis include lesion eccentricity,[8] amount of atherosclerotic plaque,[45] AHA/ACC (American Heart Association/American College of Cardiology) lesion type B2 or C,[44,45] lesion length,[45,62] residual dissection after stent placement,[44,45,63] bailout indication after failed percutaneous transluminal coronary angioplasty (PTCA),[8,39,40,62,64-66] presence of intracoronary thrombus,[35,42,62,66] and, in vessels with poor distal run-off, presence of collaterals, or vessels supplying akinetic or severely kinetic regions of myocardium.[1]

Many of the predictors of thrombosis are subject to some controversy. The presence of pre-stent thrombus is an example. There have been several reports in which presence of thrombus has not resulted in a greater risk of acute and subacute closure after stent implantation.[41,67,68] Broad classification of lesion morphology has also been suggested not to correlate with risk of thrombosis.[69] Many of these data were accumulated in the era of low pressure stent deployment. Preliminary data, much of them unpublished, using high-pressure balloon expansion without anticoagulation, suggest that low ejection fraction, the presence of residual dissections, multiple stents per lesion, plaque burden, and minimum stent diameter after final expansion remain as predictors of thrombosis while bailout stenting and pre-stent lesion characteristics are not predictive.[70-73] These findings suggest that the final result obtained post-stent is the key factor in determining predisposition to stent thrombosis. In addition to these lesion-related characteristics, stent implantation in patients with acute coronary syndromes has been associated with a higher incidence of thrombosis.[8,45,61,62,74] As the techniques of stent implantation evolve and the post-stent management improves, these markers for risk will need to be reassessed to determine whether they are still valid predictors of stent thrombosis.

Anatomic location of stent placement. The location of the stent in the coronary arterial system has been shown to influence the thrombosis rate. The risk of thrombosis has repeatedly been shown to be highest in the LAD,[63,72,75,76] and lowest in stents deployed in saphenous vein grafts.[63,77] These differences may be a result of more turbulent flow in the LAD because of frequent branch points and tortuosity of the vessel, or because the vessel dimension of the target lesion and reference segments in the LAD were smaller than in the right coronary artery. The stented saphenous vein graft, on the other hand, may be more resistant to thrombosis because of its large diameter and the absence of branch points.

Haemostatic predictors

The recognised importance of the GPIIb/IIIa fibrinogen receptor on platelets in the development of thrombotic complications led to the hypothesis that a certain subpopulation of patients may be at risk of developing thrombosis based on alterations in the expression or activation of this platelet glycoprotein. This theory has recently undergone prospective evaluation in a study examining the haemostatic markers in 140 patients undergoing Palmaz–Schatz implantation for suboptimal PTCA results.[78] Stents were expanded with high inflation pressures and all patients were treated with anticoagulation after the procedure. The expression of the GPIIb/IIIa receptor had a positive correlation with the occurrence of stent thrombosis (table 6.2). In that trial, neither plasma fibrinogen levels nor the change in level with time showed a significant relation with the risk of stent thrombosis. Similarly, neither the level of prothrombin fragment 1+2 (a marker of thrombin formation) or conventional haemostatic monitoring measurements were related to the risk of subsequent stent thrombosis. GPIIb/IIIa receptor polymorphism (PIA^2) is also associated with an increased risk of subacute thrombosis after stent implantation.[79,80]

The results of these studies are important in several respects. First, the results emphasize the importance of platelet activity on the thrombotic system relative to the coagulation system, a finding that has been realized in practice with the introduction of postprocedural ticlopidine. These data also show for the first time that a patient-related variable can modulate the risk of stent thrombosis. In clinical practice, this implies that it might be possible to identify patients who are at risk for developing stent thrombosis before the interventional procedure, and to treat them more aggressively to prevent this complication.

Technique related factors
The greatest progress in the prevention of stent thrombosis has come with the improvement of stent deployment techniques and in post-stent pharmacological management. The thrombogenicity of the stent is largely a consequence of

Table 6.2 Rate of subacute stent thrombosis in groups defined by haemostatic variables

	Above upper quartile	Below upper quartile	p value
Surface expression on platelets of glycoprotein IIb/IIIa	5/35 (14.2%)	0/105 (0%)	0.0008
Concentration of prothrombin fragments F_{1+2}	3/35 (8.6%)	2/105 (1.9%)	0.10
Fibrinogen concentration	3/35 (8.6%)	2/105 (1.9%)	0.10

Data are number (%) of patients.
(From Neumann FJ, Gawaz M, Ott I, May A, Mössmer G, Schömig A. Prospective evaluation of hemostatic predictors of subacute stent thrombosis after coronary Palmaz-Schatz stenting. *J Am Coll Cardiol* 1996; **27:** 15–21).

disturbed blood rheology resulting from stent asymmetry and gaps between the stent struts and the vessel wall. It appears that when stents are "optimally" deployed, with the stent struts well apposed to the vessel wall and in full expansion, to give a favourable milieu for laminar flow, the need for anticoagulation is abolished. This can be achieved with appropriate balloon deployment. The use of stent implantation pressures below 12 atmospheres significantly increases the risk of stent thrombosis.[81] An optimally deployed stent should restore the anatomy of the vessel as close as possible to the normal state, both in dimension and geometry, and this is the focus of research into device design and deployment.

Since platelets are the primary participant in stent thrombosis,[82] it has been proposed that with optimal stent deployment proper antiplatelet therapy should be sufficient to prevent thrombosis until neointima formation is complete. There have been more than 35 trials of reduced anticoagulation regimens after coronary stenting.[64,59–61,83–115] Each of these trials used aspirin and high-pressure balloon inflation after stent implantation, with different stent types and for different clinical indications. The subacute thrombosis rates in these trials ranged from 0 to 3.6%. From these trials, it is apparent that the regimen of aspirin plus ticlopidine in combination with high-pressure deployment techniques has resulted in a significantly lower incidence of stent thrombosis compared with earlier anticoagulation regimens, with a concomitant significant reduction in bleeding and vascular complications. What remains to be seen is whether different antiplatelet agents or adjunctive therapy with antithrombins will result in a better outcome without significantly increasing haemorrhagic side-effects.

Ticlopidine expresses its antiplatelet activity via adenosine diphosphate-mediated inhibition of platelet-fibrinogen binding, and works in synergy with aspirin.[116] Although certainly effective, the use of ticlopidine is not without its problems. In most instances, ticlopidine is started on the day of the stent procedure and its maximum pharmacological effect occurs only at 4–8 days of treatment. This is after the peak incidence of subacute thrombosis. It is interesting to note, however, that when used in combination with aspirin, the anti-ADP activity is at its maximum only after 2 days of therapy, which is in keeping with the favourable clinical data on the use of this drug.[117] The major concern about the use of ticlopidine, however, relates to its side-effect profile. Ticlopidine therapy causes gastrointestinal symptoms, cutaneous rashes, and elevations in liver-function tests, but the most significant toxic effects are the unpredictable occurrence of granulocytosis, neutropenia, and thrombocytopenia, which generally occur at about the third week of therapy.[118] It is therefore recommended that white blood cell and platelet counts be done 2 weeks after initiating therapy, and at regular intervals beyond that if treatment is continued beyond 1 month. As a result of the delayed onset of action, the side-effects and the persistent, albeit low, incidence of stent thrombosis with the use of ticlopidine, there are considerable efforts underway to identify a better postprocedural medication regimen to decrease the incidence of stent thrombosis further. The use of an aspirin/ticlopidine regimen has been supported by the Expert Consensus Committee of the American College of Cardiology only in patients undergoing elective stent implantation with 3 mm diameter arteries without evidence of thrombus, in whom the stent has been optimally deployed,[119] but since the release of this information it is becoming apparent that antiplatelet therapy may be the preferred treatment for all clinical indications for stent implantation.[120,121] We recommend that anticoagulant therapy be reserved only for those patients with atrial tachyarrythmias or prosthetic heart valves, and ticlopidine should be added with caution to the treatment regimen in these patients.

Several trials have studied whether aspirin therapy alone is adequate antiplatelet coverage, with conflicting results. In the Multicenter Ultrasound Intracoronary Stent (MUSIC) study, stents were implanted according to strict ultrasound guidance criteria.[90] Aspirin-only therapy was given to those patients meeting the MUSIC criteria, but aspirin and intravenous anticoagulation post-stenting was given to those not meeting the criteria. An overall subacute thrombosis rate of 1.3% was reported in this study, and bypass surgery was necessary in 1.3%. Similarly favourable clinical outcomes were seen in other small observational series,[122,123] but one reported a markedly inferior outcome with aspirin monotherapy.[124] In a single-centre randomized trial reported by Hall and colleagues,[86] 226 patients were randomly assigned to receive either aspirin therapy alone or a combination of aspirin and ticlopidine therapy after successful ultrasound-guided stent implantation. Primary angiographic and clinical endpoints were stent thrombosis, death, myocardial infarction, the need for coronary artery bypass surgery or repeat angioplasty, and significant side-effects of medical therapy requiring termination of the medication within the first month after a successful procedure. At 1 month, the rate of stent thrombosis was 2.9% in the aspirin-only group and 0.8% in the ticlopidine-aspirin group (p = 0.2). Cumulative major clinical events occurred in 3.9% of the patients in the aspirin-treated group and in 0.8% of the ticlopidine-aspirin group (p = 0.1). The lack of a statistically significant difference between the groups may have been due to the small size of this trial.

The results of the STARS trial conclusively ended the debate over the added benefits of ticlopidine. This trial indicated a significant benefit of combination aspirin-ticlopidine therapy over aspirin alone and an aspirin–coumadin combination, when both the primary endpoint and sub acute closure with target vessel revascularization were considered. No differences in mortality or the need for emergency bypass surgery were seen between the groups — the benefit derived mainly from a reduction in the incidence of acute Q-wave myocardial infarction (1.3% in the aspirin-only group, 0.4% in the aspirin plus coumadin group, and 0% in the aspirin plus ticlopidine group). Haematological dyscrasias with the use of ticlopidine were rare in this trial (0.4%) and reversible with short-term therapy. The contribution of ticlopidine to the inhibition of platelet activation has been examined in a randomized manner.[125]

The effectiveness of ticlopidine monotherapy has also been examined. Elsner and colleagues[126] undertook a prospective study of ticlopidine monotherapy in 263 consecutive unselected patients. All patients in this study received 250 mg ticlopidine twice daily for up to 6 months. The cumulative rate of target vessel occlusion was 2.3% at 6 months' follow-up, but the 30-day occlusion rate was only 0.8%.[126] In a large prospective observational study, Barragan and colleagues[127] treated 1051 consecutive patients with ticlopidine monotherapy by use of angiographic guidance only, without high-pressure deployment. During 30-days follow-up, stent thrombosis occurred in 11 (1.0%) patients. The results of these two studies suggest that in non-selected patients ticlopidine monotherapy is effective to prevent stent thrombosis and may be a safe alternative for patients with contraindications to aspirin.[127]

Several other adjunctive therapies are now being assessed. The benefit of subcutaneously administered low-molecular-weight heparin with aspirin and ticlopidine therapy is being compared with a standard anticoagulation regimen in the ENTICES trial.[128] Results from the IMPACT II (Integrelin to Manage Platelet Aggregation to Prevent Coronary Thrombosis) trial, which examined the use of integrelin, a GPIIb/IIIa inhibitor, in 4000 high-risk patients undergoing percutaneous intervention, indicate that GPIIb/IIIa inhibition may be of benefit in the prevention of stent thrombosis. A total of 160 patients in this trial required bailout stent implantation for failed PTCA. The use of integrelin was associated with a lower rate of myocardial infarction at 30-days clinical follow-up than in the placebo-treated group (16% vs 32%; p=0.01). Similar results were seen in the EPILOG (Evaluation of PTCA to Improve Long-term Outcome by c7E3 Glycoprotein receptor blockade) trial.[129] Although designed to assess the thrombotic and ischaemic complications after balloon angioplasty or atherectomy, stenting was used for suboptimal balloon results in 360 (13%) patients. In addition to the overall trial benefit, a significant reduction in the composite endpoint of death and myocardial infarction was seen in those patients who received abciximab, a chimeric monoclonal antibody directed against the GPIIb/IIIa receptor (figure 6.1). The EPISTENT trial[130] was designed to assess the effect on clinical outcome of GPII/IIIa inhibition with the monoclonal antibody abciximab after stenting and balloon angioplasty. Clinical events were significantly lower in those patients treated with abciximab and stent implantation compared with the balloon-treated patients. These results strongly suggest that platelet GPIIb/IIIa inhibition is effective in reducing ischaemic and thrombotic complications in high-risk patients undergoing coronary stent implantation.

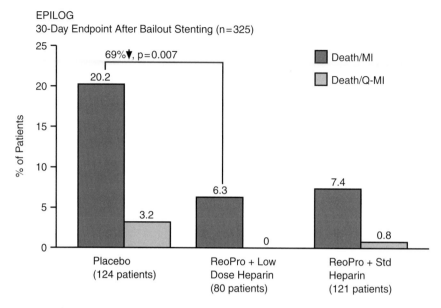

EPILOG
30-Day Endpoint After Bailout Stenting (n=325)

Figure 6.1: *30-day endpoint results of patients treated with bailout stenting in the EPILOG (Evaluation of PTCA to Improve Long-term Outcome by c7E3 Glycoprotein receptor blockade) trial.*

Prevention

The importance of avoiding stent thrombosis cannot be over-emphasized. Careful attention must be paid to stent-deployment technique and to antithrombotic therapy with or without anticoagulant therapy. Residual filling defects within the stent, which might represent extruded atheromatous tissue or thrombus, should be treated with additional high-pressure balloon inflations. Flow-limiting marginal dissections at ends of the stent should be corrected with the placement of additional stents. Patients who receive stents for high-risk indications, should be considered for more intense antithrombotic or prolonged anticoagulant therapy. It is important to realize that no antithrombotic or anticoagulant regimen has been identified to prevent thrombosis of a suboptimally deployed stent.[131]

Future strategies for the prevention of stent thrombosis may rely on the development of a thromboresistant stent. The stent surface is an important determinant of its thrombogenic potential. Treatment as simple as electrochemical polishing has been shown to decrease the thrombogenicity of metal stents.[20,21] Coating of metal stents has also been proposed as a means to passivate the stent surface. The list of materials that have been used to coat metal stents in an attempt to reduce their inherent thrombogenicity is long and is increasing[132–154] (table 6.3). Most coatings tested are designed to provide a biologically inert barrier between the stent surface and the circulating blood. Commercially available coated stents are the gold-coated InFlow and NIR stents, the silicon-carbide-coated Tensum and Tenax stents, and the diamond-like carbon (DLC) coated Diamond AS and Diamond Flex AS stents. These coatings are biologically inert.[155–156] The diamond-like coatings also reduce the release of heavy metal ions from the underlying stainless steel[162] (Figure 6.2). Heavy metal ions are known to cause endothelial damage and platelet and neutrophil activation at concentrations that can be seen in tissues surrounding implanted stainless-steel devices.[157–159] Of particular concern is the release of nickel ions. Nickel not only activates platelets and neutrophils, but it is also a potent allergen[160] and a documented carcinogen.[161] Thus, coating of stainless-steel stents with DLC not only gives the devices favourable tribological properties and improves their haemodynamic compatibility, but also improves their biocompatibility by preventing the activation of blood components such as platelets, as seen with uncoated implants.[162,163]

By contrast with barrier laminae, heparin surface coatings give a biologically active surface that interacts with the circulating blood. Many techniques have been applied to attach heparin to synthetic surfaces. The end-point attachment of heparin to polymer-coated surfaces, which preserves the activity of the antithrombin binding site, made the production of heparin-coated stents

Table 3 Coating material considered for use with metal intracoronary stents

Synthetic substances	Naturally occurring substances
Polyurethane[138–140]	Collagen/lamanin[146]
Segmented Polyurethaneurea/heparin[141]	Heparin[147–149]
Poly-L-lactic acid[142]	Fibrin[150,151,168–170]
Cellulose ester[143]	Phosphorylcholine[132–136]
Polyethylene glycol[144]	AZ1 adsorbed to cellulose[152,153]
Polyphosphate ester[145]	AZ1/UK adsorbed to cellulose[153,154]
Gold[162]	
Silicon carbide[137,156]	
Diamond-like carbon[155,162,163]	

AZ1 = monoclonal antibody directed against rabbit platelet integrin $\alpha_{IIb}\beta_{II}$,
AZ1/UK = monoclonal antibody directed against rabbit platelet integrin $\alpha_{IIb}\beta_{II}$/urokinase conjugate

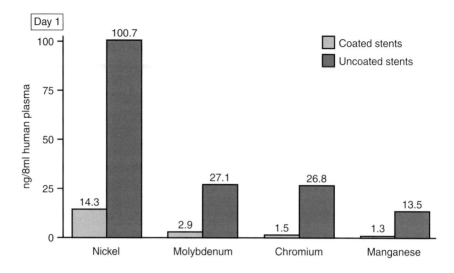

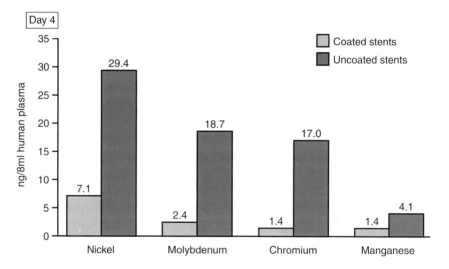

Figure 6.2: Metal ion release from diamond-like coated and uncoated stainless-steel stents. Stents were placed in human plasma, and daily aliquots were taken for analysis. Nickel and chromium analyses were performed by atomic adsorption spectrometry, and manganese and molybdenum ion concentrations were determined by mass spectroscopy. (From Beythien C, Gutensohn K, Fenner T, Padmanaban K, Köster R, Hamm CW, Terres W, Kühnl P. Diamond-like carbon coating of coronary stents: influence on platelet activation, smooth muscle cells and release of metal atoms [abstract]. Eur Heart J 1998; 19: (suppl): 497.)

feasible.[164] There are four heparin-coated stents available for clinical use, the Cordis/Johnson and Johnson heparin-coated Palmaz–Schatz stent, on which heparin is end-linked to the stent surface with a patented Carmeda coating technology (figure 6.3), the Wiktor heparin-coated stent on which heparin is also end-linked (Hepamed coating),[165] and the JOSTENT (Corline heparin coating) and PRO-STENT to which heparin is randomly attached. Covalent end-linking of heparin, as on the Palmaz–Schatz and the Wiktor stents, ensures that all of the antithrombin binding sites are exposed, whereas random covalent binding results in random exposure of antithrombin binding sites on the surface of the stent. Heparin-coated stents are effective in reducing thrombosis in rabbit peripheral vessels[147] and in porcine coronary arteries.[148,149] These encouraging results led to the evaluation of the high activity end-point attached heparin-coated stents in the BENESTENT II pilot study[166] and the BENESTENT II randomized trial.[37,167] Of the 616 patients receiving a heparinized stent in these studies, there was only one episode of subacute thrombosis (incidence <0.2%).

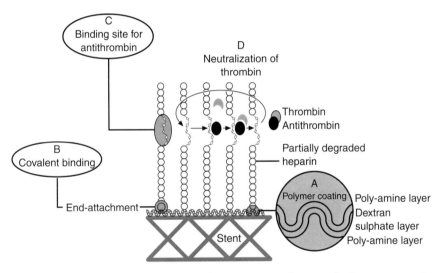

Figure 6.3: *Schematic illustrations of the prominent features of a heparin-coated stent. A. The stent is coated with a polymer made of multiple layers of polyamine and dextran sulphate. B. Depolymerized molecules of heparin are covalently bound to this polymer. C. Pentasaccharide constituting the binding site for antithrombin of each heparin molecule is depicted. D. Continuous neutralization cycle of thrombin is illustrated. (Modified from Serruys PW, Emanuelsson H, van der Giessen W et al. Heparin-coated Palmaz-Schatz stents in human coronary arteries. Early outcome of the Benestent-II pilot study. Circulation 1996; 93: 412–22.)*

229

Another commercially available coated device is the divYsio stent (Biocompatables Ltd), which is phosphorylcholine coated. Phosphorylcholine is the major phospholipid component of biological membranes. Based on promising results in vitro[132] and in vivo in animal models[133-136] it is anticipated that these coated devices will behave as intact tissue elements, a form of biomimicry, and will give a reduction in the incidence of subacute occlusion and an improvement in the long-term patency rates of treated segments. These stents are now being evaluated in clinical trials in Europe for their ability to reduce the incidence of subacute occlusion and improve the long-term outcome in stented coronary segments.

Fibrin coating of intravascular stents has been proposed as a means of passivating the stent surface and providing a platform for the recolonization of endothelial cells.[150] Fibrin coated Palmaz–Schatz stents were shown to be free of thrombus and foreign body reaction when examined 8 weeks after implantation in the peripheral arteries of dogs,[151] compared with a 45% incidence of thrombosis with the implantation of naked stents. More notable was the endothelialization of 96% of the surface of the fibrin-coated stents, whereas the uncoated controls were covered with endothelial cells over only 18% of their surface. Similarly favourable results were seen with implantation of fibrin-film covered stents in pig coronaries. No significant foreign body, giant cell, or inflammatory reaction occurred up to 1 year after stent implantation.[168] The fibrin film did not attenuate the neointimal response to vessel injury compared with that of a bare metal stent, although it may have potential as a biodegradable platform for local drug delivery.[169,170]

Investigation of stents coated with an antithrombotic drug-releasing layer is underway, and several candidate drugs for stent coatings have been considered. Undergoing clinical assessment is an InFlow stent (InFlow Dynamics AG, Munich, Germany) coated with a polylactic acid (PLA) carrier containing 5% polyethylene glycol-hirudin and 1% PGI2–analog (Iloprost). In-vitro analysis showed favourable degradation properties of the carrier and favourable time-release characteristics of the incorporated antithrombotic and platelet-inhibiting drugs.[171] Analysis of the hirudin and Iloprost eluting stents tested during stasis in a human shunt model showed a significant effect on both platelet activation and blood coagulation independent of the underlying metal surface (gold *vs* stainless steel).[172,173] When implanted in sheep coronaries these stents have shown a favourable effect on neointimal formation.[174] Another carrier/active agent system that appears promising is a cellulose polymer with passively adsorbed glycoprotein IIb/IIIa receptor antibody.[175-177] Preparation of these devices is relatively simple. Commercially available GR II stents are supplied with a proprietary cellulose polymer coating. Immersion of these devices into a solution of anti GP IIb/IIIa antibody causes the coating to swell and passively adsorb the Fab fragment as a function of the concentration of protein and the time of immersion.[178] Active compound elutes from the stents in an exponential manner, with 48% of the bound agent eluted at 12 days when studied in vitro.[179] In a rabbit iliac artery model, antibody to GP IIb/IIIa eluted from cellulose-polymer coated stents significantly reduced platelet aggregation in the stent micro-environment, reduced thrombus formation, improved blood flow and arterial patency rates, and inhibited cyclic blood-flow variation.[178] It is hoped that such coated stents, eluting GP IIb/IIIa antibody directed against human platelets, may be effective in eliminating the need for systemic antiplatelet therapy after deployment in humans.

Polymeric coating of the stent in situ has also been shown to be feasible, a technique referred to as "gel paving".[180] A recently reported trial described the application of polyethelene-glycol-lactide hydrogel polymers to the surface of Palmaz–Schatz stents implanted in a porcine femoral artery model.[180] The applied polymer was photopolymerized in situ to form a short-term semipermeable barrier. Stented segments treated in such a manner showed less overt thrombosis, less microscopic platelet adherence, and enhanced vessel patency compared with control stented segments. Much more animal data must be collected before this type of technology can be considered for clinical application.

The seeding of intravascular stents with endothelial cells to passivate the stent surface has been an area of ongoing research for over 9 years. Both self-expanding[181] and balloon expandable[182] stents have been successfully seeded with endothelial cells and have been shown to retain a significant number of viable cells after deployment in vitro.[182,183] In these early experiments, the stents were pre-coated with fibronectin matrix as a foundation for the endothelial cells. Although endothelial seeding was shown to be feasible, the clinical utility of such an approach was questionable. Fibronectin itself is thrombogenic, and the loss of attached cells on stent deployment would expose this thrombogenic surface to the circulating blood if used in vivo. The source of the endothelial cells also presented a problem: homologous tissue was necessary to prevent acute rejection of the grafted tissue on transplantation.

Recent research has addressed these two problems. Using autologous endothelial cells derived from sheep saphenous veins, a group at the National Heart, Lung, and Blood Institute (NHLBI) has successfully seeded metallic stents and implanted the stents into the femoral arteries of the donor animals.[184] The transplanted endothelial cells could be detected in six out of nine animals treated in this manner 10 days after stent implantation. Scott and colleagues[185] were also successful in identifying endothelial cells on seeded stents 3 hours after intracoronary implantation in pigs.[185] These investigators used immortalized human microvascular cells that retain the phenotypic characteristics of endothelial cells after more than 50 passages.[186] These cells were successfully seeded in vitro on an uncoated tantalum wire coil stent prior to deployment.

One stent had been frozen for 2 months, and was thawed prior to use. On explantation, retained endothelial cells could be seen predominantly on the lateral aspects of the stent.

Another approach that has been taken for the passivation of the stent surface by endothelial cells has been called cell "sodding".[187] This strategy involves the local delivery of homologous or autologous endothelial cells via a local delivery catheter to the site of stent implantation. In both pig coronaries and rabbit iliac arteries, more than 75% of the stent surface was covered with endothelial cells 4 hours after stent deployment. By 14 days, the coverage had increased to more than 90%.[187] With the recent advances in stent deployment techniques and antithrombotic therapy, thrombosis rates of less than 1% have been reported. Thus, effective stent endothelialization may be a very costly and complicated solution to the above problems. In addition, there is no evidence to suggest that rapid endothelialization of the treated arterial segment will limit in-stent restenosis. The relevance of continued investment in the development of endothelium covered stents may lie in the future possibility of seeding the stents with genetically modified endothelial cells, capable of producing compounds for the treatment of restenosis.

Genetic manipulation of the seeded endothelial cells is currently being investigated, both as a means to increase the retention of the transplanted cells,[188] and as a means of introducing genetic material for the production of bioactive proteins for the prevention of local thrombosis and late restenosis.[189,190] The local delivery of plasmid DNA encoding vascular endothelial growth factor (phVEGF$_{165}$) has recently been shown to increase stent endothelialization in situ and to reduce stent thrombosis and intimal thickening in the rabbit model.[191,192] With the recent successes in this area of research, interest in endothelial passivation of stents has been renewed.

A novel approach to stent passivation and for the treatment of vessel rupture and aneurysms has been developed by Stefanadis and Toutouzas.[193–198] Their approach involves passivation of the stent surface through the application of a segment of autologous vascular tissue. The technique utilizes a segment of cephalic vein or ulnar artery to cover the stent. A portion of the cephalic vein of appropriate size is explanted at the time of the stent procedure, and cleaned of boundary tissue so as to obtain a thin walled segment. It is then introduced into the lumen of a Palmaz–Schatz stent, and the ends of the graft are reversed upon the metallic stent struts and sutured on the external surface of the stent. The result is that both the internal and external surfaces of the stent are totally covered by the graft to create an autologous vein-graft coated stent (AVGCS) type A. Alternatively, segments of cephalic vein or radial artery can be harvested and used to cover only the external surface of a Palmaz–Schatz or a MULTI-LINK stent. The result is an AVGCS type B or an autologous arterial graft-coated stent (AAGCS). The results of the implantation of a vein graft covered stent have been reported for the treatment of total occlusions, ostial lesions, and saphenous vein grafts lesions, and in elective indications, in bailout situations, and in the setting of an acute myocardial infarction.[193-198] Radial artery covered stents have also been successfully implanted in saphenous vein bypass grafts,[199,200] as well as in both the body and ostia of native coronary vessels.[200,201] Further studies are necessary to clarify the potential of this technique.

Treatment

The clinical features of stent thrombosis usually include chest pain and ECG changes suggestive of ischaemia. Thrombosis of a previously occluded artery, however, may be clinically silent. Prompt vessel recanalization is central to the effective management of acute or subacute thrombosis. Catheter-based therapies have been most commonly used, with the goal of identifying potential causes like inadequate stent expansion, improper stent sizing, persistent dissections, or the presence of intimal flaps protruding from the stent struts. These are frequently managed by repeat balloon dilatation with or without concomitant intracoronary thrombolytic therapy, but the support for such management comes from a relatively low number of small trials.[8,44,45] In the reported series, the successful restoration of flow was achieved in 41%–80% of instances, but those that were not successfully managed percutaneously had severe adverse clinical outcomes. In a recently reported trial, the outcome of those treated with angioplasty-based procedures for stent thrombosis were retrospectively analysed.[9] In that trial, 23 patients were treated with catheter-based therapies (angioplasty alone in 14, angioplasty and intracoronary urokinase in seven, and intracoronary urokinase alone in two). TIMI grade 3 flow was restored in 21 of these patients, but only 11 had no angiographic evidence of thrombus. Of the 23 patients, two died, and nine were referred for emergent or urgent bypass surgery because of refractory angina and residual thrombosis threatening reclosure. Despite restoration of flow in most patients, 20 (87%) of the 23 patients developed an acute myocardial infarction. These findings certainly suggest that alternative or adjunctive therapies are needed to treat this disastrous complication.

Other therapies for the treatment of subacute thrombosis are being investigated. The local delivery of urokinase via local infusion or on a urokinase-hydrogel coated balloon has been proposed,[202] and uncontrolled anecdotal evidence suggests benefit for intracoronary administration of platelet disaggregators such as GPIIb/IIIa inhibitors.[203-205] One small observational trial has reported reduced bleeding and vessel complications and a reduced need for repeat PTCA and bypass surgery with the use of GPIIb/IIIa inhibitors compared with intracoronary administration of urokinase.[206,207] A newly introduced thrombectomy catheter,[208] which removes thrombus by means of high-velocity saline jets, has also proved to be effective in our hands (unpublished data).

233

Further investigations must be done before any newer therapy can be recommended.

Restenosis

The problem

Restenosis is the decrease in the vessel lumen at the site of catheter-based intracoronary therapies. With the failure of both conventional systemic and local drug therapies to reduce significantly the restenosis rate after successful balloon angioplasty, newer technologies have been touted as possibly providing the solution to this enormous problem. The demonstration by the BENESTENT[209] and the STRESS[210] trials that the rates of restenosis could be significantly, although modestly, reduced, was a major advance in the push to reduce and ultimately eliminate restenosis. What became quickly apparent after the release of the BENESTENT and STRESS results was that the beneficial effects of stent implantation on restenosis could be attributed to the larger acute lumen dimensions achieved than with balloon angioplasty, and to a decrease in the amount of vessel recoil after intervention.[211,212] Elastic recoil is reduced to 4%–18% for Palmaz–Schatz stents,[213–216] 20% for Gianturco–Roubin stents,[218] and 8%–22% for Wiktor-GX stent implantation,[215–217] and a part of this observed acute loss can be attributed to the protrusion of plaque through the stent struts.[216] More recently, the beneficial effects of coronary stent implantation for the reduction of negative (anti-Glagovian) remodeling has been shown.[219,220] What stents have failed to improve upon is the neointimal proliferative response to vessel injury, seen both in balloon angioplasty (POBA or "plain old balloon angioplasty" as it is now being referred to) and in stented vascular segments. Both experimental and clinical data have shown that stent-induced neointimal formation is more extensive and protracted than that provoked by balloon angioplasty.[221–224] Intimal hyperplasia is the major component of late lumen loss after stent implantation.[225–228] This has stimulated research into the pathobiology of the stent restenosis process — research that has revealed interesting findings that will certainly guide clinical management and prevention of restenosis.

The response to vascular injury resulting from the placement of an indwelling endovascular stent differs from that caused by balloon angioplasty alone in at least four ways.[227]

(1) *Type of injury*. Through histological examination of porcine coronary arteries it has been shown that the site of neointimal proliferation in the setting of balloon angioplasty alone occurs at the site of disruption of the internal elastic lamina.[228] When a stent of the appropriate size is placed in the pig model, the stent struts abut the vessel wall and compress the media without fracturing the

internal elastic lamina. The result is very little neointima formation. With stent strut penetration of the elastic lamina, neointimal proliferation is stimulated in accordance with the depth of penetration.[15,227] Schwartz and colleagues[228] have developed a vessel injury score to grade the degree of wall damage (table 6.4) and have shown a correlation between this score and neointimal proliferation at 4 weeks after stent implantation in a porcine model, although only a weak correlation at 12 weeks has been shown by others.[229] In an experimental model, the degree of wall injury and the subsequent neointimal response was a function of the balloon inflation pressure used to deploy the stent.[230] It is tempting to extrapolate this finding to the clinical situation, and to suggest that intentional oversizing and very high-pressure balloon post-dilatation techniques would result in increased rates of restenosis. This, however, may not be the case. One study has been reported in which high-pressure balloon inflation with pressures up to 24 atmospheres resulted in a reduction of the incidence of thrombotic events without an increase in the clinical restenosis rate as determined by the need for revascularization.[81] This may reflect enlargement of the lumen with higher pressures with accommodation of the greater neointimal burden. Angioscopic, intravascular ultrasound (IVUS) or postmortem studies need to be done to determine the ideal balloon-inflation pressure to optimize stent expansion with minimum trauma to the vessel.

(2) *Pattern of cell response.* The early events after the acute injury of the intervention differ between angioplastied lesions and stented vessels.[227,228,231] The stent struts provide a scaffold for the formation of platelet-rich thrombi, into

Table 6.4 Vessel injury score

Score	Description of vascular injury
0	Internal elastic lamina intact, endothelium denuded, media compressed (not lacterated)
1	Internal elastic lamina lacerated, media compressed (not lacerated)
2	Internal elastic lamina lacerated, media visibly lacerated, external elastic lamina intact but compressed.
3	External elastic lamina lacerated, large lacerations of the media extending through the external elastic lamina, coil wires sometimes residing in the adventitia

Values for vessel injury score (From Schwartz et al. Restenosis and proportional neointimal response to coronary artery injury: results in a porcine model. *J Am Coll Cardiol* 1992; **19:** 267–74)

which inflammatory cells from the circulation migrate. The inflammatory cell component plays a much greater part in stented lesions than in those treated with balloon angioplasty alone.[229] Reactive inflammatory infiltrates, which include lymphocytes, eosinophils, and histiocytes, extend from the luminal surface of the stented vessel, through the wall and into the adventitita.[231] Such cellular infiltrates can be seen as early as 15 minutes and as late as 56 days after stent implantation in animal models. By contrast, very early and late infiltrates are virtually absent in arteries subject to balloon angioplasty alone.[229,231] Of particular interest is the role of mononuclear cells in the pathogenesis of neointimal hyperplasia. The number of tissue monocytes rises after stent implantation, and is highest at 7 days.[232] In an experimental model, treatments that reduced adherent and tissue monocytes produced reductions in intimal cell proliferation and intimal thickening.[232] Stent geometry has also been shown to affect the degree of monocyte accumulation.[15]

The release of cytokines, mitogens, and tissue growth factors may play an important part in the later stages of stent-induced vascular injury and repair, characterized by smooth muscle cell migration, proliferation, and matrix protein secretion. Smooth muscle cells migrate from the media to the neointimal layer, where mural thrombi function as a scaffold for smooth muscle cell migration and proliferation. Direct evidence of smooth muscle cell proliferation in stent restenosis has been reported. In-stent restenotic tissue consists of larger areas of hypercellular tissue and smooth muscle cells and smaller areas of macrophages and tissue factor than in post-PTCA restenotic tissue.[233] The degree of neointimal formation and the proliferative rate of the smooth muscle cells is proportional to the early inflammatory cell involvement.[15,227,234]

(3) *Prolonged radial strain.* Balloon angioplasty applies a transient strain to the vessel wall, while permanent strain is produced by an implanted stent. This may result in a prolonged stimulus for neointimal formation. A porcine coronary model showed that with both coil and tubular stent designs histologically determined vessel wall injury progressed between weeks 1 and 12 after implantation.[229] This change was manifest as progressive laceration of the internal elastic lamina and a deeper penetration of the struts through the media. This phase of chronic injury also typically involved a chronic inflammatory response in the media, and occasionally in the intima. These inflammatory changes were never observed in balloon-treated vessels, and are thought to contribute to a derangement in the integrity of the endothelial lining.[235]

(4) *Presence of a foreign material.* The most apparent difference between balloon angioplasty and stenting may also be the most critical. The presence of a foreign body in the lumen of the vessel serves as a stimulus for intimal hyperplasia, and stent design and composition can greatly influence this process, as has been shown in animal models.[15] In vessels stented with devices with a single articulation, the pattern of lumen loss is not uniform along the stent but increases

significantly at the central articulation.[220,226,236,237] When two stents are placed in sequence without overlapping, no corresponding increase in tissue accumulation is seen.[227] The presence of a bridge, constraining one degree of freedom for the stent, seems to contribute to the restenosis process. Intuitively, it may seem that the ideal stent design would serve as a barrier to the migration of smooth muscle cells from the media, but in a study using two coiled-wire stents of identical material that differed only in the presence or absence of gaps in the design, significantly greater hyperplasia was noted in segments with gap-free stents.[238] In another report, Palmaz–Schatz slotted-tube stents were compared with both the Strecker stent (a tantalum woven mesh stent that is no longer commercially available) and the Wallstent.[239] The slotted-tube stent showed a less neointimal growth at 4 months after implantation than the other two stent designs. Low electropositivity of the stent metal also exaggerates neointimal prolilferation.[19] These data suggest that stent geometry, surface, and material may all be important determinants of stent-induced cellular proliferation and neointimal hyperplasia in humans as well.

The result of stent implantation is the production of a proliferative neointima. The layer that forms above the stent struts in humans has been shown, using atherectomy samples, to be relatively acellular, composed predominantly of extracellular matrix.[240] This is similar to animal models in which most of the late cellular activity in stented vessels can be found in the areas immediately around and beneath the stent struts.[227] The course of the stent restenosis process is similar to that reported for PTCA, with almost no significant renarrowing occurring beyond 6 months.[241]

Risk factors

Several risk factors for the development of stent restenosis have been determined by univariate and multivariate analysis of several stented populations of patients.

History of restenosis
Stent implantation at the site of a restenotic lesion is associated with a greater likelihood of stent restenosis.[242–247] This is similar to the situation seen with PTCA.[248] Arterial trauma results in a change of the smooth muscle from a contractile to an organelle-rich synthetic phenotype,[249,250] and it has been suggested that repeat trauma to an area already containing many phenotypically synthetic smooth muscle cells may heighten the risk of restenosis. The restenosis rates for patients with elective coronary stenting for post-angioplasty restenosis vary widely, with values as high as 39% with the traditional stent implantation regimen (lower pressure implantation with post-procedure anticoagulation)[243,251] and values as low as 11% with current procedural methods.[252,253] The randomized REST trial reported a restenosis rate of 18% in lesions with previous restenosis

post-angioplasty.[254] Procedural variability and differences in the populations of patients may account for the inconsistency of the results. In this regard, multivariate analysis in several trials failed to show a history of restenosis as a risk factor for subsequent clinical stent restenosis.[253,255–259]

Multiple stents
Multiple stent implantation has been shown to be a significant risk factor for stent restenosis in several studies.[48,242,244–246,253,258,260–263] It has been hypothesized that stent-on-stent trauma may prevent passivation of the stent surface, and thereby promote thrombus formation and stimulate restenosis. This has been supported by multivariate risk analysis in one small study that identified overlapping stents as an independent risk factor for restenosis.[263] A recent IVUS study however, demonstrated that the tissue growth, late lumen loss, and chronic lumen dimensions were similar at the junction of two stents regardless of whether they were overlapping or not, suggesting that stent overlap may not be responsible for the observed increase in risk.[220] Two studies have reported no differences in the clinically determined restenosis rates between patients treated with a single stent and those receiving multiple stents.[46,47] The reasons for this apparent disparity may be that multiple stents are more commonly placed in larger vessels, saphenous vein bypass grafts, and vessels which are totally occluded.[46] These differences may account for a reduced impetus for revascularization in the event of restenosis or reocclusion. One study has reported that multiple stent implantation was a risk factor for restenosis when stents were implanted with lower pressure (less than 16 atmospheres) and was not a risk factor with high-pressure implantation (16 atmospheres or greater).[264] Lesion length itself has been associated with restenosis, with longer stented lesions showing a higher rate of restenosis.[253,265–267] Multiple stent implantation has also been shown to be a risk factor for restenosis in saphenous vein graft disease.[268]

Extent of residual stenosis
The extent of residual stenosis after stenting has been shown to be correlated with the likelihood of subsequent restenosis.[242,245] This is probably because less encroachment of myointima is necessary for a greater than 50% reduction in lumen diameter (the angiographic definition of restenosis) if a significant narrowing is already present. Several reports have failed to show residual stenosis as a significant risk factor for subsequent restenosis.[253,258,263]

Stenting of total occlusions
Whether stent placement in totally occluded vessels is a risk factor for restenosis is the subject of controversy. Few reports specifically include chronic total occlusions in their statistical analysis, and have conflicting results. There are reports which show stenting of total occlusions to be a risk factor for subsequent

restenosis,[246,253] and those which do not.[258] Reported angiographic rates of restenosis from observational trials range from 19% to 76%,[269–283] and seem to depend on the clinical situation, the type of stent implanted and the location. This large variability in observed restenosis rates probably accounts for the confusing results of the studies examining risk factors.

Diabetes mellitus

A history of diabetes mellitus has been shown to correlate with the subsequent risk of developing in-stent restenosis in native coronary and saphenous vein graft lesions in several studies.[246,247,257,261–263,284–291] The mechanisms responsible for the increased proclivity for restenosis in the diabetic patient are not completely understood. It has been suggested that increased levels of growth factors such as insulin-like growth factor-1 and insulin itself may promote smooth muscle proliferation and matrix protein secretion.[292,293] This hypothesis has not been supported by the available evidence, however. It has been shown that the particular feature of atherectomy specimens retrieved from restenotic lesions in diabetic patients was not enhanced smooth muscle cell proliferation, but rather an enhanced fibrotic response that may favour vessel constriction.[294] Thus, the impact of diabetes in lesions treated with balloon angioplasty alone may be enhanced negative (anti-Glagovian) remodelling, but this does not explain the observed effect of diabetes on restenosis in stented vessels. Endothelial cell dysfunction and impaired regeneration of endothelial cells following injury may also contribute to augmented neointimal formation.[292] Two studies have failed to show diabetes as a predictor of in-stent restenosis.[253,258]

Stent deployment pressure

The effect of stent deployment pressure on the risk for restenosis is controversial. In saphenous vein grafts, high-pressure stent deployment ($\geq$16 atmospheres) is associated with a smaller minimum luminal diameter (MLD) at 6 months, which is thought to be a result of increased neointimal proliferation within the stent.[295] In native coronary arteries, higher restenosis rates have been described with low (< 12 atmospheres) stent deployment pressures.[244] Although higher pressures have been associated with a greater late loss in MLD at 6 months follow-up,[296] restenosis rates were not increased.[81,297,298] High-pressure stent deployment has been shown to have a deleterious effect on the function of the distal microcirculation.[299]

Other risk factors

Stent placement in vessels with an angiographically determined reference diameter of less than 3.0 mm is a risk factor for restenosis.[242,244,246,247,258,300] One explanation for this observation is that the absolute amount of neointima required to result in more than 50% stenosis is lower for vessels of smaller calibre. The observation that a small reference diameter was not associated with a higher late lumen loss supports this concept.[258] Other clinical and angiographic characteristics that are risk factors for stent restenosis include: (1) post-procedure lumen diameter;[246,247,257,258,292] (2) stent placement in the left anterior descending location;[246,257,285,301] (3) stent implantation in type B2 and C[262] or type C lesions[253] (according to the modified ACC/AHA classification by Ellis and colleagues);[302] (4) female gender;[253] (5) patient age of more than 63 years;[253] (6) residual dissection post-stenting;[265] and (7) restenosis of another lesion in the same patient.[303]

An interesting risk factor has been described by Ribichini and colleagues.[304] In a select cohort of patients (those with de-novo lesions in a single native coronary vessel who were treated with a Palmaz–Schatz stent deployed with high-pressure techniques) they identified high plasma levels of angiotensin converting enzyme (ACE) and the deletion/deletion (D/D) genotype of the ACE gene to be highly significant predictors for stent restenosis independent of other clinical risk factors. ACE may play an important role in the proliferation of vascular smooth muscle cells through activation of angiotensin II (an inducer of cell proliferation) and inhibition of bradykinin (an inhibitor of growth).[305] Their data indicate that with elective stent implantation in patients at low risk for restenosis, as indicated by low plasma ACE levels, restenosis rates of under 8% can be expected.

Recurrent in-stent restenosis
Very little is known about the risk factors governing the recurrence of restenosis in stents after successful treatment of in-stent restenosis. Saphenous vein graft location of the stent and vessel size less than 3 mm have been identified as risk factors in one small study.[306]

Patterns of in-stent restenosis
Evidence is accumulating that the pattern of restenosis seen on angiography may dictate the response to therapy. Several distinct patterns have been identified: (1) focal (length less than 10 mm); (2) diffuse (length greater than or equal to 10 mm, not extending beyond the stent margins); (3) proliferative (length greater than or equal to 10 mm and extending beyond the stent margins); and (4) total occlusions. The risk factors for each of these patterns may be different. Stent implantation in smaller vessels,[307] multiple stent implantation,[307] LAD location,[308] post-treatment MLD,[308] and ACE I/D polymorphism[309] have all been shown to be predictors of the diffuse or proliferative patterns of in-stent restenosis.

Prevention

The discouraging results of most trials examining the systemic administration of pharmacological agents for the prevention of restenosis in the setting of balloon angioplasty[311–314] has affected the focus of therapies directed at the improvement of the long-term outcome of stent implantation. Very few systemically administered agents have been shown to influence the clinical and angiographic rates of restenosis after PTCA. These include the prostacyclin analogue ciprostene,[314,317] GPIIb/IIIa inhibitors,[316] trapidil,[317] angiopeptin,[318] and omega-3 fatty acids.[319] These agents are also being investigated for their ability to prevent restenosis in the setting of stent implantation. Results of the randomized TRAPIST study showed the failure of trapidil to prevent in-stent restenosis.[320] Randomized trials have also shown cilostazol,[321] a 3'5'–cyclic nucleotide phosphodiesterase III inhibitor, and a combined treatment with cilstazol and probucol[322] to be successful in the prevention of in-stent restenosis.

The local delivery of therapeutic compounds using specially designed delivery catheters is being attempted as a means of obtaining high local concentrations of pharmacological agents and reducing their systemic toxicity. A small clinical study examining the local delivery of a long acting steroid (methylprednisolone) prior to elective stent implantation failed to show any beneficial effect on the rate of restenosis.[323] A randomized clinical trial examining the local delivery of antisense oligonucleotide to *c-myc* has also failed to show any benefit on the 6–months in-stent restenosis rate.[324,325] Trials are also underway in which heparin,[326] enoxaprin,[327–329] and steroids are locally delivered at the time of stent implantation. A very sophisticated approach is being tested in animals by Litvack and colleagues.[330,331] They have designed chimeric DNA–RNA hammerhead ribozymes that inhibit the expression of CDC-2 kinase and PCNA genes by cleavage at mRNA sites. Local delivery of both of these compounds at the site of stent implantation has been shown to inhibit intimal hyperplasia in a porcine coronary stent restenosis model.[330,331] The clinical potential of this novel technology is currently being assessed.

Stent coatings are also being investigated as a way of decreasing the neointimal proliferative response. Metal stents encapsulated with polytetrafluorine have been shown to reduce neointimal thickening in an animal model of vascular injury.[332] As a consequence of their long residence times, attention has become focused on endovascular stents as a platform for the delivery of therapeutic agents. This can be accomplished by coating metallic stents with controlled release matrices or by incorporating a pharmacologically active compound into a polymeric stent or a polymer-metal composite stent. Controlled-release matrices are formulated by uniform dispersion or dissolution of the drug of interest in a polymeric preparation. Drug release occurs by means of particle dissolution and diffusion through the base polymer, or by matrix breakdown and biodegradation of hydrolyzable (biodegradable) polymer. Stents can be coated with a polymeric matrix system involving either a degradable or non-degradable polymer with a dispersed pharmacological agent. Some general considerations about the choice of agents are important in formulating drug-polymer systems. For example, if non-degradable polymers are to be used for stent coatings, only water-soluble agents should be considered for incorporation, because insoluble agents could become entrapped in the polymer. Agents that are not water soluble can be incorporated easily into a biodegradable stent structure, because matrix breakdown will release these compounds. The potency of the incorporated drug is also of crucial importance because of the limited space available on the strut structure of the stent. Therefore, many of the conventionally available pharmaceuticals may not be the best available agents. Of the conventional drugs, very potent compounds with a relatively low systemic dose (compared with other drugs) offer the best possibilities. In addition, drugs rejected for human use because of systemic side-effects may, in fact, be the most suitable candidates for incorporation into pharmaceutical stents.

Drug-polymer composites are referred to as monolithic matrices. When non-degradable matrices are utilized, drug delivery is achieved through sustained release by way of particle dissolution and diffusion through the cavitating network of the matrix. Extended drug release is possible through this approach, with formulations having release durations from hours to decades in length. Examples of non-biodegradable polymers include polyurethane,[333] poly(dimethyl)-siloxane (SIL),[334] and polyethene terephthalate.[335] Biodegradable polymer systems have also been used to formulate drug delivery matrices. Biodegradable polymer matrices provide sustained delivery of pharmacological agents both by drug dissolution and by matrix degradation in vivo, leading to release of entrapped agents. Examples of some of the more widely investigated biodegradable polymers include polylactic-polyglycolic acid,[336–343] high-molecular-weight polyanhydrides,[344–346] pluronics,[347,348] chitosan,[349–352] polycaprolactone,[353,354] polyhydroxy-butyrate/-valerate copolymer (78:22),[355,356] polyorthoester[357,358], and polyethyleneoxide/polybutylene terphthalate copolymer (30:70).[359,360] The coating of a pharmaceutical stent with a biodegradable polymer also offers the attractive possibility that the drug-polymer system could disappear after a desired period of drug release.

Several candidate drugs have been considered for stent coatings. Undergoing clinical assessment is a stent coated with a polylactic acid (PLA) carrier containing 5% polyethylene glycol-hirudin and 1% prostaglandin I2 (PGI2)-analog (Iloprost). When implanted in sheep coronaries these stents have a favourable effect on neointimal formation.[174] Stents coated with dexamethasone suspended in a matrix of poly-L-lactic acid have been tested in pig coronary arteries, in an attempt to prevent the characteristic local inflammatory response seen early after stent implantation.[361] High local concentrations of dexamethasone were measured up to 28 days after stent implantation, but no reduction in the neointimal proliferative response was observed. Inhibition of neointima formation has been shown by several groups with the microtubule stabilizing agent paclitaxil incorporated into a biodegradable polymer. Significant inhibition of neointimal formation in a rabbit hind-limb model of in-stent restenosis was shown with paclitaxel incorporated in a polymer of 1% chondroitin sulfate and gelatin, which was coated on a metallic stent.[362] Similar encouraging results were reported with paclitaxel-coated GRII stents implanted in a pig coronary model.[363]

The use of gene therapy in conjunction with a pharmaceutical delivery stent could involve the transfer of a desired gene from the stent coating to the cells of the arterial wall. This should result in the expression and synthesis of a desirable product by the cells of the arterial wall. This approach would involve the incorporation of DNA or a viral vector into a polymeric matrix system under conditions that would allow cellular uptake and translation of the DNA. This task is a great challenge because of all of the complex possibilities that could interfere with efficient transfer, integration, and incorporation of DNA into a polymer stent in a biologically active form, and with the sustained release of the genetic material from the polymeric matrix.

Another possible strategy for a pharmaceutical stent approach involves the incorporation of antisense oligonucleotides into an appropriate polymeric matrix. Proof that the concept of this type of approach works has been shown by Rosenberg and colleagues[364] by the incorporation of an antisense oligonucleotide into a biodegradable polymer known as a poloxamer. In their studies, the oligonucleotide-polymer composite was injected by syringe onto the adventitia of the arterial wall of a rat carotid artery subjected to balloon injury. The biodegradable polymer released sufficient amounts of the antisense oligonucleotide specific for the *c-myb* oncogene,[365] to result in successful inhibition of proliferation of the smooth muscle cells of the arterial wall. Thus, there may be promise for the development of a stent coated with a polymeric matrix that is able to deliver antisense oligonucleotides locally.

Once a very active area of research, interest in the development of a suitable biodegradable stent with pharmacologically active agents incorporated into the polymeric matrix has waned considerably. To be effective, a drug-releasing biodegradable stent must be biocompatible, must not cause an inflammatory reaction, and the breakdown products must be non-toxic. Stent delivery must be reliable, the devices must have high radial strength, and stent degradation should occur in a reasonable time period (12–24 months). The ideal stent would deliver drugs locally that inhibit restenosis, in concentrations that are effective without inducing tissue injury. The excellent long-term biocompatability of stainless-steel stents, combined with the considerable difficulties of developing a polymeric stent with a high performance delivery system, radio-opacity, and structural characteristics competitive with stainless-steel devices (like radial hoop strength), has focused efforts away from the development of drug-releasing biodegradable stents. One such biodegradable device, however, warrants mention. The Duke Biodegradable Stent is made from a special form of poly-L-lactide (PLLA), capable of incorporating pharmacologically active agents.[366] Both self-expanding and balloon expandable versions of the Duke stent have been designed and tested in animals,[367] with promising results.

Low-power red laser light (LPRLL) is currently undergoing clinical evaluation to determine whether it can prevent in-stent restenosis. The ability of LPRLL to inhibit restenosis has been shown both in the balloon injured rabbit model[368] and in the porcine coronary stent model.[369] The mechanisms by which LPRLL reduce neointimal hyperplasia have not been fully established. It is thought that LPRLL contributes to endothelial regeneration, and, through an accelerated re-endothelialization of the denuded segment, prevents migration and proliferation of smooth muscle cells. In a observational clinical study,[370] 70 patients were treated with LPRLL with a laser power of 1.1 J/cm^2. Three groups of patients received the LPRLL; 26 patients with a suboptimal balloon angioplasty result, 24 patients with restenosis after balloon angioplasty, and 30 patients with in-stent restenosis. Overall, the restenosis rate was 21% at 6 months, indicating a potential benefit for the prevention of in-stent restenosis in these relatively high-risk patients. A randomized clinical trial is being planned to confirm these promising results.

Low-dose external beam irradiation has been shown to be a safe and effective means for the treatment of several benign proliferative disorders. The success of this approach has led to the hypothesis that brachytherapy might also result in a reduction in intimal hyperplasia when administered after percutaneous revascularization. Early results from the balloon injured porcine model of restenosis showed the efficacy of the gamma emitter iridium-192 (^{192}Ir) in limiting the formation of neointima in this model.[371,372] Endoluminal radiation in the model was delivered transiently immediately after injury, and effects of the radiation therapy persisted up to 6 months after injury. Similarly favourable results were seen with both gamma- and β-irradiation applied transiently before stent implantation in the porcine model of vascular injury.[373]

Hehrlein and colleagues[374,375] were the first to describe the use of radioactive stents, which they implanted in non-diseased rabbit iliac arteries. The stainless-steel stents were made radioactive by ion bombardment in a cyclotron, and emitted both gamma and beta radiation from the radionuclides ^{55,56,57}Co, ^{52}Mg, and ^{55}Fe. Stents with three activities (3.9–35 μCurie) were tested. At 4 weeks, exposure to the two higher doses resulted in a significant reduction in neointimal formation, while in all three groups there was a significant reduction in proliferating cell nuclear antigen positive cells and smooth muscle cell counts. Vascular re-endothelialization occurred despite prolonged irradiation, but the time to complete endothelial cell coverage was delayed in a dose-dependent manner.

Laird and colleagues[376] also assessed the effects of a radioactive coil stent. They first ion-implanted the non-radioactive element ^{31}P beneath the surface of the stent. The stents were then made radioactive by exposing them to neutron irradiation which converts a fraction of the ^{31}P atoms to ^{32}P—a pure β-particle emitter. This irradiation technique resulted in an even distribution of ^{32}P within the stent, to ensure homogenous distribution of β-particle irradiation from the stent. The technique, however, generates other short-lived radioisotopes. Intraluminal exposure to these radioactive stents for 28 days, with an initial activity of 0.14 μCurie, caused a significant reduction in neointimal area and percent area stenosis compared with the effects of non-radioactive stents.

The efficacy of a relatively low dose, pure β-emitting stent for the inhibition of intimal hyperplasia was first shown by Hehrlein and colleagues.[377] [32]P, produced by neutron bombardment, was ionized and ion-implanted beneath the outer surface of titanium-nickel stents. ^{32}P has several characteristics that make it desirable for use in stent-bound brachytherapy. The maximum energy of the β-particle is 1.709 MeV, and provides local effects with a tissue range of 5–6 mm—this minimizes the exposure of surrounding cardiac and pulmonary tissue to ionizing radiation. As a result of the low energy, shielding of the catheterization laboratory staff from radiation can be accomplished with a simple lucite case prior to stent implantation. The 14-day half-life of ^{32}P ensures a rapid decrease in radioactivity, such that there is virtually no radiation delivered several months after implantation. This allows for normal healing without persistence of the injurious effects of irradiation. In a coronary artery model, a β-emitting stent with an initial activity of 1 μCurie has been shown to provide a uniform dose to the medial layer of the vessel wall (figure 6.4). In addition to the direct effects on the medial layer, it is believed that radioactive stents cull the smooth muscle cell population as these cells pass through the "electron fence" at the plane of the stent wires.[378] ^{32}P-emitting stents with activities of 4 and 13 μCurie were implanted in rabbit iliac arteries, and histomorphometry was done at 4 and 12 weeks.[377] At 4 weeks, both groups showed significant reductions in neointimal formation, while at 12 weeks only the group receiving the highest radiation dose showed a significant reduction in neointima compared with non-radioactive stents.

Using a similar radioactive stent, the neoinitmal responses to implantation in a porcine coronary restenosis model were assessed using stents with activities from 0.15 to 23 μCuries. Neointimal formation was reduced 28 days after the implantation of low (0.15–0.5 μCuries) and high (3–23 μCuries) activity stents, but increased neointimal formation was observed with stents of 1 μCurie initial activity. These results highlight the complexity of the response of the vascular wall to ionizing radiations. The stent used in this trial has subsequently become known as the Fischell IsoStent™ (IsoStent/Cordis Corp, a Johnson and Johnson Interventional Systems Co, San Carlos, CA/Warren, NJ, USA).[379] It is a stainless-steel Palmaz–Schatz stent that has been modified to emit beta-particles by ion implantation as described above.

Bombardment of the gold-coated Inflow stents in the neutron beam of a nuclear reactor produces radioactive β-particle emitter ^{198}Au. ^{198}Au has a short half-life of 2.7 days. Implantation of radioactive Inflow stents with activities ranging from 0.2 to 20 Gray (Gy) in a porcine coronary stent model resulted in a significant, dose-dependent reduction of intimal hyperplasia.[380]

Proton activation of nitinol produces the predominantly β-emitting isotope [48]V. The Act-One™ stent (Progressive Angioplasty Systems Inc, Menlo Park, CA), the predecessor of the Paragon stent, has been made radioactive through proton activation and tested in pig coronary arteries.[381] Radioactive Act-One stents with 1.5 μCurie [48]V activity had no effect on lumen narrowing or vessel histology, but 10 μCurie [48]V stents inhibited neointimal thickening compared with non-radioactive stented control segments. Further studies are necessary to assess the effectiveness of radioactive nitinol stents for the prevention of restenosis.

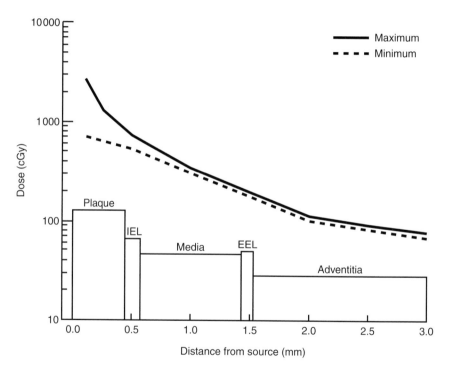

Figure 6.4: *Maximum and minimum dose after 14.3 days, and over the full area of a 3.5 mm diameter [32]P Palmaz–Schatz stent with an initial activity $A_0 = 37$ kBq (1 μCi), to a simplified stenosed artery mode consisting of plaque, internal elastic lamina (IEL), media, external elastic lamina (EEL), and adventitia. The high activity peaks are dissipated into the plaque, while the dose to the media is relatively uniform. (From Janicki C, Duggan DM, Coffey CW, Fischell DR, Fischell TA. Radiation dose from a phosphorous-32 impregnated wire mesh vascular stent. Med Phys 1997; 24: 437–45.*

A liquid-filled balloon containing the β-emitter [188]Re was effective for the prevention of restenosis in a pig coronary model of in-stent restenosis.[382] In this study, a 7 minute treatment was required to deliver a dose of 14 Gy at a 0.5 mm tissue depth. This balloon catheter is currently being used in clinical trials to assess the prevention of restenosis after balloon angioplasty.

The first study of intracoronary radiation in humans was done by Condado and colleagues.[383] In their study, a 30-mm long high activity ^{192}Ir line source was inserted by hand into a monorail closed-end catheter that was positioned in 22 lesions of 21 patients immediately after balloon angioplasty. The doses received ranged between 19 and 55 Gy. Late angiographic follow-up showed a late loss of 0.19 and a negative late loss in 10 of the 22 treated arteries. There were no adverse events reported that could be related to the radiation treatment. The SCRIPPS trial was the first randomized trial to evaluate vascular brachytherapy in patients with restenosis and stenting.[384,385] Both clinical and angiographic outcomes were significantly better in the group treated with radiation than in the control group. Prompted by the encouraging results of β-particle-emitting stents on neointimal hyperplasia in animal models,[375–377,386] a multicentre pilot study to assess the feasibility and safety of the implantation of radioactive [32]P Palmaz–Schatz stent has been completed (IRIS IA).[387,388] In that study, 30 patients with stenosis in de-novo or restenotic lesions of native coronary arteries underwent radioactive stent implantation (activity 0.5 to 1.0 μCuries). Six-months angiographic follow-up revealed a binary restenosis rate of 31% and a clinically driven target revascularization rate of 21%. The larger randomized IRIS (IsoStent for Restenosis Intervention Study) trial is now underway.

Despite the encouraging results of the feasibility and phase I trials with intracoronary brachytherapy, caution must be applied in the interpretation of the results of non-randomized trials involving small cohorts of patients. There are still many unresolved issues surrounding the use of intracoronary ionizing radiation. The therapeutic and toxic windows have not been defined, and it is unclear what the late effects of ionizing radiation will be on the patient. It has been suggested that patients who are enrolled in radiotherapy trials should be followed for years. Dosimetry is also a significant problem. It has been shown that higher dose β-emitting coronary stents (≥3 μCuries) promote the formation of an "atheromatous" neointima in a porcine model, composed of smooth muscle cells, matrix proteoglycans, calcium, foam cells, and cholesterol clefts.[389] A dose-dependent increase in neointimal area for stents with activities greater than 3.0 μCuries was also seen in this study.

Treatment

The best management for the treatment of patients with symptomatic in-stent restenosis has not been completely established. Several reports have supported the use of conventional balloon angioplasty,[225,260,390–406] but high recurrent restenosis rates of the earlier trials prompted investigations into the use of other treatments. Since the early balloon studies, stent-in-stent procedures,[404,407–411] cutting balloon angioplasty,[412] and the debulking techniques of directional atherectomy,[413,414] rotational atherectomy,[404,415–420] and eximer laser procedures[404,421–428] have been proposed as superior treatments for in-stent restenosis. The mechanism underlying the beneficial effect of the debulking procedures is relatively straightforward, while that of balloon angioplasty is less clear. One quantitative angiographic study done before the routine use of high-pressure stent deployment techniques showed that 85% of the luminal enlargement produced by balloon dilatation within stenotic stents was due to compression of protruding tissue and extrusion of hyperplastic tissue through the stent interstices, and only 15% of the enlargement was related to additional stent expansion.[429] However, the relative contribution of each mechanism seems to be device-specific.[397] More recent data obtained with the use of IVUS contradicts this finding, and shows that the predominant mechanism of lumen enlargement is through over-expansion of the stent, while the neointimal area remains unchanged.[398]

The high restenosis rates seen in the early balloon studies were probably due to an overestimation of the true restenosis rates, as a result of a low rate of angiographic follow-up.[399] For example, follow-up angiographic results at 7 months after stent redilatation were available in only 48% of the 105 patients in the US multicenter Palmaz–Schatz registry, and this series documented a recurrence of restenosis in 54% of cases.[399] A more recent study by Bauters and colleagues,[405] with 85% angiographic follow-up, reported a 22% rate of restenosis. Another study with 80% angiographic follow-up, also assessing the treatment of in-stent restenosis with balloon angioplasty, reported a 50% restenosis rate.[406] These apparently disparate results may be explained by considering the lesion characteristics in the two trials. A diffuse pattern of restenosis was present in only 29% of the patients in the former study, while those with a diffuse pattern represented 69% of the patient population in the latter. The diffuse pattern of in-stent restenosis results in the greatest recurrence of stent restenosis after balloon angioplasty.[430,431] Subgroup analysis of the results of Bauters and colleagues,[405] show a rate of recurrent restenosis of 42% in stents with a diffuse pattern of restenosis and a rate of only 14% in stents with focal recurrence. This finding suggests that stent restenosis is not a single entity and that a particular treatment may not be ideal for all patterns.

The high propensity for patients with a diffuse pattern of in-stent restenosis to develop recurrent restenosis after balloon treatment may be related to residual plaque burden after repeat angioplasty, and these patients may benefit from additional debulking strategies. One small study has used this approach. Rotational atherectomy was done on a series of 32 patients with diffuse in-stent restenosis, followed by low-pressure balloon dilatation.[420] Although there were no adverse events reported, the 6-months restenosis rate was a dissapointing 56%. Using stent implantation for focal in-stent restenosis, Mehran and colleagues[410] reported a 27% target lesion revascularization rate in their study, which is not significantly better than treatment with balloon angioplasty alone.

It must be kept in mind that all of the treatments have their own, often serious, complications. Balloon angioplasty of the stented segment is no exception, and serious dissections can result that may require emergency surgery, or, as has recently been described, stent deployment in the previously stented site.[432] Directional atherectomy may disrupt the stent struts, and there have been several reports of stent damage with its use.[433,434] Rotational atherectomy frequently results in transient hypoperfusion due to peripheral obstruction by microcavitation, atheromatous debris, release of vasoactive substances, platelet aggregation, or vessel spasm.

Although all of the techniques for the treatment of stent restenosis are feasible, only a few small studies have compared the various techniques. In a small study comparing balloon angioplasty alone with debulking using rotational or directional angioplasty plus balloon angioplasty in a series of 60 consecutive patients with diffuse in-stent restenosis, the debulking strategy resulted in a reduction in the rate of target vessel revascularization procedures at 1-year follow-up (46% for balloon alone *vs* 28% for debulking plus PTCA), although this result was not statistically significant.[435] In a study comparing the acute results of rotational atherectomy with laser angioplasty, rotational atherectomy resulted in a greater ablation efficiency.[436] This finding is difficult to interpret since the characteristics of the laser catheter were not specified. Mahdi and colleagues have reported a trial that compared PTCA, directional atherectomy, and rotational atherectomy in patients with Palmaz–Schatz in-stent restenosis.[436a] In this study, 96 patients were included, 33 treated with PTCA, 40 with directional atherectomy and 23 with rotational atherectomy. The postprocedural MLD was significantly larger in the lesions treated with directional atherectomy $(2.67 \pm 0.7 \text{ } vs \text{ } 2.15 \pm 0.6 \text{ and } 2.15 \pm 0.4 \text{ for PTCA and rotational atherectomy,}$ respectively). Cumulative event-free survival (freedom from any myocardial infarction, death, repeat intervention, and CABG) was found to be superior for directional atherectomy ($p=0.28$). Target lesion revascularization was lower in the directional atherectomy group of patients (19.5% *vs* 30% and 26% for PTCA and rotational atherectomy, respectively), although the difference was not statistically significant. Clearly, the best therapeutic approach has not yet been determined.

There have been only a few studies which reported on the long-term outcome of patients treated for in-stent restenosis. In one small study 31 patients underwent balloon angioplasty for stent restenosis.[437] The mean follow-up period in this trial was 43 ± 22 months, and 22% of patients treated with balloon angioplasty for stent restenosis required target vessel revascularization procedures. Reimers and colleagues have also reported their long-term findings for patients treated with balloon angioplasty for in-stent restenosis.[404] Clinical follow-up was obtained in 124 patients at a mean of 27 months after the procedure. Recurrence of clinical events (death, MI, target vessel revascularization, positive stress test results or recurrence of anginal symptoms) occurred in 25 patients (20%). Cumulative event-free survival at 24 months was 81%. Multivariate analysis showed lesions located in saphenous vein grafts, ejection fraction less than 30%, multivessel disease and interval between stent implantation and first in-stent restenosis $\leq$ 3 months to be significant predictors of the recurrence of a clinical event. Clinical events were observed in 17% (of 77 patients) with focal in-stent restenosis and in 25% (of 47 patients) with diffuse restenosis. Diffuse disease was not a significant predictor of clinical events in this patient cohort.

Bleeding and vascular injury

In the large randomized STRESS I and BENESTENT I trials, significant bleeding occurred in 7.3% of the stented patients and vascular complications occurred in 13.5% of the stented patients, largely due to the intensive anticoagulation regimens used.[209,210] Reduced anticoagulation regimens have had a profound impact on the reduction of local vascular complications. Major bleeding occurred in only 0.4% and major vascular complications requiring surgical repair occurred in 0.3% of 1157 patients treated without warfarin or postprocedural heparin after high-pressure stent deployment.[64] The risk factors for vascular complications which have been identified include age above 75 years, female gender, sheath size greater than 8F, duration of indwelling sheath, duration of procedure, postprocedural use of heparinoids, saphenous vein graft stenting, hypertension, and stenting for bailout indications.[438–442]

In addition to reduced anticoagulation regimens, several other approaches have been tried in an attempt to reduce the vascular complication rate further. The use of alternatives to the routine femoral access site is one strategy that has been considered. Historically, the first cardiac catheterization was done through brachial access, isolated through brachial artery cutdown.[443] One of the advantages of this approach was that the artery could be repaired with direct visualization after the procedure. The possibility of radial nerve damage, and the potentially tragic consequences of damage to the brachial artery, led to the development of the femoral access technique for cardiac catheterization by Judkins, which became the favoured approach for angioplasty procedures. The large number of femoral access site complications after stent deployment with postprocedural anticoagulation led to an assessment of the feasibility of the brachial technique for stent implantation.[444] Although the incidence of vascular complications was thought to be reduced with the use of the brachial access site, compromise of bloodflow to the hand (the consequence of brachial artery damage) limited the popularity of this approach.

The transradial approach for coronary stenting, first introduced in 1994,[445] has several advantages over femoral and brachial routes. The radial artery is superficial, therefore easily accessible, and not located near important veins or nerves. A further advantage is that occlusion of the artery does not result in significant clinical sequelae in patients who show a normal Allen's test.[446] In a comparative study of the transradial, transbrachial, and femoral approaches to coronary angioplasty in 900 patients (the ACCESS study) no entry site complications were observed in the radial group, but the incidence of complications in the brachial and femoral site groups were 2.3% and 2.0%, respectively.[447,448] An observational analysis of 377 patients, which compared radial and femoral access sites for stent implantation treated with either postprocedural anticoagulation or antiplatelet therapy only, was recently reported.[449] Vascular complications occurred in 6% of the patients treated with femoral access in both the anticoagulant and antiplatelet treated groups, but none of the patients in whom the radial approach was used showed access-site complications. With increased operator experience the radial approach for coronary stent implantation is gaining acceptance and has encouraged the development of lower-profile devices and stents.

Percutaneous vascular closure devices have also been used in patients undergoing stent implantation via the femoral route, in an attempt to reduce the vascular complication rate and promote early ambulation. The results of the effects of these devices on the vascular complication rates have been equivocal,[450–455] but further trials are needed to show this advantage.

Stent embolization

Stents may be dislodged from the delivery catheter during stent introduction, and this can result in stent embolization. The stent may embolize to the distal native coronary artery[456] or saphenous vien graft,[457] or to peripheral vessels including the aorta,[458] iliac,[459] or femoral[69] arteries. Fortunately, serious consequences of such stent embolization appear to be rare. Several successful retrieval techniques have been described that involve the use of additional balloon catheters,[457] biopsy forceps and retrieval devices,[458,460–462] and coaxial wires.[456,459,460] Although feasible, these techniques are difficult, particularly for radiolucent stents, and they require considerable operator experience.[463] With the availability of new-generation premounted stents, which are more trackable and have a lower profile, the risk of stent loss has decreased significantly.

Side-branch occlusion

Side-branch occlusion is an infrequent complication of coronary stenting,[464] with an incidence of less than 10% in one clinical series.[465] The risk of side-branch occlusion is related to the luminal diameter of the side-branch and the extent of disease within its origin. Occlusion occurs by a shift of the atherosclerotic plaque from the parent vessel into the orifice of the side-branch, by dissection at the side-branch ostium, or by mechanical obstruction of the side-branch by the stent struts.[465,466] In a study of a series of 175 patients who had stent implantation in a coronary vessel in which the stent spanned a side-branch greater than 1 mm in diameter, 19% experienced side-branch occlusion.[467] By multivariate analysis threatened side-branch morphology (greater than 50% ostial narrowing that arises from within or just beyond the diseased portion of the parent vessel) was the only predictor of side-branch occlusion. Side-branch location, target lesion characteristics, stent design, and clinical characteristics were not predictors. At 9-months follow-up there were no differences in the combined endpoints of death, myocardial infarction, need for target vessel revascularization, and myocardial infarction between patients with and without side-branch occlusion. Surprisingly, coronary stent implantation for acute or threatened closure has been shown to restore the patency of side-branches occluded by angioplasty.[468] This is thought to be a result of the re-approximation of the dissected and displaced intima towards its original position, away from the ostium of the side-branch that it is obstructing. The clinical significance of the side-branch occlusion relates to the size of the side-branch and the amount of myocardium supplied by the vessel. The management of side branch occlusion involves passage of a balloon or stent through the struts of the stent in the parent vessel. Some stent designs allow the passage of angioplasty and stent systems through their struts,[469,470] but others require selected devices.[471]

Coronary perforation

With the introduction of high-pressure balloon deployment and oversized balloon strategies for adequate stent expansion, the frequency of coronary perforation has increased, complicating 1.0% – 2.5% of stent procedures.[472–476] Features associated with perforation include complex lesion morphology, small vessel diameter, balloon to artery ratio of 1.2:1 or more, tapering vessel, need to recross a dissection with a guidewire, and heavy calcifications.[473,474,477] Reduction of the ultrasound-determined balloon artery ratio from 1.2 to 1.05 has been shown to decrease the incidence of coronary perforation from 1.2% (four ruptures in 339 lesions treated) to 0% (113 lesions treated) in one clinical series.[473] Many localized perforations can be managed with prolonged balloon inflation, and may require the administration of protamine in some instances. Successful treatment of a coronary artery perforation not responding to prolonged balloon inflation has been reported using an autologous vein-graft-covered stent.[478] The JoStent stent graft, which consists of a polytetrafluorethylene membrane interspaced between two thin metal stents, has also been used to treat coronary ruptures successfully.[479] In the event of frank or threatened tamponade, pericardiocentesis may be necessary. Despite these interventions, emergency surgery may be necessary in up to 50% of perforations, and clinical outcomes include myocardial infarction in 40% of perforations and death in 30% of perforations.[475]

Infection

A stent abscess is an extremely rare, but potentially catastrophic, complication after coronary artery stenting. There are two reports of infections complicating stent implantation. In the first report, a fatal perivascular myocardial abscess resulted from the implantation of a Palmaz–Schatz stent in the right coronary artery.[480] In the second report, a saccular aneurysm in the LAD resulted from a Pseudomonas infection, and despite surgical repair, the outcome was fatal.[481] Although there are no data to suggest the benefit of routine antibiotics in patients receiving intravascular stents, there are experimental data to show that prophylactic antibiotics should be given to those patients at risk for transient bacteraemia.[482] In a porcine stent model, systemic bacterial challenge was administered immediately after stent deployment. After 72 hours, 80% of the animals showed positive stent cultures, and at 3 weeks 60% of the cultures were positive.[482] Although not conclusive, these data support antibiotic prophylaxis for those patients who undergo dental procedures, endoscopic examinations, or other invasive procedures within 3 months of stent implantation (before neointimalization is complete).

Balloon rupture

Balloon rupture is an infrequent complication of both balloon angioplasty and stent implantation. Although most cases are without consequences, potentially serious complications such as balloon entrapment, air embolism, coronary dissection, and vessel rupture can occur. Very few studies have addressed this complication. In a retrospective analysis of 674 patients (1139 lesions) treated with stent implantation between 1990 and 1997, balloon rupture occurred in 66 (5.8%) lesions.[483] In 76% of these patients, balloon rupture did not result in any angiographic abnormality. In the remaining 24% of patients, balloon rupture caused a new coronary dissection.

Coronary artery aneurysms

Coronary artery aneurysms are defined as dilated segments whose diameters exceed 1.5 times that of the adjacent reference segment. They can occur spontaneously in a vessel segment weakened by atherosclerotic disease. When they occur after intracoronary interventions, they are likely to be a result of the weakening of the vessel wall by an intervention-related insult. True aneurysms retain the residual layers of the vessel wall (media and/or adventitia) which remain in continuity with those layers in the adjacent non-enlarged vessel wall. When an aneurysm results from deeper injury, the normal vessel layers may not be present and the integrity of the aneurysm may be maintained only by the adherent visceral pericardium, thus forming a false aneurysm. The distinction between these two forms may be important, since true aneurysms generally have a benign course and false aneurysms have the potential for progressive enlargement or eventual rupture,[484] although it has been speculated that both types of aneurysm may be prone to thrombosis and the source of emboli leading to distal infarction. IVUS investigation provides a means to distinguish these two types of aneurysms.

There have been only a few reports of aneurysm formation after stent implantation. Rab and colleagues[485] reported a 32% incidence (six of 19 patients) of aneurysm formation after Gianturco–Roubin stent implantation in patients treated with glucocorticoids as part of a restenosis prevention protocol. They proposed that steroid-mediated impairment of vascular healing might have led to weakening of the vessel wall and subsequent aneurysm formation. In a retrospective analysis of the STRESS trial, Slota and colleagues[486] reported the frequency of aneurysm formation after balloon angioplasty and stent implantation. For the entire cohort of patients, coronary artery aneurysms were observed at follow-up in 18 (5.4%) of 334 patients. The incidence of coronary artery aneurysms in the stent and PTCA groups were not different. At 1-year follow-up, coronary aneurysms were not associated with increased mortality, myocardial infarction, or the need for subsequent revascularization. This study was done before the routine use of high-pressure balloon inflation for stent implantation, and the incidence of aneurysm formation may be different with current stent-implantation techniques.

The presence of a procedural dissection has been reported to predict coronary artery aneurysm development.[487,488] There are several case reports which describe the formation of a false aneurysm after bailout stenting for coronary dissections.[498,490] One case report suggests that an angiographically inapparent edge disection may have been the trigger for the development of a resultant false aneurysm.[491] Another reports the formation of a large (6 mm × 6 mm) false aneurysm after uncomplicated primary stent implantation.[492]

254

There is no consensus on the management of coronary aneurysms. The natural history of true aneurysms appears to be benign, and they are therefore best left untreated. The management of false aneurysms is more controversial. Most authors recommend surgical intervention such as bypass grafting, resection, or ligation. Percutaneous treatments are currently being tested with the use of arterial or vein convered stents, or the recently introduced polytetrafluoroethylene stent grafts. It is hoped that with these newer treatments, surgical intervention may be avoided.

References

1. Serruys PW, Strauss BH, Beatt KJ et al. Angiographic follow-up after placement of a self-expanding coronary artery stent. *N Engl J Med* 1991; **324:** 13–17.

2. Schatz RA, Baim DS, Leon M et al. Clinical experience with the Palmaz–Schatz coronary stent. Initial results of a multicenter study. *Circulation* 1991; **83:** 148–61.

3. Lablanche J-M, McFadden EP, Bonnet J-L et al. Combined antiplatelet therapy with ticlopidine and aspirin. A simplified approach to intracoronary stent management. *Eur Heart J* 1996; **17:** 1373–80.

4. Keane D, Haase J, Slager C et al. Comparative validation of quantitative coronary angiographic systems: results and implications from a multicenter study using standardized approach. *Circulation* 1995; **91:** 2402–12.

5. Goods CM, Al-Shaibi KF, Yadav SS et al. Utilization of the coronary balloon-expandable coil stent without anticoagulation or intravascular ultrasound. *Circulation* 1996; **93:** 1803–08.

6. Mak K-H, Belli G, Ellis SG, Moliterno DJ. Subacute stent thrombosis; evolving issues and current concepts. *J Am Coll Cardiol* 1996; **27:** 494–503.

7. Fischman DL, Leon MB, Baim DS et al, for the Stent Restenosis Study investigators. A randomized comparison of coronary-stent placement and balloon angioplasty in the treatment of coronary artery disease. *N Engl J Med* 1994; **331:** 496–501.

8. Nath FC, Muller DWM, Ellis SG et al. Thrombosis of a flexible coil coronary stent: frequency, predictors and clinical outcome. *J Am Coll Cardiol* 1993; **21:** 622–27.

9. Hasdai D, Garratt K, Holmes DR, Berger PB, Schwartz RS, Bell MR. Coronary angioplasty and intracoronary thrombolytics are of limited value in resolving intracoronary stent thrombosis. *J Am Coll Cardiol* 1996; **28:** 361–67.

10. Schömig A, Kastrati A, Mudra H et al. Four-year experience with Palmaz–Schatz stenting in coronary angioplasty complicated by dissection with threatened or present vessel closure. *Circulation* 1994; **90:** 2716–24.

11. van Beusekom HMM, van der Giessen WJ, van Suylen RJ, Bos E, Bosman FT, Serruys PW. Histology after stenting of human saphenous vein bypass grafts: observations from surgically excised grafts 3 to 320 days after stent implantation. *J Am Coll Cardiol* 1993; **21:** 45–54.

12. Ueda Y, Nanto S, Komamure K, Kodama K. Neointimal coverage of stents in human coronary arteries observed by angioscopy. *J Am Coll Cardiol* 1994; **23:** 341–46.

13. Williams DF. Surface interactions. In: Sigwart U (ed.). Endoluminal Stenting. London, W.B. Saunders; 1996: 45–51.

14. Andrade JD, Hlady V. Plasma protein adsorption. The big twelve. In: Leonard EF, Turitto VT, Vroman L (eds). Blood in contact with natural and artificial surfaces. New York, New York Academy of Science; 1987: 158–72.

15. Rogers C, Edelman ER. Endovascular stent design dictates experimental restenosis and thrombosis. *Circulation* 1995; **91:** 2995–3001.

16. Baier R. Initial events in interaction of blood with a foreign surface. *J Biomed Mat Res* 1969; **3:** 191–206.

17. De Palma VE, Baier RE. Investigation of three-surface properties of several metals and their relation to blood biocompatibility. *J Biomed Mat Res* 1972; **6:** 37–75.

18. Zitter H, Plenk H Jr. The electrochemical behaviour of metallic implant materials as an indicator of their biocompatibility. *J Biomed Mat Res* 1987; **21:** 881–96.

19. Hehrlein C, Zimmerman M, Metz J, Ensinger W, Kübler W. Influence of surface texture and charge on the biocompatibility of endovascular stents. *Coron Artery Dis* 1995; **6:** 581–86.

20. De Scheerder I, Sohier J, Wang K et al. Metallic surface treatment using electrochemical polishing decreases thrombogenicity and neointimal hyperplasia after coronary stent implantation in a porcine model [abstract]. *Eur Heart J* 1997; 18 (suppl): 153.

21. De Scheerder I, Wang K, Schier J et al. Metallic surface treatment using electrochemical polishing decreases thrombogenicity and neointimal hyperplasia after coronary stent implantation in a porcine model [abstract]. *J Am Coll Cardiol* 1998; 31 (suppl): 277A.

22. Hearn JA, Robinson KA, Roubin GS. In-vitro thrombus formation of stent wires: role of metallic composition and heparin coating [abstract]. *J Am Coll Cardiol* 1991; 17 (suppl): 302A.

23. van der Giessen WJ, Serruys PW, van Beusekom HMM et al. Coronary stenting with a new radiopaque, balloon-expandable endoprosthesis in pigs. *Circulation* 1991; **83:** 1788–98.

24. Scott NA, Robinson KA, Nunes GL et al. Comparison of the thrombogenicity of stainless steel and tantalum coronary stents. *Am Heart J* 1995; **129:** 866–72.

25. Sheth S, Litvack F, Dev V, Fishbein MC, Forrester JS, Eigler N. Subacute thrombosis and vascular injury resulting from slotted-tube nitinol and stainless steel stents in a rabbit carotid artery model. *Circulation* 1996; **94:** 1733–40.

26. Sheth S, Dev V, Fishbein MC, Forrester JS, Litvack F, Eigler NL. Reduced thrombogenicity of nitinol vs stainless steel slotted stents in rabbit carotid arteries [abstract]. *J Am Coll Cardiol* 1995; 25 (suppl): 240A.

27. Murphy JG, Schwartz RS, Edwards WD, Camrud AR, Vlietstra RE, Holmes D. Percutaneous polymeric stents in porcine coronary arteries: initial experience with polyethylene terephthalate stents. *Circulation* 1992; **86:** 1596–604.

28. van Beusekom HMM, van der Giessen WJ, van Ingen Schenau D, Slager CJ. Synthetic polymers as an alternative to metal stents? In-vivo and mechanical behaviour of polyethylene-terephthalate [abstract]. *Circulation* 1992; 86 (suppl): I-731.

29. Lincoff AM, Schwartz RS, van der Giessen WJ, van Beusekom HMM, Serruys PW, Holmes DR. Biodegradable polymers can evoke a unique inflammatory response when implanted into the coronary artery [abstract]. *Circulation* 1992; 86 (suppl): I-801.

30. Zidar JP, Gammon RS, Chapman GD et al. Short- and long-term vascular tissue response to the Duke bioabsorbable stent [abstract]. *J Am Coll Cardiol* 1993; 21 (suppl): 439A.

31. Tamai H, Doi T, Hsu YS et al. Initial and long term results of biodegradable polymer stent in canine coronary artery [abstract]. *J Invas Cardiol* 1995; **7:** 9A.

32. Susawa T, Shiraki K, Shimizu Y. Biodegradable intracoronary stents in adult dogs [abstract]. *J Am Coll Cardiol* 1993; 21 (suppl): 483A.

33. Chapman GD, Gammon RS, Baumann RP et al. A bioabsorbable stent: initial experimental results [abstract]. *Circulation* 1990; 82 (suppl III): III-72.

34. Kruse KR, Tanguay J-F, Williams MS, Phillips HR, Stack RS, Zidar JP. A polymer-metal composite stent. *Semin Intervent Cardiol* 1996; **1:** 46–48.

35. Agrawal SK, Ho DSW, Lie MW et al. Predictors of thrombolytic complications after placement of the flexible coil stent. *Am J Cardiol* 1994; **73:** 1216–19.

36. Roubin GS, Cannon AD, Agrawal SK et al. Intracoronary stenting for acute and threatened closure complicating percutaneous transluminal coronary angioplasty. *Circulation* 1992; **85:** 916–27.

37. Legrand V, Serruys PW, Emanuelsson H et al. BENESTENT-II Trial – final results of visit I: a 15-day follow-up [abstract]. *J Am Coll Cardiol* 1997; 29 (suppl A): 170A.

38. Doucet S, Fajadet J, Cassagneau B, Robert G, Jordan C, Marco J. Early thrombotic occlusion following coronary Palmaz–Schatz stent implantation: frequency and clinical or angiographic predictors [abstract]. *Eur Heart J* 1992; 13 (suppl): 4.

39. Fry ET, Hermiller JB, Peters TF et al. Risks, treatment, and outcome of acute stent closure [abstract]. *Circulation* 1994; 90 (suppl): I-650.

40. Mathew V, Hasdai D, Holmes DR et al. Clinical outcome of patients undergoing endoluminal coronary artery reconstruction with three or more stents. *J Am Coll Cardiol* 1997; **30:** 676–81.

41. George BS, Voorhees WD III, Roubin GS et al. Multicenter investigation of coronary stenting to treat acute or threatened closure after percutaneous transluminal coronary angioplasty: clinical and angiographic outcomes. *J Am Coll Cardiol* 1993; **22:** 135–43.

42. Herrmann HC, Buchbinder M, Clemen MW et al. Emergent use of balloon-expandable coronary artery stenting for failed percutaneous transluminal angioplasty. *Circulation* 1992; **86:** 812–19.

43. Colombo A, Goldberg SL, Almagor Y, Maiello L, Finci L. A novel strategy for stent deployment in the treatment of acute or threatened closure complicating balloon coronary angioplasty. Use of short or standard (or both) single or multiple Palmaz–Schatz stents. *J Am Coll Cardiol* 1993; **22:** 1887–91.

44. Foley JB, Brown RIG, Penn IM. Thrombosis and restenosis after stenting in failed angioplasty: comparison with elective stenting. *Am Heart J* 1994; **128:** 12–20.

45. Haude M, Erbel R, Issa H et al. Subacute thrombotic complications after intracoronary implantation of Palmaz–Schatz stents. *Am Heart J* 1993; **126:** 15–22.

46. Kornowski R, Mehran R, Hong MK et al. Procedural results and late clinical outcomes after placement of three or more stents in single coronary lesions. *Circulation* 1998; **97:** 1355–61.

47. Eccleston DS, Belli G, Penn IM, Ellis SG. Are multiple stents associated with multiplicative risk in the optimal stent era? [abstract]. *Circulation* 1996; 94 (suppl): I-454.

48. Pulsipher MW, Baker WA, Sawchak SR et al. Outcomes in patients treated with multiple coronary stents [abstract]. *Circulation* 1996; 94 (suppl): I-332.

49. Rolland PH, Charifi AB, Friggi A et al. Hemodynamic consequences and wall rheologic properties of endovascular stent implantation in the iliac artery in the minipig [abstract]. *Circulation* 1997; 96 (suppl): I-136.

50. Xu XY, Collins MW. Fluid dynamics in stents. In: Sigwart U (ed.). Endoluminal stenting. London, W.B. Saunders; 1996: 52–59.

51. Brown CH, Leverett LB, Lewis CE. Morphological, biochemical and functional changes in human platelets subject to shear stress. *J Lab Clin Med* 1975; **86:** 462–71.

52. Woscoboinik JR, Gordov EP, Boussignac G et al. Difference in flow characteristics for different stent models: implications for stent design from results of an in vitro study [abstract]. *Circulation* 1996; 94 (suppl): I-260.

53. Goy JJ, Eeckhout E, Debbas N, Stauffer JC, Vogt P. Stenting of the right coronary artery for de novo stenosis. A comparison of the Wiktor and the Palmaz–Schatz stents [abstract]. *Circulation* 1995; 92 (suppl I): I-596.

54. Macisaac AI, Ellis SG, Muller DW, Topol EJ, Whitlow PL. Comparison of three coronary stents: clinical and angiographic outcome after elective placement in 134 patients. *Cathet Cardiovasc Diagn* 1994; **33:** 199–204.

55. Goy J-J, Eeckhout E, Stauffer J-C, Vogt P, Kappenberger L. Emergency endoluminal stenting for abrupt vessel closure following coronary angioplasty: a randomized comparison of the Wiktor and Palmaz–Schatz stents. *Cathet Cardiovasc Diagn* 1995; **34:** 128–32.

56. Chan CNS, Tan ATH, Koh TH et al. Intracoronary stenting in the treatment of acute or threatened closure in angiographically small coronary arteries (<3.0 mm) complicating percutaneous transluminal coronary angioplasty. *Am J Cardiol* 1995; **75:** 23–25.

57. Savage MP, Fischman DL, Rake R et al, for the Stent Restenosis Study (STRESS) Investigators. Efficacy of coronary stenting versus balloon angioplasty in small coronary arteries. *J Am Coll Cardiol* 1998; **31:** 307–11.

58. Teirstein P, Schatz R, Russo R, Guarneri E, Stevens M. Coronary stenting of small diameter vessels: is it safe? [abstract]. *Circulation* 1995; 92 (suppl): I-281.

59. Hall P, Colombo A, Itoh A et al. Gianturco–Roubin stent implantation in small vessels without anticoagulation [abstract]. *Circulation* 1995; 92 (suppl): I-795.

60. Koning R, Cribier A, Chan C, Eltchaninoff H, Tron C, Letac B. Palmaz–Schatz coronary stenting for de novo lesions in small coronary arteries: clinical and quantitative angiographic results of a prospective pilot study [abstract]. *Circulation* 1996; 94 (suppl): I-685.

61. Morice M-C, Amor M, Beneviste E et al. Coronary stenting without coumadin phase II,III,IV,V [abstract]. *Circulation* 1995; 92 (suppl); I-795.

62. Yokoi H, Nobuyoshi M, Nosaka H et al. Coronary stent thrombosis: pattern, management and long term follow-up result [abstract]. *Circulation* 1996; 94 (suppl): I-332.

63. Liu MW, Voorhees WD, Agrawal S, Dean LS, Roubin GS. Stratification of the risk of thrombosis after intracoronary stenting for threatened or acute closure complicating coronary balloon angioplasty: a Cook registry study. *Am Heart J* 1995; **130:** 8–13.

64. Karrillon GJ, Morice MC, Benveniste E et al. Intracoronary stent implantation without ultrasound guidance with replacement of conventional anticoagulation therapy by antiplatelet therapy. 30–day clinical outcome of the French Multicenter Registry. *Circulation* 1996; **94:** 1519–27.

65. Shaknovich A, Moses JW, Bailey S et al, for STRESS Investigators. Subacute stent thrombosis in the STent REstenosis Study (STRESS); clinical impact and predictive factors [abstract]. *Circulation* 1994; 90 (suppl); I-650.

66. Schömig A, Kastrati A, Dietz R et al. Emergency coronary stenting for dissection during percutaneous transluminal coronary angioplasty: angiographic follow-up after stenting and after repeat angioplasty of the stented segment. *J Am Coll Cardiol* 1994; **23**: 1053–60.

67. Neumann F-J, Walter H, Richardt G, Schmitt C, Schömig A. Coronary Palmaz–Schatz stent implantation in acute myocardial infarction. *Heart* 1996; **75**: 121–26.

68. Grinstead WC, Raizner AE, Churchill DA et al, for the Cook Stent Investigators. Intracoronary thrombosis prior to stenting: impact on angiographic success and clinical outcome. *J Am Coll Cardiol* 1993; 21 (suppl): 30A.

69. Rocha-Singh KJ, Fischman DL, Savage MP, Goldberg S, Teirstein PS, Schatz RA. Influence of angiographic lesion characteristics on early complication rates after Palmaz–Schatz stenting [abstract]. *J Am Coll Cardiol* 1993; 21 (suppl): 292A.

70. Moussa I, Di Mario C, Francesco LD et al. Stents don't require systemic anticoagulation . . . but the technique (and results) must be optimal. *J Invas Cardiol* 1996; 8 (suppl E): 3E–7E.

71. Moussa I, Di Mario C, Francesco LD et al. Subacute stent thrombosis in the era of intravascular ultrasound-guided coronary stenting without anticoagulation: frequency, predictors and clinical outcome. *J Am Coll Cardiol* 1997; **29**: 6–12.

72. Werner GS, Gastmann O, Ferrari M et al. Risk factors for acute and subacute stent thrombosis after high-pressure stent implantation: a study by intracoronary ultrasound. *Am Heart J* 1998; **135**: 300–09.

73. Baim DS, Cutlip DE, Zhang Y, Mehran R, Abizaid AS, Fitzpatrick M. Characteristics and predictors of stent thrombosis from the stent anticoagulation regimen study (STARS) [abstract]. *Circulation* 1997; 96 (suppl): I-653.

74. Karrillon GJ, Morice MC, Benveniste E et al. Intracoronary stent implantation without ultrasound guidance with replacement of conventional anticoagulation therapy by antiplatelet therapy. 30-day clinical outcome of the French Multicenter Registry. *Circulation* 1996; **94**: 1519–27.

75. Schömig A, Kastrati A, Mudra H et al. Four-year experience with Palmaz–Schatz stenting in coronary angioplasty complicated by dissection with threatened or present vessel closure. *Circulation* 1994; **90**: 2716–24.

76. Eeckhout E, Stauffer J-C, Vogt P, Kappenberger L, Goy J-J. Can early closure and restenosis following endoluminal stenting be predicted from clinical and angiographic variables at the time of intervention? [abstract]. *J Invas Cardiol* 1995; **7**: 7A.

77. Serruys PW, Emanuelsson H, van der Giessen W et al, on behalf of the BENESTENT II Study Group. Heparin coated Palmaz–Schatz stents in human coronary arteries. Early outcome of the BENESTENT II Pilot Study. *Circulation* 1996; **93:** 412–22.

78. Neumann FJ, Gawaz M, Ott I, May A, Mössmer G, Schömig A. Prospective evaluation of hemostatic predictors of subacute stent thrombosis after coronary Palmaz–Schatz stenting. *J Am Coll Cardiol* 1996; **27:** 15–21.

79. Walter DH, Schächinger V, Reyes-Araiza R, Dimmeler S, Ficus S, Zeiher AM. Platelet glycoprotein IIb/IIIa polymorphism is a risk factor for subacute coronary stent thrombosis [abstract]. *Eur J Cardiol* 1997; 18 (suppl): 69.

80. Walter DH, Schachinger V, Elsner M, Gotte S, Dimmeler S, Zeiher AM. Platelet glycoprotein IIb/IIIa polymorphism is a potent risk factor for stent vessel occlusion [abstract]. *Circulation* 1997; 96 (suppl): I-23.

81. Waksman R, Shen Y, Ghazzi Z, Scott NA, Douglas Jr JS, King III SB. Optimal balloon inflation pressures for stent deployment and correlates of stent thrombosis and in-stent restenosis [abstract]. *Circulation* 1996; 94 (suppl): I-258.

82. Jeong MH, Owen WG, Srivatsa SS et al. Platelets are the primary component of acute stent thrombosis [abstract]. *J Invas Cardiol* 1995; **7:** 11A.

83. Colombo A, Hall P, Nakamura S et al. Intracoronary stenting without anticoagulation accomplished with intravascular ultrasound guidance. *Circulation* 1995; **91:** 1676–88.

84. Morice MC, Zemour G, Beneviste E et al. Intracoronary stenting without coumadin: one month results of a French multicenter study. *Cathet Cardiovasc Diagn* 1995; **35:** 1–7.

85. Schömig A, Neumann FJ, Kastrati A et al. A randomized comparison of antiplatelet and anticoagulant therapy after the placement of coronary-artery stents. *N Engl J Med* 1996; **334:** 1084–89.

86. Hall P, Nakamura S, Maiello L et al. A randomized comparison of combined ticlopidine and aspirin therapy versus aspirin therapy alone after successful intravascular ultrasound-guided stent implantation. *Circulation* 1996; **93:** 215–22.

87. Brodie RR, Grines CL, Ivanhoe R et al. Six-month clinical and angiographic follow-up after direct angioplasty for acute myocardial infarction. Final results from the primary angioplasty registry. *Circulation* 1994; **90:** 156–62.

88. Goods CM, Al-Shaibi KF, Yadav SS et al. Utilization of the coronary balloon-expandable coil stent without anticoagulation or intravascular ultrasound. *Circulation* 1996; **93:** 1803–08.

89. Morice MC, Valeix B, Marco J et al. Preliminary results of the MUST trial. Major clinical events during the first month [abstract]. *J Am Coll Cardiol* 1996; 27 (suppl): 137A.

90. de Jaegere P, Mudra H, Figulla H et al. Intravascular ultrasound-guided optimized stent deployment. Immediate and 6 months clinical and angiographic results from the Multicenter Ultrasound Stenting in Coronaries study (Music study). *Eur Heart J* 1998; **19:** 1214–23.

91. Morice MC, Breton C, Bunouf P et al. Coronary stenting without intravascular ultrasound. Results of the French Registry [abstract]. *Circulation* 1995; 92 (suppl): I-796.

92. Goods CM, Al-Shabi KF, Iyer SS et al. Flexible coil stenting without anticoagulation or intravascular ultrasound: a prospective observational study [abstract]. *Circulation* 1995; 92 (suppl): I-795.

93. Wong SC, Hong MK, Chuang YC et al. The Anti-PLatelet treatment After intravascular Ultrasound guided optimal Stent Expansion (APPLAUSE) trial [abstract]. *Circulation* 1995; 92 (suppl): I-795.

94. Fernández-Avilés F, Alonso J, Durán JM et al. Subacute occlusion, bleeding complications, hospital stay and restenosis after Palmaz–Schatz coronary stenting under a new antithrombotic regimen. *J Am Coll cardiol* 1996; **27:** 22–29.

95. Blasini R, Mudra H, Schühlen H et al. Intravascular ultrasound guided optimized emergency coronary Palmaz–Schatz stent placement without post procedural systemic anticoagulation [abstract]. *J Am Coll Cardiol* 1995; 25 (suppl): 197A.

96. Colombo A, Nakamura S, Hall P et al. A prospective study of Gianturco–Roubin coronary stent implantation without anticoagulation [abstract]. *J Am Coll Cardiol* 1995; 25 (suppl): 197A.

97. Russo R, Schatz RA, Sklar MA, Johnson AD, Tobis M, Teirstein PS. Ultrasound guided coronary stent placement without prolonged systemic anticoagulation [abstract]. *J Am Coll Cardiol* 1995; 25 (suppl): 197A.

98. Colombo A, Nakamura S, Hall P, Maiello L, Finci L, Martini G. A prospective study of Wiktor coronary stent implantation without anticoagulation [abstract]. *J Am Coll Cardiol* 1995; 25 (suppl): 239A.

99. Van Belle E, McFadden EP, Bauters C, Harmon M, Bertrand ME, Lablanche J-M. Combined antiplatelet therapy without anticoagulation: an effective alternative to prevent subacute thrombosis after coronary stenting? A 3 month follow-up [abstract]. *J Am Coll Cardiol* 1995; 25 (suppl): 197A.

100. Barragan P, Silvestri M, Sainsous J et al. Prevention of subacute occlusion after coronary stenting with ticlopidine regimen without intravascular ultrasound guided stenting [abstract]. *J Am Coll Cardiol* 1995; 25 (suppl): 182A.

101. Buszman P, Clague J, Gibbs S et al. Improved post stent management: high gain at low risk [abstract]. *J Am Coll Cardiol* 1995; 25 (suppl): 182A.

102. Van Belle E, McFadden EP, Lablanche J-M, Bauters C, Hamon M, Bertrand ME.

Two-pronged antiplatelet therapy with aspirin and ticlopidine without systemic anticoagulation: an alternative therapeutic strategy after bailout stent implantation. *Coron Artery Dis* 1995; **6**: 341–45.

103. Lablanche J-M, Grollier G, Bonnet J-L et al. Ticlopidine aspirin stent evaluation (TASTE); a French multicenter study [abstract]. *Circulation* 1995; 92 (suppl): I-476.

104. Lablanche J-M, Bonnet J-L, Grollier G et al. Combined antiplatelet therapy without anticoagulation after stent implantation; the Ticlopidine Aspirin Stent Evaluation (TASTE) Study [abstract]. *J Am Coll Cardiol* 1996; 27 (suppl): 137A.

105. Belli G, Whitlow P, Gross L et al. Intracoronary stenting without oral anticoagulation: the Cleveland Clinic Registry [abstract]. *Circulation* 1995; 92 (suppl): I-796.

106. Saito S, Kim K, Hosokawa G, Hatano K, Tanaka S. Primary Palmaz–Schatz stent implantation without coumadin in acute myocardial infarction [abstract]. *Circulation* 1995; 92 (suppl): I-796.

107. Haase J, Reifart N, Baier T et al. Bail-out stenting (Palmaz–Schatz) without anticoagulation [abstract]. *Circulation* 1995; 92 (suppl): I-795.

108. Galli S, Trabattoni D, Loaldi A et al. Comparison of anticoagulation, combined ticlopidine and aspirin, and aspirin alone therapy following coronary stenting [abstract]. *Circulation* 1996; 94 (suppl): I-684.

109. Sainsous J, Silvestri M, Bayet G et al. Coronary artery stenting without anticoagulation, intravascular ultrasound or high pressure balloon: immediate results of one month follow-up [abstract]. *Circulation* 1996; 94 (suppl): I-262.

110. The STRESS Investigators. Early outcomes after coronary stent placement with high pressure inflation and antiplatelet therapy: interim results of the STRESS III Trial [abstract]. *Circulation* 1996; 94 (suppl): I-684.

111. Lablanche J-M, Gauthier L, McFadden EP et al. In-hospital and six month outcome after bailout stenting managed with antiplatelet therapy alone [abstract]. *Circulation* 1996; 94 (suppl): I-684.

112. Leon MB, Ellis SG, Moses J et al. Interim report from the reduced anticoagulation VEin Graft Stent (RAVES) Study [abstract]. *Circulation* 1996; 94 (suppl): I-683.

113. Dirschinger J, Schühlen H, Walter H et al. Intracoronary stenting and antithrombotic regimen trial: one year clinical follow-up [abstract]. *Circulation* 1996; 94 (suppl): I-683.

114. Hong MK, Wong SC, Pichard AD et al. Long term results of patients enrolled in the anti-platelet treatment after intravascular ultrasound guided optimal stent expansion (APPLAUSE) trial [abstract]. *Circulation* 1996; 94 (suppl): I-686.

115. Strain JE, Rehman DE, Fischman D, Cohen N, Moses JW, for the STRESS III

Investigators. STRESS III: preliminary acute results of IVUS vs non-IVUS stenting [abstract]. *Circulation* 1996; 94 (suppl): I-686.

116. Darius H, Veit K, Rupprecht H-J. Synergistic inhibition of platelet aggregation by ticlopidine plus aspirin following intracoronary stent placement [abstract]. *Circulation* 1996; 94 (suppl): I-257.

117. Preiss JP, Lecompte T, Alnot Y et al. Serial antiplatelet effects of combined treatment with ticlopidine and aspirine after stent implantation [abstract]. *Circulation* 1996; 94 (suppl): I-685.

118. Rodriguez JN, Fernandez-Jurado A, Dieguez JC, Amian A, Prados D. Ticlopidine and severe aplastic anemia [letter]. *Am J Haematol* 1994; **47:** 332.

119. Pepine CJ, Holmes DR, Block PC et al, and the cardiac catheterization committee. ACC expert consensus document. *J Am Coll Cardiol* 1996; **28:** 782–94.

120. Schühlen H, Hadamitzky M, Walter H, Ulm K, Schömig A. Major benefit from antiplatelet therapy for patients at high risk for adverse cardiac events after coronary Palmaz–Schatz stent placement. Analysis of a prospective risk stratification protocol in the intracoronary stenting and antithrombotic regimen (ISAR) trial. *Circulation* 1997; **95:** 2015–21.

121. Schühlen H, Hadamitzky M, Kastrati A et al. Grading the risk for restenosis after coronary stent placement. Analysis of a prospective risk stratification protocol in the ISAR-trial [abstract]. *Circulation* 1996; 94 (suppl): I-91.

122. Mehan VK, Salzmann C, Kaufmann U, Meier B. Coronary stenting without anticoagulation. *Cathet Cardiovas Diagn* 1995; **34:** 137–40.

123. Albiero R, Hall P, Itoh A et al. Results of a consecutive series of patients receiving only antiplatelet therapy after optimized stent implantation. *Circulation* 1997; **95:** 1145–56.

124. Goods CM, al-Shaibi KF, Liu MW et al. Comparison of aspirin alone versus aspirin plus ticlopidine after coronary artery stenting. *Am J Cardiol* 1996; **78:** 1042–44.

125. Neumann F-J, Gawaz M, Dickfeld T et al. Antiplatelet effect of ticlopidine. *J Am Coll Cardiol* 1997; **29:** 1515–19.

126. Elsner M, Peifer A, Drexler M, Wenzel C, Hebbeker C, Kasper W. Clinical outcome at six months of coronary stenting followed by ticlopidine monotherapy. *Am J Cardiol* 1998; **81:** 147–51.

127. Barragan P, Sainsous J, Silvestri M et al. Coronary artery stenting without anticoagulation, aspirin, ultrasound guidance, or high pressure: prospective study of 1,051 consecutive patients. *Cathet Cardiovasc Diagn* 1997; **42:** 367–73.

128. Kruse KR, Greenberg CS, Tanguay J-F et al. Thrombin and fibrin activity in patients treated with enoxaprin, ticlopidine and aspirin versus the conventional coumadin regimen after elective stenting: the ENTICES trial [abstract]. *J Am Coll Cardiol* 1996; 27 (suppl A): 334A.

129. The EPILOG Investigators. Platelet glycoprotein IIb/IIIa receptor blockade and low-dose heparin during precutaneous coronary revascularization. *N Engl J Med* 1997; **336:** 1689–96.

130. The EPISTENT Investigators. Randomised placebo-controlled and balloon angioplasty controlled trial to assess safety of coronary stenting with use of platelet glycoprotein-IIb/IIIa blockade. *Lancet* 1998; **352:** 87–92.

131. Bittl JA. Coronary stent occlusion; thrombus horribilis [editorial]. *J Am Coll Cardiol* 1996; **28:** 368–70.

132. Chronos NAF, Robinson KA, Kelly AB et al. Thromboresistant phosphorylcholine coatings for coronary stents [abstract]. *Circulation* 1995; 92 (suppl I): I-685.

133. Malik N, Gunn J, Shepard L, Newman CMH, Crossman DC, Cumberland DC. Phosphorylcholine-coated stents in porcine coronary arteries: angiographic and morphometric assessment. *Eur J Cardiol* 1997; 18 (suppl): 152.

134. Bonan R, Paiement P, Tanguay JF et al. Recoil evaluation of a new stent with phosphorylcholine coating in porcine coronary arteries. *Eur J Cardiol* 1997; 18 (suppl): 153.

135. Gunn J, Malik N, Holt C et al. The BioDivYsio® stent: morphometric superiority to the Palmaz–Schatz stent in the porcine coronary model [abstract]. *Am J Cardiol* 1997; 80 (suppl 7A): 29S.

136. Beusekom HMM, Whelan DM, Krabbendam SC et al. Biocompatibility of phosphorylcholine coated stents in a porcine coronary model [abstract]. *Circulation* 1998; 96 (suppl): I-289.

137. Heublein B, Pethig K, Elsayed A-M. Silicon carbide coating – a semiconducting hybrid design of coronary stents – a feasibility study. *J Invas Cardiol* 1998; **10:** 255–62.

138. De Scheerder IK, Wilczek K, Van Dorpe J et al. Ampiphilic polyurethane coating of intracoronary stents decreases mortality due to subacute thrombosis in porcine coronary model [abstract]. *Circulation* 1993; 88 (suppl): I-645.

139. De Scheerder IK, Wilczek K, Verbeken E et al. Ampiphilic polyurethane coating of intracoronary stents decreases mortality due to subacute thrombosis in porcine coronary model [abstract]. *J Am Coll Cardiol* 1994; 23 (suppl): 186A.

140. Holmes DR, Camrud AR, Jorgenson MA, Edwards WD, Schwartz RS. Polymeric stenting in the porcine coronary artery model: differential outcome of exogenous fibrin sleeves versus polyurethane-coated stents. *J Am Coll Cardiol* 1994; **24:** 525–31.

141. Sheth S, Dev V, Jacobs H, Forrester JS, Litvack F, Eigler N. Prevention of subacute stent thrombosis by polymer-polyethylene oxide-heparin coating in the rabbit carotid artery [abstract]. *J Am Coll Cardiol* 1995; 25 (suppl): 348A.

142. Staab ME, Holmes DR Jr, Schwartz RS. Polymers. In: Sigwart U (ed.). Endoluminal Stenting. London, W.B. Saunders; 1996: 34–44.

143. Cox DA, Anderson PG, Roubin GS, Chou CY, Agrawal SK, Cavender JB. Effects of local delivery of heparin and methotrexate on neointimal proliferation in stented porcine coronary arteries. *Coron Art Dis* 1992; **3:** 237–48.

144. Slepian MJ, Roth L, Wesselcouch E, Massia S, Khosravi F. Gel paving of intra-arterial stents: a method for reducing stent and adjacent arterial wall thrombogenicity [abstract]. *J Invas Cardiol* 1995; **7:** 5A.

145. Schwartz RS, Murphy JG, Edwards WD, Holmes DR. Bioabsorbable, drug-eluting, intracoronary stents: design and future applications. In: Sigwart U, Frank GI (eds). Coronary Stents. Berlin, Springer-Verlag; 1992: 135–54.

146. van Beusekom HMM, van Vleit HHDM, van der Giessen WJ. Fibrin and basement membrane components as a biocompatible and thromboresistant coating for metal stents. *Circulation* 1993; 88 (suppl): I-645.

147. Bailey SR, Paige S, Lunn A, Palmaz J. Heparin coating of endovascular stents decreases subacute thrombosis in a rabbit model [abstract]. *Circulation* 1992; 86 (suppl): I-186.

148. van der Giessen WJ, Härdhammar PA, van Beusekom HMM et al. Prevention of (sub)acute thrombosis using heparin-coated stents [abstract]. *Circulation* 1994; 90 (suppl): I-650.

149. Härdhammar PA, van Beusekom HMM, Emanuelsson HU et al. Reduction in thrombotic events with heparin-coated Palmaz–Schatz stents in normal porcine coronary arteries. *Circulation* 1996; **93:** 423–30.

150. Kipshidze N, Baker JE, Nikolaychik V. Fibrin coated stents as an improved vehicle for endothelial cell seeding [abstract]. *Circulation* 1994; 90 (suppl): I-597.

151. Baker JE, Horn JB, Nikolaychik V, Kipshidze NN. Fibrin stent coatings. In: Sigwart U (ed.). Endoluminal Stenting. London, W.B. Saunders; 1996: 84–89.

152. Aggarwal RK, Martin W, Ireland DC, Azrin MA, de Bono DP, Gershlick AH. Effects of polymer-coated stents eluting antibody to platelet integrin glycoprotein IIb/IIIa on platelet deposition and neointima formation [abstract]. *Eur J Cardiol* 1996; 17 (suppl): 176.

153. Aggarwal RK, Martin WA, Azrin MA, Ezekowitz MD, de Bono DP, Gershlick AH. Effects of platelet GPIIb/IIIa antibody and antibody-urokinase conjugate adsorbed to stents on platelet deposition and neointima formation [abstract]. *Circulation* 1996; 94 (suppl): I-258.

154. Aggarwal RK, Ireland DC, Ragheb A, de Bono DP, Gershlick AH. Reduction in thrombogenicity of polymer-coated stents by immobilization of platelet-targeted urokinase [abstract]. *Eur J Cardiol* 1996; 17 (suppl): 177.

155. Lu L, Jones MW. Diamond-like carbon as biological compatible material for cell culture and medical applications. *Bio Med Mat Engin* 1993; **3**: 223–28.

156. Amon M, Bolz A, Schaldach M. Improvement of stenting therapy with a silicon carbide coated tantalum stent. *J Mater Sci Mater Med* 1996; **7**: 273–78.

157. Wataha JC, Sun ZL, Hanks CT, Fang DN. Effect of Ni ions on expression of intracellular adhesion molecule 1 by endothelial cells. *J Biomed Mat Res* 1997; **36**: 145–51.

158. Klein CL, Köhler H, Kirkpatrick CJ. Increased adhesion and activation of polymorphonuclear neutrophil granulocytes to endothelial cells under heavy metal exposure in vitro. *Pathobiology* 1994; **62**: 90–98.

159. Klein CL, Köhler H, Kirkpatrick CJ. The role of metal corrosion in inflammatory processes: induction of adhesion molecules by heavy metals. *J Mater Sci Mater Med* 1994; **5**: 798–807.

160. Hildebrand HF, Vernon C, Martin P. Nickel, chromium, cobalt dental alloys and allergic reactions: an overview. *Biomaterials* 1989; **10**: 545–48.

161. Costa M. Molecular mechanisms of nickel carcinogenesis. *Ann Rev Pharmacol* 1991; **31**: 321–27.

162. Beythien C, Gutensohn K, Kühnl P, Hamm CW, Alt E, Terres W. Influence of "diamond-like" and gold coating on platelet activation: a flow cytometry analysis in a pulsed floating model [abstract]. *J Am Coll Cardiol* 1998; 31 (suppl): 413A.

163. Beythien C, Gutensohn K, Fenner T, Padmanaban K, Köster R, Hamm CW, Terres W, Kühnl P. Diamond-like carbon coating of coronary stents: influence on platelet activation, smooth muscle cells and release of metal atoms [abstract]. *Eur J Cardiol* 1998; 19 (suppl): 497

164. Larm O, Larsson R, Olsson P. A new non-thrombogenic surface prepared by selective covalent binding of heparin via a reducing terminal residue. *Biomat Med Dev Artif Org* 1983; **11**: 161–74.

165. Vrolix MC, Grolier G, Legrand V et al. Heparin-coated wire coil (Wiktor) for elective stent placement—the MENTOR Trial [abstract]. *Eur Heart J* 1997; 18 (suppl): 152.

166. Serruys PW, Emanuelsson H, van der Giessen W et al, on behalf of the BENESTENT II Study Group. Heparin coated Palmaz–Schatz stents in human coronary arteries. Early outcome of the BENESTENT II Pilot Study. *Circulation* 1996; **93**: 412–22.

167. Garcia E, Serruys PW, Dawkins K et al. BENESTENT-II trial: final results of visit II & III: a 7 month follow-up [abstract]. *Eur Heart J* 1997; 18 (suppl): 350.

168. McKenna CJ, Camrud AR, Wolff R, Edwards WD, Holmes DR, Schwartz RS. Evaluation of the biocompatability and safety of fibrin-film stenting up to one year post deployment in a porcine coronary injury model [abstract]. *Am J Cardiol* 1997; 80 (suppl 7A): 155.

169. McKenna CJ, Camrud AR, Sangiorgi G et al. Fibrin-film stenting in a porcine coronary injury model: efficacy and safety compared with uncoated stents. *J Am Coll Cardiol* 1998; **31:** 1434–38.

170. McKenna CJ, Camrud AR, Wolff R, Edwards WD, Schwartz RS. Fibrin-film stenting in a porcine coronary injury model: efficacy and safety compared to uncoated stents [abstract]. *Circulation* 1997; 96 (suppl): I-15.

171. Alt E, Beilharz C, Preter D et al. Biodegradable stent coating with polylactic acid, hirudin and prostacyclin reduces restenosis [abstract]. *J Am Coll Cardiol* 1997; 29 (suppl A): 238A.

172. Schmidmaier G, Stemberger A, Alt E, Gawaz M, F-J Neumann, Schömig A. A new biodegradable polylactic acid coronary stent-coating, releasing PEG-hirudin and a prostacycline analog, reduces both platelet activation and plasmatic coagulation [abstract]. *J Am Coll Cardiol* 1997; 29 (suppl A): 354A.

173. Herrmann RA, Schmidmaier G, Resch A et al. Comparison of the thrombogenicity of steel and gold-surface coronary stents with a biodegradable, drug releasing coating in a human stasis model [abstract]. *Circulation* 1997; 96 (suppl): I-722.

174. Schmidmaier G, Stemberger A, Alt E, Gawaz M, Schömig A. Non-linear time release characteristics of a biodegradable polylactic acid coating releasing PEG-hirudin and a PGI2 analog [abstract]. *Eur Heart J* 1997; 18 (suppl): 571.

175. Aggarwal RK, Martin W, Ireland DC, Azrin MA, de Bono DP, Gershlick AH. Effects of polymer-coated stents eluting antibody to platelet integrin glycoprotein IIb/IIIa on platelet deposition and neointima formation [abstract]. *Eur Heart J* 1996; 17 (suppl): 176.

176. Aggarwal RK, Martin WA, Azrin MA, Ezekowitz MD, de Bono DP, Gershlick AH. Effects of platelet GPIIb/IIIa antibody and antibody-urokinase conjugate adsorbed to stents on platelet deposition and neointima formation [abstract]. *Circulation* 1996; 94 (suppl): I-258.

177. Aggarwal RK, Ireland DC, Azrin MA, Ezekowitz MD, de Bono DP, Gershlick AH. Antithrombotic potential of polymer-coated stents eluting platelet glycoprotein IIb/IIIa receptor antibody. *Circulation* 1996; **94:** 3311–17.

178. Baron JH, de Bono DP, Azrin MA, Ezekowitz MD, Gershlick AH. Adsorption and elution of c7E3Fab from polymer-coated stents in vitro: local delivery of an anti-thrombotic agent that also may inhibit restenosis [abstract]. *Circulation* 1997; 96 (suppl): I-402.

179. Baron JH, Aggrawal R, de Bono D, Gershlick AH. Adsorption and elution of c7E3 Fab from polymer-coated stents in-vitro [abstract]. *Eur Heart J* 1997; 18 (suppl): 503.

180. Slepian MJ, Khosravi F, Massia SP, Kieras M, Khera GS, Hubbell JA. Gel paving of intrarterial stents in vivo reduces stent and adjacent arterial wall thrombogenicity [abstract]. *J Vasc Interven Radiol* 1995; **6:** 50.

181. van der Giessen WJ, Serruys PW, Visser WJ, Verdouw PD, van Schalkwijk WP, Jongkind JF. Endothelialization of intravascular stents. *J Intervent Cardiol* 1988; **1:** 109–20.

182. Dichek DA, Neville RF, Zwiebel JA, Freeman SM, Leon MB, Anderson WF. Seeding of intravascular stents with genetically engineered endothelial cells. *Circulation* 1989; **80:** 1347–53.

183. Flugelman MY, Virmani R, Leon MB, Bowman RL, Dichek DA. Genetically engineered endothelial cells remain adherent and viable after stent deployment and exposure to flow in vitro. *Circ Res* 1992; **70:** 348–54.

184. Flugelman MY, Rome JJ, Virmani R, Neuman KD, Dichek DA. Detection of genetically engineered endothelial cells seeded on endovascular prosthesis ten days after in vivo deployment [abstract]. *J Mol Cell Cardiol* 1993; 25 (suppl I): S-83.

185. Scott NA, Candal FJ, Robinson KA, Ades EW. Seeding of intracoronary stents with immortalized human microvascular endothelial cells. *Am Heart J* 1995; **129:** 860–66.

186. Ades EW, Candal FJ, Swerlick RA et al. HMEC-1: establishment of an immortalized human microvascular endothelial cell line. *J Invest Dermatol* 1992; **99:** 683–90.

187. Bailey SR. Endothelial "SODDING": intraprocedural replacement of endothelial cells on endovascular stents [abstract]. *Circulation* 1996; 94 (suppl): I-261.

188. Vinogradsky B, Sawa H, Guala A, Lundgren C, Fuji S. Seeding of stents with genetically modified endothelial cells: overexpression of urokinase receptor results in increased seeded cell retention [abstract]. *Circulation* 1996; 94 (suppl): I-261.

189. Dichek DA, Nussbaum O, Degen SJF, Anderson WF. Enhancement of the fibrinolytic activity of sheep endothelial cells by retroviral vector-mediated gene transfer. *Blood* 1991; **77:** 533–541.

190. Flugelman MY. Inhibition of intravascular thrombosis and vascular smooth muscle cell proliferation by gene therapy. *Thromb Haemost* 1995; **74:** 406–10.

191. Van Belle E, Chen D, Tio FO, Maillard L, Passeri J, Isner JM. Accelerated endothelialization improves stent biocompatibility: feasibility and effects of VEGF-gene transfer. *Circulation* 1996: 94 (suppl): I-259.

192. Van Belle E, Tio FO, Chen D et al. Passivation of metallic stents after arterial gene transfer of phVEGF$_{165}$ inhibits thrombus formation and intimal thickening. *J Am Coll Cardiol* 1997; **29:** 1371–79.

193. Stefanadis C, Toutouzas P. Percutaneous implantation of autologous vein graft stent for the treatment of coronary artery disease. *Lancet* 1995; **345:** 1509.

194. Stefanadis C, Eleftherios T, Toutouzas K et al. Autologous vein graft-coated stent

for the treatment of coronary artery disease: immediate results after percutaneous placement in humans [abstract]. *J Am Coll Cardiol* 1996; 27 (suppl): 179A.

195. Stefanadis C, Toutouzas K, Tsiamis E et al. The clinical experience using the autologous vein graft-coated stent for the treatment of coronary artery disease [abstract]. *Eur Heart J* 1997; 18 (suppl): 154.

196. Toutouzas K, Stefanadis C, Tsiamis E et al. The clinical experience using the autologous vein graft-coated stent for the treatment of coronary artery disease [abstract]. *Am J Cardiol* 1997; 80 (suppl 7A): 27S.

197. Toutouzas K, Stefanadis C, Tsiamis E et al. Primary autologous vein graft-coated stent in acute myocardial infarction: immediate and short-term results [abstract]. *Circulation* 1996; 94 (suppl): I-576.

198. Toutouzas K, Stefanadis H, Tsiamis L et al. Experience with the autologous vein graft-coated stent for the treatment of coronary artery disease [abstract]. *Circulation* 1997; 96 (suppl): I-275.

199. Tsiamis E, Stefanadis C, Toutouzas K et al. Autologous arterial graft-coated stent implantation in diseased saphenous by-pass grafts: immediate results and mid-term outcome [abstract]. *Eur Heart J* 1997; 18 (suppl): 154.

200. Stefanadis C, Toutouzas K, Tsiamis E et al. Preliminary results by using the autologous arterial graft-coated stent for the treatment of coronary artery disease [abstract]. *Eur Heart J* 1997;18 (suppl): 154.

201. Toutouzas K, Stefanadis C, Tsiamis E et al. Stents coated by an autologous arterial graft: the first application in human coronary arteries [abstract]. *J Am Coll Cardiol* 1998; 31 (suppl): 351A.

202. Mitchel JF, McKay RG. Treatment of acute stent thrombosis with local urokinase therapy using catheter based, drug delivery systems: a case report. *Cathet Cardiovasc Diagn* 1995; **39:** 149–54.

203. Robinson NMK, Thomas MR, Wainwright RJ, Jewitt DE. Is unstable angina a contraindication to intracoronary stent insertion? *J Invas Cardiol* 1996; **8:** 351–56.

204. Casserly IP, Hasdai D, Garratt KN, Bell MR. Improved clinical outcome after abciximab therapy in patients with early intracoronary stent thrombosis [abstract]. *Circulation* 1997; 96 (suppl): I-594.

205. Rozenman YR, Mosseri M, Mereuta A, Gotsman MS. Monoclonal antibodies against the IIb/IIIa platelet receptor to treat acute thrombotic occlusion of a coronary stent. *J Invas Cardiol* 1998; **10:** 42–44.

206. Maimaitiming A, Rupprecht HJ, Voigtländer T, Nowak B, Meyer J. Comparison of "rescue"-ReoPro with "rescue"-lysis for acute stent thrombosis [abstract]. *Eur Heart J* 1997; 18 (suppl): 380.

207. Maimaitiming A, Rupprecht HJ, Nowak B, Voigtlander T, Meyer J. Comparison of

Reopro vs intracoronary thrombolysis for acute coronary stent thrombosis [abstract]. *Circulation* 1997; 96 (suppl): I-640.

208. Hamburger JN, de Feyter PJ, de Mario C et al. Preliminary experience with the coronary angiojet rheolytic thrombectomy catheter: a preamble to the Euro-ARTS study [abstract]. *Eur Heart J* 1996; 17 (suppl): 181.

209. Serruys PW, de Jaegere P, Kiemeneij F et al, for the Benestent Study Group. A comparison of balloon-expandable-stent implantation with balloon angioplasty in patients with coronary artery disease. *N Engl J Med* 1994; **331:** 489–95.

210. Fischman DL, Leon MB, Baim DS et al, for the Stent Restenosis Study investigators. A randomized comparison of coronary-stent placement and balloon angioplasty in the treatment of coronary artery disease. *N Engl J Med* 1994; **331:** 496–501.

211. Kuntz RE, Gibson CM, Nobuyoshi M, Baim DS. Generalized model of restenosis after conventional balloon angioplasty, stenting and directional atherectomy. *J Am Coll Cardiol* 1993; **21:** 15–25.

212. Kuntz RE, Safian RD, Carozza JP Jr, Fischman RF, Mansour M, Baim DS. The importance of acute luminal diameter in determining restenosis after coronary atherectomy or stenting. *Circulation* 1992; **86:** 1827–35.

213. Leon MB, Popma JF, Fischman DL et al. Vascular recoil immediately after implantation of tubular slotted metallic coronary stent [abstract]. *J Am Coll Cardiol* 1992; 19 (suppl): 109A.

214. Rechavia E, Litvack F, Macko G, Eigler N. Influence of expandable balloon diameter on Palmaz–Schatz stent recoil. *Cathet Cardiovasc Diagn* 1995; **36:** 11–15.

215. White CJ. Stent recoil: comparison on the Wiktor-GX coil and the Palmaz–Schatz tubular coronary stent. *Cathet Cardiovasc Diagn* 1997; **41:** 1–3.

216. Bermejo J, Botas J, García E et al. Mechanisms of residual lumen stenosis after high-pressure stent implantation. A quantitative coronary angiography and intrtavascular ultrasound study. *Circulation* 1998; **98:** 112–18.

217. de Jaegere P, Serruys PW, van Es GA et al. Recoil following Wiktor stent implantation for restenotic lesions of coronary arteries. *Cathet Cardiovasc Diagn* 1994; **32:** 147–56.

218. Popina JJ, White CH, Pinkerton CA et al. Effect of balloon expandable stent design on vascular recoil and lesion-site morphology after intracoronary placement [abstract]. *Circulation* 1992; 86 (suppl): I–321.

219. Painter JA, Mintz GS, Wong SC et al. Serial intravascular ultrasound studies fail to show evidence of chronic Palmaz–Schatz stent recoil. *Am J Cardiol* 1995; **75:** 398–400.

220. Hoffmann R, Mintz GS, Dussaillant GR et al. Patterns and mechanisms of in-stent restenosis. A serial intravascular ultrasound study. *Circulation* 1996; **94:** 1247–54.

221. Schwartz RS. Characteristics of an ideal stent based upon restenosis pathology. *J Invas Cardiol* 1996; **8**: 386–87.

222. Hanke H, Kamenz J, Hassenstein S et al. Prolonged proliferative response of smooth muscle cells after experimental intravascular stenting. *Eur Heart J* 1995; **16**: 785–93.

223. Karas SP, Gravanis MB, Santoian EC, Robinson KA, Andernerg KA, King SB III. Coronary intimal proliferation after balloon injury and stenting in swine: an animal model of restenosis. *J Am Coll Cardiol* 1992; **20**: 467–74.

224. Rogers C, Karnovsky MJ, Edelman EP. Inhibition of experimental neointimal hyperplasia and thrombosis depends on the type of vascular injury and the site of drug administration. *Circulation* 1993; **88**: 1215–21.

225. Gordon PC, Gibson CM, Cohen DJ, Carrozza JP, Kunz RE, Baim DS. Mechanism of restenosis and redilatation within coronary stents: quantitative angiographic assessment. *J Am Coll Cardiol* 1993; **21**: 1166–74.

226. Dussaillant GR, Mintz GS, Pichard AD et al. Small stent size and intimal hyperplasia contribute to restenosis: a volumetric intravascular ultrasound analysis. *J Am Coll Cardiol* 1995; **26**: 720–24.

227. Edelman ER, Rogers C. Hoop dreams. Stents without restenosis [editorial]. *Circulation* 1996; **94**: 1199–1202.

228. Schwartz RS, Huber KC, Murphy JG et al. Restenosis and proportional neointimal response to coronary artery injury: results in a porcine model. *J Am Coll Cardiol* 1992; **19**: 267–74.

229. Hofma SH, Whelan DMC, van Beusekom HMM, Verdouw PD, van der Giessen WJ. Increasing arterial wall injury after long-term implantation of two types of stent in a porcine coronary model. *Eur Heart J* 1998; **19**: 601–09.

230. De Scheerder IK, Wang K, Verbeken EV, Zhou XR, Piessens JH, Van de Werf F. Stent deployment pressure defines the stent/vessel wall relationship and has important implications for early and late outcome. *J Invas Cardiol* 1998; **10**: 151–57.

231. Carter AJ, Laird JR, Farb A, Kufs W, Wortham DC, Virmani R. Morphologic characteristics of lesion formation and time course of smooth muscle proliferation in a porcine proliferative restenosis model. *J Am Coll Cardiol* 1994; **24**: 1398–405.

232. Rogers C, Welt FGP, Karnovsky MJ, Edelman ER. Monocyte recruitment and neointimal hyperplasia in rabbits. Coupled inhibitory effects of heparin. *Arterioscler Thromb Vasc Biol* 1996; **16**: 1312–18.

233. Moreno PR, Palacios IF, Pathan A, Fuster V, Fallon JT. Histological comparison of in-stent and post-PTCA restenotic tissue [abstract]. *Circulation* 1997; **96**: I-591.

234. Kornowski R, Hong MK, Tio FO, Bramwell O, Wu H, Leon MB. In-stent restnosis: contributions of inflammatory responses and arterial injury to neointimal hyperplasia. *J Am Coll Cardiol* 1998; **31**: 224–30.

235. van Beusekom HMM, Whelan DM, Hofma SH, Verdouw PD, van der Giessen WJ. Stents but not balloon angioplasty induce chronic neointimal permeability [abstract]. *Circulation* 1995; 92 (suppl): I-87.

236. Penn IM, Galligan L, Brown RIG, Murray-Parson N, Foley JB, White J. Restenosis at the stent articulation: is this a design flaw? [abstract] *J Am Coll Cardiol* 1992; 19 (suppl): 291A.

237. Ikari Y, Hara K, Tamura T, Saeki F, Yamaguchi T. Luminal loss and site of restenosis after Palmaz–Schatz coronary stent implantation. *Am J Cardiol* 1995; **76:** 117–20.

238. Tominaga R, Kambic HE, Emoto H, Harasaki H, Sutton C, Hollman J. Effects of design geometry of endovascular prostheses on stenosis rate in normal rabbits. *Am Heart J* 1992; **123:** 21–28.

239. Barth KH, Virmani R, Froelich J et al. Paired comparison of vascular wall reactions to Palmaz stents, Streker tantalum stents, and Wallstents in canine iliac and femoral arteries. *Circulation* 1996; **93:** 2161–69.

240. Chung I-M, Reidy MA, Schwartz SM, Wight TN, Gold HK. Enhanced extracellular matrix synthesis may be important for restenosis of arteries after stent deployment [abstract]. *Circulation* 1996; 94 (suppl): I-349.

241. Kastrati A, Schömig A, Dietz R, Neumann FJ, Richart G. Time course of restenosis during the first year after emergency coronary stenting. *Circulation* 1993; **87:** 1498–505.

242. Ellis SG, Savage M, Fischman D et al. Restenosis after placement of Palmaz–Schatz stents in native coronary arteries. Initial results of a multicenter experience. *Circulation* 1992; **86:** 1836–44.

243. Savage MP, Fischman DL, Schatz RA et al. Long-term angiographic and clinical outcome of a balloon-expandable stent in the native coronary circulation. *J Am Coll Cardiol* 1994; **24:** 1207–12.

244. Lablanche J-M, Danchin N, Grollier G et al. Factors predictive of restenosis after stent implantation managed by ticlopidine and aspirin [abstract]. *Circulation* 1996; 94 (suppl): I-256.

245. Mittal S, Weiss DL, Hirshfield JW, Kolansky DM, Herrmann HC. Restenotic lesions have a worse outcome after stenting [abstract]. *Circulation* 1996; 94 (suppl): I-131.

246. Kastrati A, Schömig A, Elezi S et al. Predictive factors of restenosis after coronary stent placement. *J Am Coll Cardiol* 1997; **30:** 1428–36.

247. Mehran R, Abizaid AS, Hoffman RH et al. Clinical and angiographic predictors of target lesion revascularization after stent placement in native coronary lesions [abstract]. *Circulation* 1997; 96 (suppl): I-472.

248. Black AJR, Anderson HV, Roubin GS, Powelson SW, Douglas JS, King III SB. Repeat coronary angioplasty: correlates of a second restenosis. *J Am Coll Cardiol* 1988; **11:** 714–18.

249. Manderson JA, Mosse PRL, Safstrom JA, Young SB, Campbell GR. Balloon catheter injury to rabbit carotid artery. I. Changes in smooth muscle phenotype. *Arteriosclerosis* 1989; **9:** 289–98.

250. Simon M, Leclerc G, Safian RD, Isner JM, Weir L, Baim DS. Relation between activated smooth-muscle cells in coronary artery lesions and restenosis after atherectomy. *N Engl J Med* 1993; **328:** 608–13.

251. de Jaegere P, Serruys PW, Bertrand M et al. Angiographic predictors of recurrence of restenosis after Wiktor stent implantation in native coronary arteries. *Am J Cardiol* 1993; **72:** 165–70.

252. Colombo A, Ferraro M, Itoh A, Martini G, Blengino S, Finci L. Results of coronary stenting for restenosis. *J Am Coll Cardiol* 1996; **28:** 830–36.

253. Antoniucci D, Valenti R, Santoro GM et al. Restenosis after coronary stenting in current clinical practice. *Am Heart J* 1998; **135:** 510–18.

254. Erbel R, Haude M, Höpp HW et al, on behalf of the REST Study Group. REstenosis ST (REST)-Study: randomized trial comparing stenting and balloon angioplasty for treatment of restenosis after balloon angioplasty. *J Am Coll Cardiol* 1996; 27 (suppl A): 139A.

255. Strauss BH, Serruys PW, de Scheerder IK et al. Relative risk analysis of angiographic predictors of restenosis within the coronary Wallstent. *Circulation* 1991; **84:** 1636–43.

256. Hong MK, Kent KM, Satler LF et al. Are long-term results different when stents are used in de novo versus restenotic lesions? [abstract]. *Circulation* 1996; 94 (suppl): I-131.

257. Moscucci M, Piana RN, Kuntz RE et al. Effect of prior coronary restenosis on the risk of subsequent restenosis after stent placement or directional atherectomy. *Am J Cardiol* 1994; **73:** 1147–53.

258. Bauters C, Hubert E, Prat A et al. Predictors of restenosis after coronary stent implantation. *J Am Coll Cardiol* 1998; **31:** 1291–98.

259. Kuntz RE, Ki Ho K, Senerchia C et al. Prior restenosis does not increase the risk of restenosis following coronary stenting: an analysis from the stent anticoagulation regimen study (STARS) trial [abstract]. *Circulation* 1997; 96 (suppl): I-471.

260. Haude M, Erbel R, Straub U, Dietz U, Meyer J. Short and long term results after intracoronary stenting in human coronary arteries: monocentre experience with the balloon-expandable Palmaz–Schatz stent. *Br Heart J* 1991; **66:** 337–45.

261. Alonso JJ, Durán JM, Gimeno F et al. Clinical and angiographic restenosis after coronary stenting. incidence and predictors [abstract]. *J Am Coll Cardiol* 1997; 29 (suppl A): 239A.

262. Gaxiola E, Vlietstra RE, Brenner AS, Browne KF, Ebersole DG. Diabetes and multiple stents independently double the risk of short-term revascularisation [abstract]. *Circulation* 1997; 96 (suppl): I-649.

263. Dirschinger J, Hausleiter J, Schuehlen H et al. Predictive factors of restenosis after coronary stent placement [abstract]. *Circulation* 1997; 96 (suppl): I-472.

264. Haude M, Caspari D, Baumgart D, Welge D, Liu F, Erbel R. Risk factor analysis for the development of restenosis after intracoronary stent implantation with adjunct high pressure stent dilatation [abstract]. *J Am Coll Cardiol* 1998; 31 (suppl): 139A.

265. Hamasaki N, Nosaka H, Kimura T et al. Influence of lesion length on late angiographic outcome and restenostic process after successful stent implantation [abstract]. *J Am Coll Cardiol* 1997; 29 (suppl A): 239A.

266. Pomerantsev EV, Juergens CP, Gerckens U, Grube E, Oesterle SN, Stertzer SH. Angiographic predictors of restenosis after optimal coronary stent deployment [abstract]. *Circulation* 1997; 96 (suppl): I-473.

267. Kobayashi Y, DeGregario J, Reimers B, DiMario C, Finci L, Colombo A. The length of the stented segment is an independent predictor of restenosis [abstract]. *J Am Coll Cardiol* 1998; 31 (suppl): 366A.

268. Khosla S, White CJ, Collins TJ et al. Predictors of angiographic restenosis following stent revascularization of aorto-coronary saphenous vein grafts [abstract]. *Circulation* 1997; 96 (suppl): I-473.

269. Medina A, Melian F, Suarez de Lezo J et al. Effectiveness of coronary artery stents for the treatment of chronic total occlusion in angina pectoris. *Am J Cardiol* 1994; **73:** 1222–24.

270. Ozaki Y, Violaris AG, Hamburger J et al. Short- and long-term clinical and quantitative angiographic results with the new less shortening Wallstent for vessel reconstruction in chronic total occlusion: a quantitative angiographic study. *J Am Coll Cardiol* 1996; **28:** 354–60.

271. Goldberg SL, Colombo A, Maiello L, Borrione M, Finci L, Almagor Y. Intracoronary stent insertion after balloon angioplasty of chronic total occlusions. *J Am Coll Cardiol* 1995; **26:** 713–19.

272. Almagor Y, Borrione M, Maiello L, Khlat B, Finci L, Colombo A. Coronary stenting after recanalisation of chronic total coronary occlusions [abstract]. *Circulation* 1993; 88 (suppl): I-504.

273. Bilodeau L, Iyer SS, Cannon AD et al. Stenting as an adjunct to balloon angioplasty for recanalization of totally occluded coronary arteries: clinical and angiographic follow-up [abstract]. *J Am Coll Cardiol* 1993; 21 (suppl): 292A.

274. Etsuo T, Osamu K, Masanobu F, Satoru O, Hitone T, Tohru K. Impact of stenting on PTCA of chronic total occlusions [abstract]. *Circulation* 1996; 94 (suppl): I-249.

275. Suttorp MJ, Mast G, Plokker HWT, Kelder JC, Ernst SMPG, Bal E. Primary coronary stenting after successful balloon angioplasty of chronic total occlusions: a single-center experience [abstract]. *Circulation* 1996; 94 (suppl): I-687.

276. Suttorp MJ, Mast G, Plokker HWT, Kelder JC, Ernst SMPG, Bal E. Primary coronary stenting after successful balloon angioplasty of chronic total occlusions: A single-center experience. *Am Heart J* 1998; **135:** 318–22.

277. Nienaber CA, Fratz S, Lund GK, Stiel GM. Primary stent placement or balloon angioplasty for chronic coronary occlusions: a matched pair analysis in 100 patients [abstract]. *Circulation* 1996; 94 (suppl): I-686.

278. Moussa I, di Mario C, Moses J et al. Comparison of angiographic and clinical outcomes of coronary stenting of chronic total occlusions versus subtotal occlusions. *Am J Cardiol* 1998; **81:** 1–6.

279. Gambhir DS, Sudha R, Singh S et al. Elective coronary stenting after recanalization for chronic total occlusion: clinical and angiographic follow-up results. *Indian Heart J* 1997; **49:** 163–68.

280. Anzuini A, Rosanio S, Legrand V et al. Wiktor stent for treatment of chronic total coronary occlusions: short- and long-term clinical and angiographic results from a large multicenter expreience. *J Am Coll Cardiol* 1998; **31:** 281–88.

281. Rau T, Schofer J, Schlüter M, Seidensticker A, Berger J, Mathey DG. Stenting of nonacute total coronary occlusions: predictors of late angiographic outcome. *J Am Coll Cardiol* 1998; **31:** 275–80.

282. Mori M, Kurogane H, Hayashi T et al. Comparison of results of intracoronary implantation of the Palmaz–Schatz stent with conventional balloon angioplasty in chronic total coronary arterial occlusion. *Am J Cardiol* 1996; **78:** 985–89.

283. Anzuini A, Legrand VM, Kulbertus H et al. Medtronic™ Wiktor stent implantation in chronic coronary total occlusions: in-hospital and long term outcomes [abstract]. *Circulation* 1997; 96 (suppl): I-268.

284. Wong SC, Baim DS, Schatz RA et al, for the Palmaz–Schatz Stent Study Group. Acute results and late outcomes after stent implantation in saphenous vein graft lesions: the multicenter U.S. Palmaz–Schatz stent experience. *J Am Coll Cardiol* 1995; **26:** 704–12.

285. Carrozza JP, Kuntz RE, Levine MJ et al. Angiographic and clinical outcome of intracoronary stenting: immediate and long-term results from a large single center experience. *J Am Coll Cardiol* 1992; **20:** 328–37.

286. Carrozza JP, Kuntz RE, Fishman RF, Baim DS. Restenosis after arterial injury caused by coronary stenting in patients with diabetes mellitus. *Ann Intern Med* 1993; **118:** 344–49.

287. Abizaid A, Mehran R, Bucher TA et al. Does diabetes influence clinical recurrence after coronary stent implantation? [abstract]. *J Am Coll Cardiol* 1997; 29 (suppl A): 188A.

288. Elezi S, Schühlen H, Wehinger A et al. Stent placement in diabetic versus non-diabetic patients. Six-month angiographic follow-up [abstract]. *J Am Coll Cardiol* 1997; 29 (suppl A): 188A.

289. Joseph T, Loubeyre Ch, Fajadet J et al. Reconstruction of diffusely degenerated stenosed or occluded saphenous vein grafts with less-shortening Wallstents after aggressive antiplatelet-anticoagulant pre-treatment [abstract]. *Eur Heart J* 1997; 18 (suppl): 383.

290. van Belle E, Bauters C, Hubert E et al. Restenosis rates in diabetic patients. A comparison of coronary stenting and balloon angioplasty in native coronary vessels. *Circulation* 1997; **96:** 1454–60.

291. Kornowski R, Mintz GS, Kent KK et al. Increased restenosis in diabetes mellitus after coronary interventions is due to exaggerated intimal hyperplasia. A serial intravascular ultrasound study. *Circulation* 1997; **95:** 1366–69.

292. St Claire DA Jr, King SB III. Effect of diabetes mellitus on outcome after percutaneous transluminal coronary angioplasty. *Coron Artery Dis* 1996; **7:** 744–52.

293. Aronson D, Bloomgarden Z, Rayfield EJ. Potential mechanisms promoting restenosis in diabetic patients. *J Am Coll Cardiol* 1996; **27:** 528–35.

294. Moreno P, Murcia AM, Fallon JT, Fuster V. Smooth muscle cell proliferation does not account for restenosis in diabetic patients [abstract]. *Circulation* 1996; 94 (suppl): I-619.

295. Savage MP, Fischman DL, Douglas JS Jr et al, for the SAVED Investigators. The dark side of high pressure stent deployment [abstract]. *J Am Coll Cardiol* 1997; 29 (suppl A): 368A.

296. Fernández-Avilés F, Alonso JJ, Durán JM et al. High pressure impairs restenotic process after coronary stenting [abstract]. *Circulation* 1997; 96 (suppl): I-87.

297. Hausleiter J, Schühlen H, Elezi S et al. Impact of high inflation pressures on six-month angiographic follow-up after coronary stent placement [abstract]. *J Am Coll Cardiol* 1997; 29 (suppl A): 369A.

298. Fernández-Avilés, Alonso JJ, Durán JM et al. High pressure increases late loss after coronary stenting [abstract]. *J Am Coll Cardiol* 1997; 29 (suppl A): 369A.

299. Metzger JP, Catuli D, Le Feuvre C et al. Impact of high pressure inflation on coronary stent deployment: an intracoronary blood flow analysis [abstract]. *Circulation* 1997; 96 (suppl): I-403.

300. Azar AJ, Detre K, Goldberg S, Kiemeneij F, Leon MB, Serruys PW, on behalf of the Benestent and Stent Restenosis Study. A meta-analysis on the clinical and angiographic outcomes of Stents vs PTCA in the different coronary vessel sizes in the Benestent-1 and Stress-1/2 trials [abstract]. *Circulation* 1995; 92 (suppl): I-475.

301. Koostra JJ, Serruys PW, Morel MA. Ultimate clinical and procedural predictors of

the long-term outcome of patients treated with either balloon or Palmaz–Schatz stent [abstract]. *Eur Heart J* 1998; 19 (suppl): 570.

302. Ellis SG, Vandormael MG, Cowley MJ et al. Coronary morphologic and clinical determinants of procedural outcome with angioplasty for multivessel coronary disease: implication for patient selection. *Circulation* 1990; **82:** 1193–202.

303. Kastrati A, Schömig A, Elizi S, Schühlen H, Wilhelm M, Dirschinger J. Interlesion dependence of the risk for restenosis in patients with coronary stent placement in multiple lesions. *Circulation* 1998; **97:** 2396–401.

304. Ribichini F, Steffenino G, Dellavalle A et al. Plasma activity and insertion/deletion polymorphism of angiotensin I-converting enzyme. A major risk factor and a marker of risk for coronary stent restenosis. *Circulation* 1998; **97:** 147–54.

305. Itoh H, Mukoyama M, Pratt RE, Gibbons GH, Dzau VJ. Multiple autocrine growth factors modulate vascular smooth muscle cell growth response to angiotensin II. *J Clin Invest* 1993; **91:** 2268–74.

306. Jolly N, Ellis SG, Franco I, Raymond RE, Jolly M, Whitlow PL. Determinants of recurrent in stent restenosis-insights from clinical follow-up [abstract]. *Circulation* 1997; 96 (suppl): I-472.

307. Hoffmann R, Keers B, Oljaca B et al. Predictors of diffuse in-stent restenosis [abstract]. *Circulation* 1997; **96:** I-472–I-473.

308. Loussararian AH, Akiyama T, Kobayshi Y et al. Diffuse vs focal in-stent restenosis: clinical, angiographic and procedural determinants [abstract]. *Circulation* 1997; 96 (suppl): I-591.

309. Bodart J-C, Amant C, Bauters C et al. The D allele of the angiotensin converting enzyme is associated with diffuse in-stent restenosis [abstract]. *J Am Coll Cardiol* 1998; 31 (suppl): 356A.

310. Herrman J-PR, Hermans WRM, Vos J, Serruys PW. Pharmacological approaches to the prevention of restenosis following angioplasty. The search for the Holy Grail? (Part I). *Drugs* 1993; **46:** 18–52.

311. Herrman J-PR, Hermans WRM, Vos J, Serruys PW. Pharmacological approaches to the prevention of restenosis following angioplasty. The search for the Holy Grail? (Part II). *Drugs* 1993; **46:** 249–62.

312. Kutryk MJB, Serruys PW. Prevention of restenosis after PTCA. *Vessels* 1996; **2:** 4–12.

313. Dangas G, Fuster V. Management of restenosis after coronary intervention. *Am Heart J* 1996; **132:** 428–36.

314. Raizner AE, Hollman J, Abukhail J, Demke D for the Ciprostene Investigators. Ciprostene for restenosis revisited: quantitative analysis of angiograms. *J Am Coll Cardiol* 1993; **21:** 321A.

315. Darius H, Nixdorff U, Zander J. Effects of ciprostene on restenosis rate during therapeutic transluminal coronary angioplasty. *Agents Actions Suppl* 1992; **37:** 305–11.

316. Topol EJ, Califf RM, Weisman HF et al, on behalf of the EPIC Investigators. Randomized trial of coronary intervention with antibody against platelet IIb/IIIa integrin for reduction of clinical restenosis: results at six months. *Lancet* 1994; **343:** 881–86.

317. Maresta A, Balducelli M, Cantini L et al, for the STARC Investigators. Trapidil (Triazolopyrimidine), a platelet-derived growth factor antagonist, reduces restenosis after percutaneous transluminal coronary angioplasty. Results of the randomized, double-blind STARC study. *Circulation* 1994; **90:** 2710–15.

318. Emanuelsson H, Beatt KJ, Bagger JP et al, for the European Angiopeptin Study Group. Long-term effects of angiopeptin treatment in coronary angioplasty. Reduction of clinical events but not restenosis. European Angiopeptin Study Group. *Circulation* 1995; **91:** 1689–96.

319. Dehmer GJ, Popma JJ, van den Berg EK et al. Reduction in the rate of early restenosis after coronary angioplasty by a diet supplemented with n-3 fatty acids. *N Engl J Med* 1988; **319:** 733–40.

320. Serruys PW, Pieper M, van den Bos A et al. TRAPIST study: a randomized double-blind study to evaluate the efficacy of trapidil on restenosis after successful elective coronary stenting [abstract]. *Eur Heart J* 1998; **19:** 568.

321. Kunishima T, Musha H, Eto F et al. A randomized trial of aspirin versus cilostazol after successful coronary stent implantation. *Clin Ther* 1997; **19:** 1058–66.

322. Sekiya M, Funada J, Watanabe K, Miyagawa M, Akutsu H. Effects of probucol and cilostazol alone and in combination on frequency of poststenting restenosis. *Am J Cardiol* 1998; **82:** 144–47.

323. Reimers B, Akiyama T, Moussa I, Blengino S, Di Francesco L. Persistent high restenosis after local delivery of long acting steroids prior to coronary stent implantation [abstract]. *Circulation* 1997; 96 (suppl): I-710.

324. Kutryk MJB, Serruys PW, Bruining N et al. Randomized trial of antisense oligonucleotide therapy for the prevention of restenosis after stenting: results of the Thoraxcenter "ITALICS" trial [abstract]. *Eur Heart J* 1998; 19 (suppl): 569.

325. Kutryk MJB, de Groot MR, van den Brand M et al. Feasibility of the local delivery of antisense oligonucleotide against *c-myc* for the prevention of in-stent restenosis: acute results of the "ITALICS" trial [abstract]. *Eur Heart J* 1997; 18 (suppl): 507.

326. Wilensky RL, Tanguay J-F, Ito S et al. The Heparin Infusion Prior to Stenting (HIPS) trial: Procedural, in-hospital, 30 Day, and six month clinical, angiographic and IVUS results [abstract]. *J Am Coll Cardiol* 1998; 31 (suppl): 457A.

327. Kiesz RS, Deutsch E, Buszman P et al. Prospective randomized study of local

enoxaparin delivery versus systemic heparin for NIR stent placement [abstract]. *Am J Cardiol* 1997; 80 (suppl 7A): 19S.

328. Kiesz RS, Deutsch E, Buszman P et al. Results of prospective randomized study of local enoxaparin delivery versus systemic heparinization for NIR stent placement [abstract]. *J Am Coll Cardiol* 1998; 31 (suppl): 495A.

329. Kiesz RS, Deutsch E, Buszman P et al. Prospective randomized study of local enoxaparin delivery vs systemic heparinization for NIR stent placement [abstract]. *Circulation* 1997; 96 (suppl): I-654.

330. Frimerman A, Eigler N, Makkar RR, Forrester JS, Litvack F. Chimeric DNA-RNA hammerhead ribozymes to CDC-2 Kinase and PCNA reduce stent induced stenosis in a porcine coronary model [abstract]. *Circulation* 1997; 96 (suppl): I-87.

331. Frimerman A, Honda H, Makkar N et al. Ribozymes to conserved human-porcine PCNA reduce in-stent restenosis in a porcine model [abstract]. *J Am Coll Cardiol* 1998; 31 (suppl): 145A.

332. Rogers C, Tseng DY, Gingras PH, Karwoski T, Martakos P, Edelman ER. Expanded polytetrafluoroethylene stent graft encapsulation reduces intimal thickening regardless of stent design [abstract]. *J Am Coll Cardiol* 1998; 31 (suppl): 413A.

333. Coury AJ, Slaikeu PC, Cahalan PT, Stokes KB. Medical applications of implantable polyurethanes: current issues. *Prog Rubber Plastics Tech* 1987; **3**: 24–37.

334. Frisch EE. Silicones in artificial organs. In: Gebelein CG (ed.). Polymeric materials and artificial organs. Washington, DC, American Chemical Society; 1984: 63–97.

335. Goidoin R, Couture J. Polyester prostheses: the outlook for the future. In: Sharma CP, Szycher M (eds). Blood compatible materials and devices. Lancaster PA, Technomic Publishing Co Inc; 1991: 221–37.

336. Lin SY, Ho LT, Chiou HL. Microencapsulation and controlled release of insulin from polylactic acid microcapsules. *Biomater Med Devices Artif Organs* 1985; **13**: 187.

337. Miyamoto S, Takaoka K, Okada T et al. Evaluation of polylactic acid homopolymers as carriers for bone morphogenetic protein. *Clin Orthop* 1992; **278**: 274.

338. Aguado MT, Lambert PH. Controlled-release vaccines - biodegradable polylactide/polyglycolide (PL/PG) microspheres as antigen vehicles. *Immunobiology* 1992; **184**: 113.

339. Bötman OM. Absorbable implants for the fixation of fractures. *J Bone Joint Surg Am* 1991; **73–A**: 148–53.

340. Chegini N, Hay DL, von Fraunhofr JA, Masterson BJ. A comparative scanning electron microscopic study on degradation of absorbable ligating clips in vivo and in vitro. *J Biomed Mater Res* 1988; **22**: 71–79.

341. Rosilio V, Benoit JP, Deyme M, Thies C, Madelmont G. A physiochemical study of the morphology of progesterone-loaded microspheres fabricated from poly(d,l-lactide-co-glycolide). *J Biomed Mater Res* 1991; **25**: 667–82.

342. Frazza EJ, Schmitt EE. A new absorbable suture. *J Biomed Mater Res* 1971; **4**: 43–58.

343. Miller RA, Brady JM, Cutright DE. Degradation rates of oral resorbable implants (polylactates and polyglycolates): rate modification with changes in PLA/PGA copolymer ratios. *J Biomed Mater Res* 1977; **11**: 711–19.

344. Bindschaedler C, Leong K, Mathiowitz E et al. Polyanhydride microsphere formulation by solvent extraction. *J Pharm Sci* 1988; **77**: 696.

345. Mathiowitz E, Kline D, Langer R. Morphology of polyanhydride microsphere delivery systems. *Scanning Microsc* 1990; **4**: 329.

346. Brem H, Mahaley MS Jr, Vick NA et al. Interstitial chemotherapy with drug polymer implants for the treatment of recurrent gliomas. *J Neurosurg* 1991; **74**: 441.

347. Fults KA, Johnston RP. Sustained-release of urease from a poloxamer gel matrix. *J Parenter Sci Technol* 1990; **44**: 58.

348. Johnston TP, Punjabi MA, Froelich CJ. Sustained delivery of interleukin-2 from a poloxamer 407 gel matrix following intraperitoneal injection in mice. *Pharm Res* 1992; **9**: 425.

349. Sawayanagi Y, Nambu N, Nagai T. Use of chitosan for sustained-release preparations of water-soluble drugs. *Chem Pharm Bull* (Tokyo) 1982; **30**: 4213.

350. Hassan EE, Parish RC, Gallo JM. Optimized formulation of magnetic chitosan microspheres containing the anticancer agent, oxantrazole. *Pharm Res* 1992; **9**: 390.

351. Miyazaki S, Yamguchi H, Yokouchi C et al. Sustained release of indomethacin from chitosan granules in beagle dogs. *J Pharm Pharmacol* 1988; **40**: 642.

352. Chandy T, Sharma CP. Biodegradable chitosan matrix for the controlled release of steroids. *Biomater Artif Cells Immobiliz Biotechnol* 1991; **19**: 745.

353. Pitt CG. Poly-γ-caprolactone and its copolymers. In: Chaisin M, Langer R, (eds). Biodegradable polymers as drug delivery systems. Marcel Dekker, New York, NY: 1990.

354. Woodward SC, Brewer PS, Moatamed F, Schindler A, Pitt CG. The intracellular degradation of poly (γ-caprolacton). *J Biomed Mater Res* 1985; **19**: 437–44.

355. Miller ND, Williams DF. On the biodegradation of poly-8–hydroxy-butyrate (PHB) homopolymer and poly-8–hydroxybutyrate-hydroxyvalerate copolymers. *Biomaterials* 1987; **8**: 129–37.

356. Koosha F, Muller RH, Davis SS. Polyhydroxybutyrate as a drug carrier. *Crit Rev Ther Drug Carrier Syst* 1989; **6**: 117–30.

357. Bora FW, Bednar JM, Osterman AL, Brown MJ, Sumner AJ. Prosthetic nerve grafts: a resorbable tube as an alternative to autogenous nerve grafting. *J Hand Surg (Am)* 1987; 12A(pt I): 685–92.

358. Heller J, Fritzinger BK, Ng SY, Pendale DWH. In vitro and in vivo release of levonorgestrel from poly(orthoesters). *J Controlled Release* 1985; **1:** 225–32.

359. Bakker D, van Blitterswijk CA, Daems WT, Grote JJ. Biocompatibility of six elastomers in vitro. *J Biomed Mater Res* 1988; **22:** 423–29.

360. Bakker D, van Blitterswijk CA, Hesseling SC, Koerten HK, Kuijpers W, Grote JJ. Biocompatability of a polyether urethane, polypropylene oxide, and a polyether polyester copolymer: a qualitative and quantitative study of three alloplastic tympanic membrane materials in the rat middle ear. *J Biomed Mater Res* 1990; **24:** 489–515.

361. Lincoff MA, Furst JG, Ellis SG, Tuch RJ, Topol EJ. Sustained local delivery of dexamethasone by a novel intravascular eluting stent to prevent restenosis in the porcine coronary injury model. *J Am Coll Cardiol* 1997; **29:** 808–10.

362. Farb A, Heller PF, Carter AJ et al. Paclitaxel polymer-coated stents reduce neointima [abstract]. *Circulation* 1997; 96 (suppl): I-608.

363. Kornowski R, Hong MK, Ragheb AO, Bramwell O, Leon MB. Slow-release taxol coated GRII™ stents reduce neointima formation in a porcine coronary in-stent restenosis model [abstract]. *Circulation* 1997; 96 (suppl): I-341.

364. Simons M, Rosenberg RD. Antisense nonmuscle myosin heavy chain and c-myb oligonucleotides suppress smooth muscle cell proliferation in vitro. *Circ Res* 1992; **70:** 835–43.

365. Simons M, Edelman ER, DeKeyser JL et al. Antisense c-myb oligonucleotides inhibit intimal arterial smooth muscle cell accumulation in vivo. *Nature* 1992; **359:** 67–70.

366. Gammon RS, Chapman GD, Agrawal GM et al. Mechanical features of the Duke biodegradable intravascular stent [abstract]. *J Am Coll Cardiol* 1991; 17 (suppl): 235A.

367. Labinaz M, Zidar JP, Stack RS, Phillips HR. Biodegradable stents: the future of interventional cardiology? *J Intervent Cardiol* 1995; **8:** 395–405.

368. Kipshidze NN, Keelan MH Jr, Sahota H et al. Photostimulation of wound healing following angioplasty: impact of red laser light on endothelial regeneration and late restenosis following balloon dilatation in atherosclerotic rabbits [abstract]. *Circulation* 1995; 92 (suppl): I-33.

369. De Scheerder IK, Wang K, Zhou XR et al. Intravascular low power red laser light as an adjunct to coronary stent implantation evaluated in a porcine coronary model. *J Invas Cardiol* 1998; **10:** 263–68.

370. De Scheerder IK, Wang K, Keelan MH, Kipshidze N. First clinical experience with

intravascular low power red laser light therapy for prevention of restenosis following coronary stenting [abstract]. *J Am Coll Cardiol* 1998; **31:** 143A.

371. Waksman R, Robinson KA, Crocker IR, Gravanis MB, Cipolla GD, King SB III. Endovascular low-dose irradiation inhibits neointima formation after coronary artery balloon injury in swine: a possible role for radiation therapy in restenosis prevention. *Circulation* 1995; **91:** 1553–59.

372. Mazur W, Ali MN, Dabaghi SF et al. High dose rate intracoronary radiation suppresses neointimal proliferation in the stented and ballooned model of porcine restenosis [abstract]. *Circulation* 1994; 90 (suppl): I-652.

373. Waksman R, Robinson KA, Crocker IR et al. Intracoronary radiation before stent implantation inhibits neointima formation in stented porcine coronary arteries. *Circulation* 1995; **92:** 1383–86.

374. Hehrlein C, Zimmerman M, Metz J, Fehsenfeld P, von Hodenberg E. Radioactive coronary stent implantation inhibits neointimal proliferation in non-atherosclerotic rabbits [abstract]. *Circulation* 1993; 88 (suppl): I-651.

375. Hehrlein C, Gollan C, Donges K et al. Low-dose radioactive endovascular stents prevent smooth muscle cell proliferation and neointimal hyperplasia in rabbits. *Circulation* 1995; **92:** 1570–75.

376. Laird JR, Carter AJ, Kufs WM et al. Inhibition of neointimal proliferation with low-dose irradiation from a β–particle-emitting stent. *Circulation* 1996; **93:** 529–36.

377. Hehrlein C, Stintz M, Kinscherf R et al. Pure β–particle-emitting stents inhibit neointima formation in rabbits. *Circulation* 1996; **93:** 641–45.

378. Fischell TA, Kharma BK, Fischell DR et al. Low-dose β-particle emission from "stent" wire results in complete, localized inhibition of smooth muscle proliferation. *Circulation* 1994; **90:** 2956–63.

379. Fischell TA, Carter AJ, Laird JR. The β-particle-emitting radioisotope stent (Isostent): animal studies and planned clinical trials. *Am J Cardiol* 1996; 78 (suppl 3A): 45–50.

380. Alt E, Hermann RA, Rybnikar A et al. Reduction of neointimal proliferation after implantation of a beta particle emitting gold Au 198 coated stent [abstract]. *J Am Coll Cardiol* 1998; 31 (suppl): 350A-351A.

381. Eigler N, Whiting J, Makkar R et al. Effects of β$^+$ emitting V^{48} Act-One nitinol stents on neointimal proliferation in pig coronary arteries [abstract]. *J Am Coll Cardiol* 1997; 29 (suppl A): 237A.

382. Makkar R, Whiting J, Li A et al. A β-emitting liquid isotope filled balloon markedly inhibits restenosis in stented porcine coronary arteries [abstract]. *J Am Coll Cardiol* 1998; 31 (suppl): 350A.

383. Condado JA, Waksman R, Gurdiel O et al. Long-term angiographic and clinical

outcome after percutaneous transluminal coronary angioplasty and intracoronary radiation therapy in humans. *Circulation* 1997; **96:** 727–32.

384. Teirstein PS, Massullo V, Jani S et al. Radiation therapy following coronary stenting - 6 month follow-up of a randomized clinical trial [abstract]. *Circulation* 1996; 94 (suppl): I-210.

385. Teirstein PS, Massullo V, Jani S et al. Catheter-based radiotherapy to inhibit restenosis after coronary stenting. *N Engl J Med* 1997; **336:** 1697–1703.

386. Rivard A, Leclerc G, Bouchard M et al. Low-dose β-emitting radioactive stents inhibit neointimal hyperplasia in porcine coronary arteries: an histological assessment [abstract]. *J Am Coll Cardiol* 1997; 29 (suppl A): 238A.

387. Moses JW, Ellis SG, Bailey SR et al, for the IRIS investigators. Short-term (1 month) results of the dose response IRIS fesibility study of a beta-particle emitting radioisotope stent [abstract]. *J Am Coll Cardiol* 1998; 31 (suppl): 350A.

388. Baim DS, Fischell T, Weissman NJ, Laird JR, Marble SJ, Ki Ho K. Short-term (1 month) results of the IRIS feasibility study of a beta-particle emitting radioisotope stent [abstract]. *Circulation* 1997; 96 (suppl): I-218.

389. Carter AJ, Scott D, Bailey LR, Jones R, Fischell TA, Virmani R. High activity 32P stents promote the development of atherosclerosis at six months in a porcine coronary model [abstract]. *Circulation* 1997; 96 (suppl): I-607.

390. Levine MJ, Leonard BM, Burke JA et al. Clinical and angiographic results of balloon-expandable intracoronary stents in right coronary stenoses. *J Am Coll Cardiol* 1990; **16:** 332–39.

391. Fajadet JC, Marco J, Cassagneau G et al. Restenosis following successful Palmaz–Schatz intracoronary stent implantation [abstract]. *J Am Coll Cardiol* 1991; 17 (suppl): 346A.

392. Roubin G, Hearn J, Carlin S, Lembo J, Douglas J, King S. Angiographic and clinical follow-up in patients receiving a balloon-expandable, stainless steel stent (Cook, Inc.) for prevention or treatment of acute closure after PTCA [abstract]. *Circulation* 1990; 82 (suppl): III-191.

393. Colombo A, Maiello L, Almagor Y et al. Coronary stenting: single institutional experience with the initial 100 cases using the Palmaz–Schatz stent. *Cathet Cardiovasc Diagn* 1992; **26:** 171–76.

394. Levine M, Lemen M, Schatz R, Buchbinder M, Erbel R, Baim D. Management of restenosis following Palmaz–Schatz intracoronary stenting: multicenter results [abstract]. *Circulation* 1990; 82 (suppl): III-657.

395. Macander PJ, Agrawal SK, Cannon AD et al. Is PTCA within the stenotic coronary stent safer than routine angioplasty [abstract]. *Circulation* 1991; 84 (suppl): II-199.

396. Garratt K, Holmes D, Schwartz R, Camrud A, Jorgenson M. Balloon dilatation of

restenotic lesions within metallic coronary stents: initial clinical and histopathologic observations [abstract]. *J Am Coll Cardiol* 1992; 19 (suppl): 109A.

397. Macander PJ, Roubin GS, Agrawal SK, Cannon AD, Dean LS, Baxley WA. Balloon angioplasty for treatment of in-stent restenosis: feasibility, safety, and efficacy. *Cathet Cardiovasc Diagn* 1994; **32:** 125–31.

398. Schiele F, Meneveau N, Vuillemenot A et al. Assessment of balloon angioplasty in intrastent restenosis with intracoronary ultrasound [abstract]. *J Am Coll Cardiol* 1998; 31 (suppl): 495A.

399. Baim DS, Levine MJ, Leon MB. Management of restenosis within the Palmaz–Schatz coronary stent (the U.S. multicenter experience). *Am J Cardiol* 1993; **71:** 364–66.

400. Tan H-C, Sketch MH, Tan ME, Wah L-WS, Tcheng JE, Zidar JP. Is there an optimal treatment strategy for stent restenosis? [abstract]. *Circulation* 1996; 94 (suppl): I-91.

401. Houplon P, Jullière Y, Selton-Suty C et al. Absence of risk of conventional balloon angioplasty for treatment of coronary in-stent restenosis [abstract]. *Eur Heart J* 1997; 18 (suppl): 498.

402. Vahdat B, Bonan R, Paiement P, Bilodeau L, Doucet S, Pagé D. Management of coronary in-stent restenosis by balloon angioplasty [abstract]. *Eur Heart J* 1997; 18 (suppl): 498.

403. Eltchaninoff H, Cribier A, Koning R, Tron C, Letac B. Balloon angioplasty for in-stent restenosis: immediate and 6–months clinical and angiographic results [abstract]. *Eur Heart J* 1997; 18 (suppl): 498.

404. Reimers B, Moussa I, Akiyama T et al. Long-term clinical follow-up after successful repeat percutaneous intervention for stent restenosis. *J Am Coll Cardiol* 1997; **30:** 186–92.

405. Bauters Ch, Banos JL, Van Belle E, McFadden EP, Lablanche JM, Bertrand ME. Six-month angiographic outcome after successful repeat percutaneous intervention for in-stent restenosis. *Circulation* 1998; **97:** 318–21.

406. Eltchaninoff H, Cribier A, Koning R, Tron C, Letac B. Balloon angioplasty for in-stent restenosis : 6-months angiographic follow-up [abstract]. *Circulation* 1997; 96 (suppl): I-88.

407. Lefevre T, Louvard Y, Morice MC, Karrillon G, Dumas P, Loubeyre C. In-stent restenosis: should we stent the stent? A single center prospective study [abstract]. Circulation 1997; 96 (suppl): I-88.

408. Goldberg SL, Loussararian AH, Di Mario C et al. Stenting for in-stent restenosis [abstract]. *Circulation* 1997; 96 (suppl): I-88.

409. Elezi S, Kastrati A, Schuhlen H, Hausleiter, Alt E, Wehinger A. Stenting for restenosis of stented lesions: acute and 6 months clinical and angiographic follow-up [abstract]. *Circulation* 1997; 96 (suppl): I-88.

410. Mehran R, Abizaid AS, Mintz GS et al. Mechanisms and results of additional stent implantation to treat focal in-stent restenosis [abstract]. *J Am Coll Cardiol* 1998; 31 (suppl): 455A.

411. Lefèvre T, Louvard Y, Morice MC et al. New device for in-stent restenosis: stenting of the stent. A single center prospective study [abstract]. *Am J Cardiol* 1997; 80 (suppl 7A): 10S.

412. Nakamura M, Suzuki T, Matsubura T et al. Results of cutting balloon angioplasty for stent restenosis. Japanese multicenter registry [abstract]. *J Am Coll Cardiol* 1998; 31 (suppl): 235A.

413. Cattelaens N, Gerckens U, Mueller R, Gerlach J, Grube E. Directional atherectomy for treatment of stent restenosis—feasibility and histopathological findings in 28 patients [abstract]. *J Am Coll Cardiol* 1998; 31 (suppl): 142A.

414. Strauss B, Umans V, van Suylen R-J et al. Directional atherectomy for treatment of restenosis within coronary stents: clinical, angiographic and histologic results. *J Am Coll Cardiol* 1992; **20:** 1465–73.

415. Sharma SK, Duvvuri S, Kakarala V et al. Rotational atherectomy (RA) for in-stent restenosis (ISR): intravascular ultrasound (IVUS) and quantitative coronary analysis (QCA) [abstract]. *Circulation* 1996; 94 (suppl): I-454.

416. Buchbinder M, Goldberg SL, Fortuna R et al. Rotational atherectomy for intra-stent restenosis: initial experience [abstract]. *Circulation* 1996; 94 (suppl): I-621.

417. Sharma SK, Duvvuri S, Dangas G et al. Rotational atherectomy for in-stent restenosis: acute and long-term results of the first 100 cases [abstract]. *Eur Heart J* 1997; 18 (suppl): 497.

418. Schiele F, Meneveau N, Vullemenot A, Gupta S, Xu C, Bassand JP. Rotational atherectomy followed by balloon angioplasty for treatment of intrastent restenosis. A pilot study with quantitative angiography and intracoronary ultrasound [abstract]. *Eur Heart J* 1997; 18 (suppl): 499.

419. Sharma SK, Duvvuri S, Kini A et al. Rotational atherectomy for in-stent restenosis: acute and long term results of first 100 cases [abstract]. *Circulation* 1997; 96 (suppl): I-88.

420. Büttner HJ, Müller C, Hodgson JMcB et al. Rotational ablation with adjunctive low-pressure ballooon dilatation in diffuse in-stent restenosis: immediate and follow-up results [abstract]. *J Am Coll Cardiol* 1998; 31 (suppl): 141A.

421. Goy J-J, Sigwart U, Vogt P et al. Long-term follow-up of the first 56 patients treated with intracoronary self-expanding stents (the Lausanne experience). *Am J Cardiol* 1991; **67:** 569–72.

422. Köster RP, Koschyk DH, Kähler J, Steffan W, Terres W, Hamm CW. Laser angioplasty of in-stent restenosis [abstract]. *Circulation* 1996; 94 (suppl): I-621.

423. Hamm CW, Seabra-Gomes R, Bonnier J et al, on behalf of the LARS study group. Laser angioplasty of within-stent restenosis—results of the LARS surveillance study [abstract]. *Eur Heart J* 1997; 18 (suppl): 497.

424. Margolis J, Bejarano J, Diaz P. Laser approach for coronary artery or vein graft in-stent restenosis [abstract]. *Eur Heart J* 1997; 18 (suppl): 497.

425. Mehran R, Mintz GS, Satler LF et al. Treatment of in-stent restenosis with eximer laser coronary angioplasty. Mechanisms and results compared with PTCA alone. *Circulation* 1997; **96:** 2183–89.

426. Köster R, Hamm CW, Terres W et al. Treatment of in-stent coronary restenosis by excimer laser angioplasty. *Am J Cardiol* 1997; **80:** 1424–28.

427. Köster R, Hamm CW, Terres W et al. Long term results of laser angioplasty for in-stent restenosis [abstract]. *J Am Coll Cardiol* 1998; 31 (suppl): 141A.

428. Hamm CW, Simon R, Seabra Gomes RJ et al. Laser angioplasty for within stent restenosis - final results of the LARS surveillance study [abstrtact]. *J Am Coll Cardiol* 1998; 31 (suppl): 143A.

429. MacDonald RG, O'Neill BJ, Creighton JE, Brown RIG, Slivocka JE, Penn IM. Is coronary stent expansion the mechanism for the successful dilatation of stent restenosis? A quantitative angiographic study [abstract]. *Circulation* 1991; 84 (suppl): II-196.

430. Yokoi H, Kimura T, Nobuyoshi M. Palmaz–Schatz coronary stent restenosis: pattern and management [abstract]. *J Am Coll Cardiol* 1994; 25 (suppl): 117A.

431. Yokoi H, Tamura T, Kimura T, Nosaka H, Nobuyoshi M. Clinical and angiographic predictors of diffuse type in-stent restenosis [abstract]. *J Am Coll Cardiol* 1998; 31 (suppl): 140A.

432. Morís C, Alfonso F, Lambert J et al. Stenting for coronary dissection after balloon dilatation of in-stent restenosis: stenting a previously stented site. *Am Heart J* 1996; **131:** 834–36.

433. Bowerman RE, Pinkerton CA, Kirk B, Waller BF. Disruption of a coronary stent during atherectomy for restenosis. *Cathet Cardiovasc Diagn* 1991; **34:** 248–51.

434. Meyer T, Schmidt T, Buchwald A, Wiegand V. Stent wire cutting during coronary directional atherectomy. *Clin Cardiol* 1993; **16:** 450–52.

435. Dauerman HL, Baim DS, Sparano AM et al. Balloon angioplasty versus debulking for treatment of diffuse in-stent restenosis [abstract]. *J Am Coll Cardiol* 1998; 31 (suppl): 455A.

436. Mehran R, Mintz GS, Abizaid A et al. Mechanistic comparison of rotational atherectomy and eximer laser angioplasty in the treatment of in-stent restenosis: a volumetric ultrasound study [abstract]. *J Am Coll Cardiol* 1998; 31 (suppl): 103A.

436a. Mahdi NA, Leon M, Mikulic M et al. PTCA, directional and rotational coronary atherectomy in the management of Palmaz–Schatz instent restenosis [abstract]. *J Am Coll Cardiol* 1998; 31 (suppl): 275A.

437. Sridhar K, Teefy PJ, Almond DG, Penn IM, Brown RG. Long-term clinical outcomes of patients with in-stent restenosis [abstract]. *Circulation* 1996; 94 (suppl): I-454.

438. Oweida SW, Roubin GS, Smith RB III, Salam AQA. Postcatheterization vascular complications associated with percutaneous transluminal coronary angioplasty. *J Vasc Surg* 1990; **12**: 310–15.

439. McCann RL, Schwartz LB, Pieper KS. Vascular complications of cardiac catheterization. *J Vasc Surg* 1991; **14**: 375–81.

440. Muller DW, Shamir KJ, Ellis SG, Topol EJ. Peripheral vascular complications after conventional and complex percutaneous coronary interventional procedures. *Am J Cardiol* 1992; **69**: 63–68.

441. Berge PG, Winter UJ, Hoffmann M, Albrecht D, Hopp HW, Hilger HH. Local vascular complications in heart catheter studies. *Z Kardiol* 1993; **82**: 449–56.

442. Mansour KA, Moscucci M, Kent C et al. Vascular complications following directional coronary atherectomy or Palmaz–Schatz stenting [abstract]. *J Am Coll Cardiol* 1994; 23 (suppl): 136A.

443. Sones FM Jr, Shirey EK, Proudfit WL, Westcott RN. Cine-coronary arteriography [abstract]. *Circulation* 1959; 20 (suppl): 773.

444. Resar JR, Wolff MR, Blumenthal RS, Coombs V, Brinker JA. Brachial approach for intracoronary stent implantation: a feasibility study. *Am Heart J* 1993; **126**: 300–04.

445. Kiemeneij F, Laarman GJ. Bailout techniques for failed coronary angioplasty using 6 french guiding catheters. *Cathet Cardiovasc Diagn* 1994; **32**: 359–66.

446. Arnold AM. Hemostasis after radial artery cardiac catheterization. *J Invas Cardiol* 1996; 8 (suppl D): 26D-29D.

447. Kiemeneij F. Transradial artery coronary angioplasty and stenting: history and single center experience. *J Invas Cardiol* 1996; 8 (suppl D): 3D-8D.

448. Kiemeneij F, Laarman GJ, Odekerken D, Slagboom T, van der Wieken R. A randomized comparison of percutaneous transluminal coronary angioplasty by the radial, brachial and femoral approaches: the ACCESS study. *J Am Coll Cardiol* 1997; **29**: 1269–75.

449. Mann JT III, Cubeddu G, Schneider JE et al. Clinical evaluation of current stent deployment strategies. *J Invas Cardiol* 1996; 8 (suppl D): 30D-35D.

450. Bartorelli AL, Sganzerla P, Fabbiocchi F et al. Prompt and safe femoral hemostasis with a collagen device after intracoronary implantation of Palmaz–Schatz stents. *Am Heart J* 1995; **130**: 26–32.

451. Kiemeniej F, Laarman GJ. Improved anticoagulation management after Palmaz–Schatz coronary stent implantation by sealing the arterial puncture site with a vascular hemostasis device. *Cathet Cardiovasc Diagn* 1993; **30:** 317–22.

452. Webb JG, Carere RA, Dodek AA. Collagen plug hemostatic closure of femoral arterial puncture sites following implantation of intracoronary stents. *Cathet Cardiovasc Diagn* 1993; **30:** 314–16.

453. von Hoch F, Neumann F-J, Theiss W, Kastrati A, Schömig A. Efficacy and safety of collagen implants for hemostasis of the vascular access site after coronary balloon angioplasty and coronary stent placement: a randomized study. *Eur Heart J* 1995; **16:** 640–46.

454. Camenzind E, Grossholz M, Urban P et al. Mechanical compression (Femostop) alone versus combined collagen application (Vasoseal) and Femostop for arterial puncture site closure after coronary stent implantation: a randomized trial [abstract]. *J Am Coll Cardiol* 1994; 25 (suppl): 355A.

455. Sridhar K, Porter K, Gupta B et al. Reduction in peripheral vascular complications after coronary stenting by the use of a pneumatic vascular compression device [abstract]. *Circulation* 1994; 90 (suppl): I-621.

456. Veldhuijzen FLMJ, Bonnier HJRM, Michels HR, El Gamal MIH, van Gelder BM. Retrieval of undeployed stents from the right coronary artery: report of two cases. *Cathet Cardiovac Diagn* 1993; **30:** 245–48.

457. Rozenman Y, Burstein M, Hasin Y, Gotsman M. Retrieval of occluding unexpanded Palmaz–Schatz stent from a saphenous aorto-coronary vein graft. *Cathet Cardiovasc Diagn* 1995; **34:** 159–61.

458. Berder V, Bedossa M, Gras D, Paillard F, Le Breton H, Pony JC. Retrieval of a lost coronary stent from the descending aorta using a PTCA balloon and biopsy forceps. *Cathet Cardiovasc Diagn* 1993; **28:** 351–53.

459. Cishek MB, Laslett L, Gershony G. Balloon catheter retrieval of dislodged coronary artery stents: a novel technique. *Cathet Cardiovasc Diagn* 1995; **34:** 350–52.

460. Eeckhout E, Stauffer JC, Goy JJ. Retrieval of a migrated coronary stent by means of an alligator forceps catheter. *Cathet Cardiovasc Diagn* 1993; **30:** 166–68.

461. Foster Smith KW, Garratt KN, Higano ST, Holmes DR. Retrieval techniques for managing flexible intracoronary stent misplacement. *Cathet Cardiovasc Diagn* 1993; **30:** 63–68.

462. Wong PH. Retrieval of undeployed intracoronary Palmaz–Schatz stents. *Cathet Cardiovasc Diagn* 1995; **35:** 218–23.

463. Mohiaddin RH, Roberts RH, Underwood R, Rothman M. Localization of a misplaced coronary artery stent by magnetic resonance imaging. *Clin Cardiol* 1995; **18:** 175–77.

464. Iniguez A, Macaya C, Alfonso F, Goicolea J. Early angiographic changes of side

branches arising from a Palmaz–Schatz stented segment: results and clinical implications. *J Am Coll Cardiol* 1994; **23:** 911–13.

465. Fischman DL, Savage MP, Leon MB et al. Fate of lesion-related side branches after coronary artery stenting. *J Am Coll Cardiol* 1993; **22:** 1641–46.

466. Pan M, Medina A, Suarez de Lezo J. Follow-up patency of side branches covered by intracoronary Palmaz–Schatz stent. *Am Heart J* 1995; **129:** 436–40.

467. Aliabadi D, Tilli FV, Bowers TR et al. Incidence and angiographic predictors of side branch occlusion following high-pressure intracoronary stenting. *Am J Cardiol* 1997; **80:** 994–97.

468. Mazur W, Grinstead C, Hakim A et al. Fate of side branches after intracoronary implantation of the Gianturco–Roubin flex-stent for acute or threatened closure after percutaneous transluminal coronary angioplasty. *Am J Cardiol* 1994; **74:** 1207–10.

469. Nakamura S, Hall P, Maiello L, Colombo A. Techniques for Palmaz–Schatz stent deployment in lesions with a large side branch. *Cathet Cardiovasc Diagn* 1995; **34:** 353–61.

470. Lowe HC. New balloon expandable stent for bifurcation lesions. *Cathet Cardiovasc Diagn* 1997; **42:** 235–36.

471. Erminia M, Sklar MA, Russo RJ, Claire D, Schatz RA, Teirstein PS. Escape from stent jail: an in vitro model [abstract]. *Circulation* 1995; 92 (suppl): I-688.

472. Goldberg SL, Colombo A, Nakamura S, Almagor Y, Maiello L, Tobis J. Benefit of intracoronary ultrasound in the deployment of Palmaz–Schatz stents. *J Am Coll Cardiol* 1994; **24:** 996–1003.

473. Colombo A, Hall P, Nakamura S et al. Intracoronary stenting without anticoagulation accomplished with intravascular ultrasound guidance. *Circulation* 1995; **91:** 1676–88.

474. Benzuly KH, Glazier S, Grines CL, O'Neill WW, Safian RD. Coronary perforation: an unreported complication after intracoronary stent implantation [abstract]. *J Am Coll Cardiol* 1996; 27 (suppl): 252A.

475. Hall P, Nakamura S, Maiello L, Blengino S, Martini G, Colombo A. Factors associated with procedural complications during high pressure optimized Palmaz–Schatz intracoronary stent implantation [abstract]. *Circulation* 1994; 90 (suppl): I-612.

476. Shah MS, Raymond RE. Coronary perforations: a persistent problem in interventions [abstract]. *J Am Coll Cardiol* 1998; 31 (suppl): 493A.

477. Reimers B, von Birgelen C, van der Giessen WJ, Serruys PW. A word of caution on optimizing stent deployment in calcified lesion: acute coronary rupture with cardiac tamponade. *Am Heart J* 1996; **131:** 192–94.

478. Chae J-K, Park S-W, Kim Y-H, Hong MK, Park S-J. Successful treatment of coronary artery perforation during angioplasty using autologous vein graft-coated stent. *Eur Heart J* 1997; **18:** 1030–32.

479. Elsner M, Auch-Schwelk W, Walter DH, Schächinger V. Evolving coronary application of stent-grafts containing a polytetrafluoroethylene-membrane [abstract]. *Eur Heart J* 1998; 19 (suppl): 497.

480. Gunther HU, Strupp G, Volmar J, von Korn H, Bonzel T, Stegmann T. Koronare stentimplantation: infektion and abszedierung mit lentalem ausgang. *Z Kardiol* 1993; **82:** 521–25.

481. Leroy O, Martin E, Prat A et al. Fatal infection of coronary stent implantation. *Cathet Cardiovasc Diagn* 1996; **39:** 168–70.

482. Thibodeaux LC, James KV, Lohr JM, Welling HM, Roberts WH. Infection of endovascular stents in a swine model. *Am J Surg* 1996; **172:** 151–54.

483. Alfonso F, Pérez-Vizcayno MJ, Hernández R et al. Clinical and angiographic implications of balloon rupture during coronary stenting. *Am J Cardiol* 1997; **80:** 1077–80.

484. Bal ET, Thijs Plokker HW, van den Berg EMJ et al. Predictability and prognosis of PTCA-induced coronary artery aneurysms. *Cathet Cardiovasc Diagn* 1991; **22:** 85–88.

485. Rab ST, King SB III, Roubin GS, Carlin S, Hearn JA, Douglas JS. Coronary aneurysms after stent placement: a suggestion of altered vessel wall healing in the presence of anti-inflammatory agents. *J Am Coll Cardiol* 1991; **18:** 1524–28.

486. Slota PA, Fischman DL, Savage MP, Rake R, Goldberg S, for the STRESS Trial Investigators. Frequency and outcome of development of coronary artery aneurysm after intracoronary stent placement and angioplasty. *Am J Cardiol* 1997; **79:** 1104–06.

487. Vassanelli C, Turri M, Morando G, Menegatti G, Zardini P. Coronary arterial aneurysms after percutaneous transluminal coronary angioplasty—a not uncommon finding at elective follow-up angiography. *Int J Cardiol* 1989; **22:** 151–56.

488. Bell MR, Garratt KN, Bresnahan JF, Edwards WD, Holmes DR. Relation of deep arterial resection and coronary artery aneurysms after directional coronary atherectomy. *J Am Coll Cardiol* 1992; **20:** 1474–81.

489. Voigtänder T, Rupprecht HJ, Stähr P, Nowak B, Kupferwasser I, Meyer J. Development of a coronary aneurysm 6 months after stent implantation assessed by intracoronary ultrasound. *Am Heart J* 1996; **131:** 833–34.

490. Regar E, Klauss V, Henneke KH, Werner F, Thisen K, Mudra H. Coronary aneurysm after bailout stent implantation: diagnosis of a false lumen with intravascular ultrasound. *Cathet Cardiovasc Diagn* 1997; **41:** 407–10.

491. Kitzis I, Kornowski R, Miller HI. Delayed development of a pseudoaneurysm in the left circumflex artery following angioplasty and stent placement, treated with intravascular guided stenting. *Cathet Cardiovasc Diagn* 1997; **42**: 51–53.

492. Nisanci Y, Coskun I, Oncul A, Umman S. Coronary artery aneurysm development after successful primary stent implantion. *Cathet Cardiovasc Diagn* 1997; **42**: 420–22.

7. LONG-TERM FOLLOW-UP

Although the number of stenting procedures is increasing at a very rapid rate, very little information is available on the long-term outcome of these patients and the integrity of the implanted devices. Serial angiographic studies with long-term follow-up clinical data has recently been reported. A total of 143 patients were followed for up to 3 years, with angiography being performed at 6, 12, and 36 months after Palmaz–Schatz stent implantation in native coronary arteries.[1] Complete angiographic data was available in roughly half of the patients at all time points. Follow-up coronary angiography revealed a decrease in minimal luminal diameter from 2.54 ± 0.44 mm immediately after stent implantation to 1.87 ± 0.56 mm at 6 months. Significant late improvement in luminal diameter was observed at 3 years (1.94 ± 0.48 mm at 6 months and 2.09 ± 0.48 mm at 3 years, $p < 0.001$ in patients with paired angiograms) (figure 7.1). The rate of survival, free of myocardial infarction, bypass surgery, and repeat coronary angioplasty at 3 years in this group of patients was 74.6%, which compared well with similar follow-up data for balloon angioplasty.[2] Later lumen enlargement at the stented site was also noted in two other series.[3,4]

The mechanism for this late remodeling process is probably through regression of the neointima with time. It is possible that this occurs in the same way in which scar tissue contracts during the late stages of wound healing. This phenomenon of in-stent neointimal regression was studied in a porcine coronary model of stent restenosis.[5] In this study, stents were explanted at 2 and 6 months after placement. A significant reduction was seen in the neointima at 6 months. Histopathological assessment showed that the regression was accompanied by a reduction in proteoglycan, an increase in collagen I and III, and no change in smooth muscle cell density.

Three years event-free survival results have also been presented for 65 patients treated with elective Palmaz–Schatz stent implantation.[6] Three years event-free survival was 56% in this group, with the majority of events occurring within the first year after stenting. Long-term clinical follow-up results up to 104 months have also been reported for patients with stents (Palmaz–Schatz, Wiktor and Wallstent) implanted for the treatment of restenosis.[7] In this series, 70% of the patients remained event free, with a survival rate of 95%. Long-term follow-up results 9 years after implantation of the Wallstent for restenosis, bailout indications and in saphenous vein grafts demonstrated a 75% event-free survival

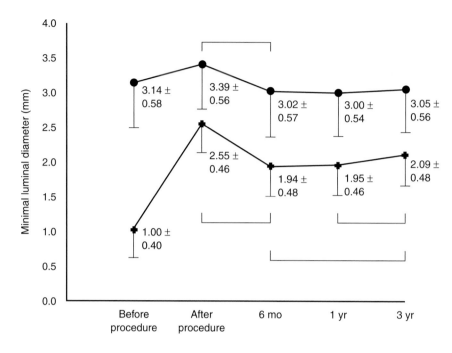

Figure 7.1: *Serial changes in the mean (± SD) minimal luminal diameter of 72 lesions for which sequential studies over a 3-year period were completed (+), as compared with a reference diameter (•). There was a significant improvement in minimal luminal diameter during the period from 1 year to 3 years after implantation of the stent. p < 0.001 for the comparison between the points indicated by brackets. (From Kimura T, Yokoi H, Nakagawa Y et al. Three-year follow-up after implantation of metallic coronary artery stents. N Eng J Med 1996; 334: 561–6).*

rate in 131 stents implanted in 105 patients.[8] Although these first results are encouraging, the number of reports is small and the patient population consists of those patients stented with early low pressure balloon dilatation techniques. More data at longer follow-up periods are required in order to advocate the continued long-term efficacy of coronary stent implantation.

References

1. Kimura T, Yokoi H, Nakagawa Y et al. Three-year follow-up after implantation of metallic coronary artery stents. N Eng J Med 1996; **334:** 561–6.

2. King SB III, Schlumpf M. Ten-year completed follow-up of percutaneous transluminal coronary angioplasty: the early Zurich experience. *J Am Coll Cardiol* 1993; **22:** 353–60.

3. Foley JB, White J, Teefy P et al. Late angiographic follow-up after Palmaz–Schatz stent implantation. *Am J Cardiol* 1995; **76:** 76–7.

4. Hermiller JB, Fry ET, Peters TF et al. Late coronary artery stenosis regression with the Gianturco–Roubin intracoronary stent. *Am J Cardiol* 1996; **77:** 247–51.

5. Hong MK, Virmani R, Kornowski R et al. Histologic responses during in-stent neointimal regression in a porcine coronary model [abstract]. *J Am Coll Cardiol* 1998; **31** (SupplA): 365

6. Klugherz BD, DeAngelo D, Kim BK et al. Three-year clinical follow-up after Palmaz–Schatz stenting. *J Am Coll Cardiol* 1996; **27:** 1185–91.

7. Debbas NMG, Sigwart U, Eeckhout E et al. Intracoronary stenting for restenosis: long-term follow-up: a single center experience. *J Invas Cardiol* 1996; **8:** 241–8.

8. Debbas N, Sigwart U, Eeckhout E et al. Late clinical follow-up 9 years after intracoronary stenting with the Wallstent [abstract]. *Circulation* 1995; **92** (Suppl): I-280.

8. Cost Considerations

As health care resources undergo persistent constraint, decisions regarding the use of new technologies must reflect an assessment of cost as well as clinical benefit. The concept of cost effectiveness ratios have been introduced to allow comparison of a new treatment modality to an accepted current standard. Using this comparison it is possible to decide whether the new treatment represents an efficient use of limited resources. A description of these principles of medical economics and cost effectiveness analyses is beyond the scope of this chapter and have been reviewed elsewhere.[1-4] Applied to the role of coronary stenting in interventional cardiology, these principles simply stated, consider the cost of stent implantation with respect to the quality of life benefits achieved with the use of this technology.

A number of comparative studies to evaluate the cost-effectiveness of stenting and other forms of percutaneous revascularization have been performed. When used with intense anticoagulation regimens, these studies have shown that elective stenting results in higher hospital costs due to the initial cost of the stent, higher vascular bleeding complications, and a prolonged hospital stay.[5-11] These results appeared to be consistent despite differences in patient population and disparate health care systems. In an analysis of a substudy of the STRESS trial involving 207 patients, this increased cost of coronary stenting persisted despite consideration of the savings accrued by the avoidance of subsequent revascularization procedures.[8] Since the publication of these analyses however, the practice of coronary stenting has changed dramatically with the adoption of less intense anticoagulation regimens and high pressure balloon deployment techniques. These changes have resulted in a significant reduction in the vascular complication rate and the length of hospital stay. Concomitant with changes in the techniques of stent implantation, balloon angioplasty techniques have also evolved. Only very limited information on cost comparisons are currently available with the implementation of these matured interventional approaches.[12-14] Results from the randomized BENESTENT II trial indicate that the initial costs of elective stenting with a heparin coated Palmaz–Schatz stent are significantly higher than the intial costs of a percutaneous transluminal coronary-angioplasty (PTCA) strategy.[9] The differences were mainly related to the use of more balloons and the cost of the stent itself. Part of the additional costs were recouped during the follow-up period due to a significantly lower number of revascularization procedures. The end result was equivalent cost—effectiveness ratios for the two approaches.

A clinical and economic outcomes prediction model has been described which was developed to compare the clinical effects and health costs of different strategies for treating patients with single-vessel and multi-vessel coronary disease.[15] These models have been tailored to the specific economic environments of several European countries including France,[16] Germany,[17] Italy,[18] The Netherlands,[19] and Spain.[20] The application of these models indicates that stenting is cost-effective at 1 and 3 years compared with balloon angioplasty in single-vessel disease, and that coronary bypass surgery is the preferred treatment in patients with three-vessel disease. These findings are relevant for current practice since estimates of procedural outcome from contemporary stent trials were used and country-specific data were incorporated into the models.

Before conclusions can be reached concerning cost effectiveness, several issues must be considered. Unlike balloon angioplasty procedures, the techniques of coronary stenting are still being developed, and improvements in the methods are ongoing, which will certainly affect cost effectiveness. With the reduction in vascular complications, the cost of the stent device has become a major contributor to the initial hospitalization costs of the stenting procedure. As the major stent suppliers recoup their research and development costs, and as competition between the stent manufacturers and the number of new stents being introduced to the market increases, it is likely that stent prices will fall. A re-intervention rate (PTCA and coronary artery bypass graft surgery (CABG)) of 14% (per patient analysis) in the BENESTENT II trial also introduces an interesting twist for future cost analyses. Considering this low number, it may be reasonable to eliminate non-invasive post-procedural testing and reduce follow-up in patients undergoing elective stent implantation in a de-novo lesion. This would certainly contribute to the cost effectiveness of the procedure compared with other revascularization techniques. Finally, it must be borne in mind that stent implantation is not the only revascularization technology being improved. Other techniques such as minimally invasive surgical procedures and adjunctive mechanistic and pharmacological therapies to balloon angioplasty are also being developed. As the indications for coronary stenting are expanded to include problems such as multi-vessel, ostial and bifurcation disease, stenting techniques will have to be compared in a randomized fashion with other developing therapies to ensure relative cost effectiveness.

References

1. Doubilet P, Weinstein MC, McNeil BJ. Use and misuse of the term "cost effective" in medicine. *N Engl J Med* 1986; **314**: 253–56.

2. Weinstein MC. Principles of cost-effective resource allocation in health care organizations. *Int J Technol Assess Health Care* 1990; **6:** 93–103.

3. Johannesson M. The concept of cost in the economic evaluation of health care. *Int J Technol Assess Health Care* 1994; **10:** 675–82.

4. Cohen EJ, Schwartz L. Coronary artery stenting: indications and cost implications. *Progr Cardiovasc Dis* 1996; **39:** 83–110.

5. Dick RJ, Popma JJ, Muller DW et al. In-hospital costs associated with new percutaneous coronary devices. *Am J Cardiol* 1991; **68:** 879–85.

6. Lazzam C, Lazzam L, McLaughlin PR et al. Implications of higher initial in-hospital costs on restenosis rates with new devices [abstract]. *Circulation* 1992; 86 (Suppl): I-513.

7. Cohen DJ, Breall JA, Ho KKL et al. Economics of elective coronary revascularization. Comparison of costs and charges for conventional angioplasty, directional atherectomy, stenting and bypass surgery. *J Am Coll Cardiol* 1993; **22:** 1052–9.

8. Cohen DJ, Krumholz HM, Sukin CA et al, for the Stent Restenosis Study Investigators. In-hospital and one-year economic outcomes after coronary stenting or balloon angioplasty: results from a randomized clinical trial. *Circulation* 1995; **92:** 2480–87.

9. Cohen DJ, Gordon PC, Friedrich SP et al. The cost-effectivemness of selective adjunctive balloon dilatation after successful (but suboptimal) directional coronary atherectomy: a decision-analytic model [abstract]. *Circulation* 1993; 88 (Suppl): I-602.

10. Cohen DJ, Breall JA, Ho KKL et al. Evaluating the potential cost-effectiveness of stenting as a treatment for symptomatic single-vessel coronary disease. Use of a decision-analytic model. *Circulation* 1994; **89:** 1859–74.

11. Ellis SG, Miller DP, Brown KJ et al. In-hospital cost of percuataneous coronary revascularization. Critical determinants and implications. *Circulation* 1995; **92:** 741–47.

12. Goods CM, Liu MW, Iyer SS et al. A cost analysis of coronary stenting without anticoagulation versus stenting with anticoagulationn using warfarin. *Am J Cardiol* 1996; **73:** 334–36.

13. Kiemeneij F, Hofland J, Laarman GJ et al. Cost comparison between two modes of Palmaz-Schatz coronary stent implantation: transradial bare stent technique vs. transfemoral sheath protected stent technique. *Cathet Cardiovasc Diagn* 1995; **35:** 301–8.

14. Serruys PW, van Hout B, Bonnier H et al. Effectiveness, costs and cost-effectiveness of a strategy of elective heparin-coated stenting compared to balloon angioplasty in selected patients with coronary artery disease: The Benestent II Study. *Lancet* 1998 (in press).

15. Schwicker D, Banz K. New perspectives on the cost-effectiveness of Palmaz–Schatz™ coronary stenting, balloon angioplasty, and coronary artery bypass surgery - a decision model analysis. *J Invas Cardiol* 1997; 9 (Suppl A): 7A–16A.

16. Banz K, Schwicker D. Cost-effectiveness of Palmaz–Schatz stenting for patients with coronary artery disease in France. *J Invas Cardiol* 1997; 9 (Suppl A): 17A–22A

17. Banz K, Schwicker D. Cost-effectiveness of Palmaz–Schatz stenting for patients with coronary artery disease in Germany. *J Invas Cardiol* 1997; 9 (Suppl A): 23A–28A.

18. Banz K, Schwicker D. Cost-effectiveness of Palmaz–Schatz stenting for patients with coronary artery disease in Italy. *J Invas Cardiol* 1997; 9 (Suppl A): 29A–34A.

19. Banz K, Schwicker D. Cost-effectiveness of Palmaz–Schatz stenting for patients with coronary artery disease in The Netherlands. *J Invas Cardiol* 1997; 9 (Suppl A): 35A–40A.

20. Banz K, Schwicker D. Cost-effectiveness of Palmaz–Schatz stenting for patients with coronary artery disease in Spain. *J Invas Cardiol* 1997; 9 (Suppl A): 41A–46A.

9. Future Trends

It is clear that the use of coronary stents will continue to increase in the near future as the indications expand and the results of randomized trials become available. Advances in device technology will certainly play a major part in determining the future role of stenting techniques. The field of stent coatings is a subject of intense investigation with new biocompatible polymers and drug eluting polymers being developed for application to the metal stent scaffold. Polymeric stents are also being developed with the ongoing search for a biocompatible and biodegradable polymer capable of being loaded with antiproliferative or antithrombotic drugs. Composite stents, composed of metal-augmented polymers are also being developed in an attempt to combine the mechanical strength of metal with the biocompatible or drug eluting properties of a polymer in order to minimize local tissue reaction. A promising advance has been the development of stents which provide locally active ionizing radiation. These devices have the potential to inhibit the restenosis process completely, although long-term effects of these devices must be carefully analysed. Modifications in stent design are also proceeding at an unprecedented rate. Novel "rotating" and "locking" mechanisms are being incorporated into stent designs affording them high flexibility when unexpanded and remarkable rigidity when expanded. Stents designed for specific indications are quickly being introduced, with stents configured specifically for small vessels, bifurcation lesions, ostial stenosis, aneurysms and vessel rupture currently available. When considering stent restenosis, the previous decade focused on standard pharmacological approaches, the current decade has been the era in which efforts have been directed towards developing new mechanistic means of preventing and treating restenosis, while the next decade promises to be the most exciting, with the development of gene therapy strategies to address this vexing problem. With these continued developments and refinements, stenting will continue to be an important part of the interventionalist's armamentarium for the management of coronary artery disease.

Appendix A LIST OF ABBREVIATIONS

AAGCS Autologous arterial graft-coated stent
ACS Advanced Cardiovascular Systems
AMI acute myocardial infarction
ASA acetyl salycylic acid
AVE Applied Vascular Engineering
AVGCS Autologous vein graft-coated stent
BEIG balloon expandable intraluminal graft
BEL beStent large
BES beStent small
BX balloon expandable
CABG coronary artery bypass graft surgery
CAVD Cardiac allograft vascular disease
CCS Canadian Cardiovascular Society
CFR Coronary flow reserve
cGy centiGray
CI confidence interval
CIA coronary improved architecture
CVD CardioVascular Dynamics
CVR coronary velocity reserve
DCA direct coronary atherectomy
DLC diamond-like carbon
ELCA Eximer laser coronary angioplasty
EPILOG Evaluation of PTCA to Improve Long-term Outcome with abciximab
    GPIIb/IIIa blockade
ECG electrocardiogram
EXTRA Evaluation of the XT stent for restenosis – native arteries
FDA Food and Drug Administration
GR Gianturco–Roubin
Gy Gray
ICUS intracoronary ultrasound
INR International Normalized Ratio
IVT Interventional Technologies
IVUS intravascular ultrasound
LAD left anterior descending artery

LMCA left main coronary artery
LPRLL Low power red laser light
MACE major adversity cardiac event rate
MI myocardial infarction
MLD minimum luminal diameter
MSA Minimun stent area
MUSIC Multicentre Ultrasound Stenting in Coronaries
OTW over-the-wire
PAIR Pullback Atherectory for In-stent Restenosis
PASS Progressive Angioplasty System
PLA Polylactic acid
PS Palmaz–Schatz
PSJ Parallel-Serial-Jang
PTCA percutaneous transluminal coronary angioplasty
PTFE Polytetrafluoroethylene
QCA quantitative coronary angiography
RX rapid exchange
SAVED SAphenous VEin graft de novo
SOS Stent or Surgery
SPACTO Wiktor Stent Implantation in Chronic Total Occlusions
STAMI Stenting in Acute Myocardial Infarction
STARS Stent Anticoagulation Regimen Study
START Stent versus Angioplasty Restenosis Trial
STENT-BY
STENTIM Stent in Acute Myocardial Infarction
STOP Stents in Total Occlusion and restenosis Prevention
STRESS Stent Restenosis Study
TASC Trial of Angioplasty and Stents in Canada
TEC Transluminal extractional atherectomy
TIMI Thrombolysis in Myocardial Infarction
TM trademark
ULTIMA Unprotected Left Main Trunk Intervention Multicentre Assessment
WEST Western European Stent Trial
WIN Wallstent In Native Vessels
WRIST Washington Radiation for In-Stent Restenosis Trial

Appendix B LIST OF CLINICAL TRIALS

ADVANCE Additional Value of NIR stents for treatment of long coronary lesions

ARTS Arterial Revascularization Therapies Study

ASCENT

AVID Angiography Versus Intravascular Ultrasound Directed Coronary Stent Placement

BENESTENT Belgium Netherlands Stent

BESSAMI Berlin Stent in Acute Myocardial Infarction

BOSS Balloon Optimization versus Stent Study

BRAFE Brachial Radial Femoral

CADILLAC Controlled Abciximab and Device Investigation to Lower Late Angioplasty CASS Complications

CORSICA Chronic Occlusion Revascularization with Stent Implantation versus Coronary Angioplasty

DISTRESS Dispatch Stent Restenosis Study

Edres

ENTICESS Enoxaprin, Ticlopidine and Aspirin versus the Conventional Regimen after Elective Stenting

EPISTENT Evaluation of Platelet IIb/IIIa Inhibitor for Stenting

ERASER Evaluation of ReoPro and Stenting to Eliminate Restenosis

ESCOBAR Emergency Stenting Compared to Conventional Balloon Angioplasty Randomized trial (now called The Zwolle Myocardial Infarction Study)

FANTASTIC Full Anticoagulation versus Ticlopidine plus Aspirin after Stent Implantation

FRESCO Florence Randomized Elective Stenting in Acute Coronary Occlusions

FROST French Randomized Optimal Stenting

GISSOC Grupo Italiano di Studio sullo Stent nelle Occlusioni Coronariche

GRACE Gianturco–Roubin Stent Acute Closure Evaluation

GRAMI GR II in Acute Myocardial Infarction

HIPS Heparin Infusion Prior to Stenting

IMPACT II Integrelin to Manage Platelet Aggregation to Prevent Coronary Thrombosis

IRIS IsoStent for Restenosis Intervention Study

ISAR Intracoronary Stenting and Antithrombotic Regimen

ITALICS Investigation by the Thoraxcenter on Antisense DNA Given by Local Delivery and Assessed by IVUS after Coronary Stenting
MATTIS Multi-centre Aspirin and Ticlopidine after Intracoronary Stenting
MUSCAT Music Using CAT
NIRVANA NIR Vascular Advanced North American
OCBAS Optimal Coronary Balloon Angioplasty versus Stent
OPTICUS Optimization with Intracoronary Ultrasound to Reduce Stent Restenosis
OSTI Optimal Stent Implantation
PAMI Primary Angioplasty in Myocardial Infarction
PASTA Primary Angioplasty versus Stent in Acute Myocardial Infarction
PRISAM Primary Stenting for Acute Myocardial Infarction
RENEW
RESIST
REST Stent versus PTCA Restenosis
ROSTER Rotablator versus Balloon for Stent Restenosis
RotaStent
SALTS Strategic Alternatives with Ticlopidine in Stenting Study
SAVED Saphenous Vein Graft De Novo
SCORES Stent Comparative Restenosis
SCRIPPS Scripps Coronary Radiation to Prevent Restenosis
SICCO Stenting in Chronic Coronary Occlusion
SIMA Stenting vs Internal Mammary Artery
SIPS Strategy of Intracoronary Ultrasound Guided PTCA and Stenting
SMART Study of AVE-Micro Stent Ability to Limit Restenosis Trial
TRAPIST TRAPIDIL on Restenosis After Stenting

Index

Note: Italic page numbers refer to illustrations.

307